Encyclopedia of Parkinson's Disease: Therapeutics

Volume VI

Encyclopedia of Parkinson's Disease: Therapeutics

Volume VI

Edited by **Kate White**

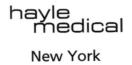

New York

Published by Hayle Medical,
30 West, 37th Street, Suite 612,
New York, NY 10018, USA
www.haylemedical.com

Encyclopedia of Parkinson's Disease: Therapeutics
Volume VI
Edited by Kate White

International Standard Book Number: 978-1-63241-194-5 (Hardback)

Printed in the United States of America.

Contents

Preface

Various therapeutic modalities and treatments of Parkinson's disease (PD) have been described in this book. This disease is caused mainly due to the death of dopaminergic neurons in the substantia nigra. Recent PD medications treat symptoms; though none decrease the rate of dopaminergic neuron degeneration. The primary problem in development of neuroprotective therapies is a restricted comprehension of the crucial molecular mechanisms that incite neurodegeneration. The discovery of PD genes has led to the hypothesis that dysfunction of the ubiquitin-proteasome pathway and misfolding of proteins are both critical to pathogenesis of the disease. Oxidative stress and mitochondrial dysfunction, earlier labeled as responsible in the neurodegeneration of this disease, may also act in part by causing the collection of misfolded proteins, along with the production of other harmful events in dopaminergic neurons. PD models based on the manipulation of PD genes should prove crucial in explaining significant characteristics of the disease, like selective vulnerability of substantia nigra dopaminergic neurons to the degenerative process. Some important topics include theoretical model for PD, PD in drosophila, animal models of PD, etc.

All of the data presented henceforth, was collaborated in the wake of recent advancements in the field. The aim of this book is to present the diversified developments from across the globe in a comprehensible manner. The opinions expressed in each chapter belong solely to the contributing authors. Their interpretations of the topics are the integral part of this book, which I have carefully compiled for a better understanding of the readers.

At the end, I would like to thank all those who dedicated their time and efforts for the successful completion of this book. I also wish to convey my gratitude towards my friends and family who supported me at every step.

Editor

Targeting Tyrosine Hydroxylase to Improve Bradykinesia

Michael F. Salvatore
Louisiana State University Health Sciences Center-Shreveport
USA

1. Introduction

The product of the tyrosine hydroxylase (TH) catalyzed conversion of L-tyrosine, L-DOPA, has been the gold standard for treating Parkinson's disease (PD) for half a century (Birkmayer and Hornykiewicz, 1961; Calne and Sandler, 1970). While L-DOPA therapy can improve locomotor disability in PD, it does not arrest the course of PD progression. Furthermore, dyskinesia is a debilitating side-effect of L-DOPA use over time. There have been promising results from preclinical and clinical studies for PD treatment. In fact, preclinical work indicates that enhanced TH protein expression accompanies locomotor improvements. Furthermore, the fact that L-DOPA treatment alone can improve locomotor dysfunction in PD is, by itself, a testimony to the critical importance of TH function in the nigrostriatal pathway for maintaining the capacity for initiating and maintaining normal locomotor activity. Clearly the major loss of TH, the rate-limiting enzyme of DA biosynthesis, in PD diminishes the capacity for locomotor activity. Surprisingly, efforts to treat PD symptoms have not deliberately focused on restoration of TH protein or its activity. Nonetheless, the rationale to focus on improving TH function to reduce the motor deficits associated with PD has been developed serendipitously over the past decade. Notably, research studying the neurobiological basis of how growth factors can improve locomotor activity in both Parkinson's disease and aging-related bradykinesia has revealed that increasing TH protein and its activity, through enhanced phosphorylation, should be a central feature of therapies intended to restore locomotor function in PD and aging-related Parkinsonism. Furthermore, these studies have led to the prospect that increasing DA tissue content in the substantia nigra alone could improve locomotor activity. Taken together, the possibility that increasing TH protein and activity in the substantia nigra could, by itself, restore locomotor deficits must be explored and no longer ignored.

2. The importance of tyrosine hydroxylase in Parkinson's disease

Undoubtedly, research in Parkinson's disease (PD) is flourishing on multiple fronts and substantial progress has been made in understanding PD and determining rationale for its treatment. Numerous studies have produced intriguing results on PD etiology from environmental, genetic, and aging-related associations. There has also been considerable focus upon PD treatment, from restoration of nigrostriatal neuropil function by increasing the expression of dopamine (DA)-regulating proteins with growth factors to understanding the impact of extrinsic forces (such as the physical activity and diet) on PD prevention or improvement of symptoms. There is also a rich literature on defining the role of not only DA regulation in PD, but also the involvement of other neurotransmitters, particularly glutamate, in PD progression. The awesome breadth and depth of this work precludes discussion for the purposes of this chapter. The goal of the chapter is to provide evidence that one way to understand PD and determine an accurate treatment is to examine post-translational events in the nigrostriatal pathway and its allied tissue during PD progression. Defining these cellular and biochemical processes could unravel a therapeutic avenue that would facilitate these post-translational events, which may already be at work to correct PD-related deficiencies in the nigrostriatal pathway. The brain is indeed a robust organ capable of plasticity to accommodate insults in order to maintain as normal of function that is possible. During PD progression, there is evidence of dopaminergic compensation which may maintain sufficient levels of DA necessary for normal locomotor activity until major loss of TH (>70%) occurs. Thus, a major theme of this article is to focus on how the dopamine-regulating proteins of the nigrostriatal pathway, in particular tyrosine hydroxylase (TH), are functioning during PD progression and to propose that targeting TH should be a major priority in treating the PD patient. It will be proposed that the insights gained, and still to be gained, from understanding TH regulation during PD progression or in aging-related Parkinsonism will yield molecular targets for accurate treatment of the locomotor dysfunction accompanying these conditions.

The theme of this chapter does not infer that PD can be simply resolved by targeting TH. Certainly there are a number of molecular events and deficiencies that occur in PD, including the devastating non-motor symptoms of PD, as highlighted in several recent and comprehensive reviews (Obeso et al., 2010; Lim and Lang, 2010). However, with regard to the goal of improving compromised locomotor activity and execution, it cannot be ignored that, at the very least, a partial restoration of the expression or enhancement of function of the dopamine-regulating proteins (TH, dopamine transporter, and vesicular monoamine transporter) is important to reclaim a normal locomotor phenotype in the PD patient. This should be obvious since DA has an established role in the modulation of locomotor activity (Rech et al., 1966; Calne and Sandler, 1970; Brown and Robbins, 1991).

The dopaminergic neuropil of the nigrostriatal pathway modulates the basal ganglia circuitry to affect locomotor activity. The modulation of DA signaling in the striatum, the terminal field region of the nigrostriatal pathway, has engaged most research efforts to define the role of DA in locomotor activity. Thus the current model of how DA modulates basal ganglia output to impact locomotor activity is based upon DA release and modulation of post-synaptic DA receptor-regulation of the activity of the striatal medium spiny neurons. Conversely, the attention paid to DA in the somatodendritic region has been spent on measures of viability of the nigrostriatal neuropil in post-mortem tissue from PD patients, models of PD, and in aging related Parkinsonism by quantification of TH protein levels in the substantia nigra (SN). In subsequent sections, it should become evident to the reader that measures of nigral TH should not be considered to be static index of nigrostriatal viability, but rather a possible measure of the remaining functional capacity of DA biosynthesis that could affect locomotor capacity. Indeed, a distinct minority of studies have shown that interference with dopamine signaling in the somatodendritic region of the nigrostriatal pathway in the SN does not impact locomotion.

This chapter is also intended to present and discuss research of TH, an extraordinary enzyme with regard its multiple phosphorylation sites, and what phosphorylation of TH does to modulate its activity. Tyrosine hydroxylase is a vastly studied enzyme and its function in the CNS has been of great interest in the neurosciences. It is well known that TH protein levels precipitously decrease in PD progression. However, this decline is considerable prior to the presentation of PD symptoms (Bernheimer et al., 1973). While this curious observation led to examination of TH function in PD models, it has been a rather neglected area of study since. It is a major intent of this chapter to re-energize interest in studying the importance of TH function, through its post-translational modifications in PD progression and in aging-related Parkinsonism or bradykinesia, and how agents such as growth factors mechanistically improve its activity. There is a caveat in these studies of TH protein and function in the CNS, largely because we simply do not know at the present time (2011) the extent that site-specific phosphorylation of TH affects its activity *in vivo*. However, strides have been made to identify the post-translational changes in TH function, through phosphorylation assessment, that are associated with behavioral outcomes. However, the role TH phosphorylation may play in compensating for TH loss occurring during PD progression is poorly understood. This is ultimately a vital question for accurate therapies for PD and aging-related Parkinsonism because it may define what phosphorylation site could be targeted to enhance synthesis capabilities. Certainly, increasing TH protein expression is also a vital goal, at least in PD. Again, the fact that L-DOPA, the product of TH catalysis of tyrosine, is an effective treatment for PD symptoms belies the critical importance of TH in maintaining dopamine in quantities sufficient for normal locomotor activity.

3. Site-specific tyrosine hydroxylase phosphorylation *in vivo:* current status

The phosphorylation of TH is a well-established mechanism of regulating its activity. It is unique in that there are three physiologically-regulated sites in brain, ser19, ser31, and ser40 (Haycock and Haycock, 1991). As to be discussed, there is plenty of evidence from cellular work that increased phosphorylation at ser40 can regulate L-DOPA biosynthesis. However, there is also evidence that ser31 also plays a role and furthermore, there is recent evidence that ser31 phosphorylation status has a significant role in regulating basal levels of DA in terminal field and somatodendritic regions of DA pathways (including the nigrostriatal pathway) in brain (Salvatore et al., 2009b). Yet, the question remains today as to how phosphorylation at each site can regulate its activity *in vivo*. The answer to this question will provide insight in how to most efficiently activate TH in the face of its progressive loss as seen in PD. Significant momentum and insight to answer this question has been gained from growth factor studies, as to be discussed in later sections. If TH activity can be enhanced from a treatment, then perhaps only partial restoration of TH protein in PD may be sufficient to maintain the levels of DA that are necessary for locomotion. However, again, the questions are 1) at which phosphorylation site can or should this be achieved and, 2) as recent work is telling us, where, neuroanatomically, should this restoration of DA biosynthesis capabilities be targeted: the terminal fields in striatum or somatodendritic region on the substantia nigra?

The discovery of cAMP-dependent protein kinase (PKA) in brain (Miyamoto et al., 1969) and that PKA could activate TH in brain homogenates (Morgenroth et al. 1975) set forth an explosion of research to identify TH-phosphorylating protein kinases and TH phosphorylation sites that were later characterized to be ser8, ser19, ser31, and ser40; with ser40 being a PKA-phosphorylation site (Haycock, 1990). However, the focus of TH activation has predominated around PKA-mediated ser40 phosphorylation, with the long-standing assumption that any increase in ser40 phosphorylation increases TH activity. One could argue that because of the dominating attention the PKA-targeted phosphorylation site received, it has became virtual dogma that this phosphorylation site is the most critical site for regulation of TH activity. Yet it was also apparent, as studies went forward, that TH activation could occur on one of these phosphorylation sites not associated with PKA-mediated phosphorylation. Shortly after the discovery of ser31 as a TH phosphorylation site (Haycock, 1990), evidence suggested its phosphorylation could affect TH activity (Haycock et al., 1992). This supported an earlier observation, before ser31 was identified, that the peptide fragment associated with TH activation had ser31 in the sequence (Tachikawa et al., 1987). Indeed, increased ser31 phosphorylation, alone from NGF treatment or in conjunction with depolarization-stimulated ser19 phosphorylation, enhances L-DOPA accumulation and is independent of any affect on ser40 phosphorylation (Mitchell et al., 1990; Harada et al., 1996; Salvatore et al., 2001).

There certainly is substantial evidence that ser40 phosphorylation can modulate TH activity from *in vitro* and *in situ* work. Phosphorylation at ser40 reduces catecholamine-influenced end-product inhibition of TH (Fitzpatrick et al., 1999). It was also shown that the temporal dynamics of VIP-stimulation of PKA-activation and the associated increase in TH phosphorylation and activation were matched in chromaffin cells (Waymire et al., 1991), one of several studies to show that PKA activity could enhance TH activity. The identification of ser40 phosphorylation as the PKA-targeted site (Haycock, 1990) then firmly established the notion that ser40 phosphorylation was the key regulatory site of TH. The notion that ser40 is the sole regulator of TH activity has expanded into *in vivo* and *in situ* studies, as there are numerous reports detailing phosphorylation assessment only at ser40, to the exclusion of ser31 and ser19. While evidence supports that ser40 phosphorylation can regulate TH activity, including *in vivo* (Leviel et al., 1991), a critical threshold of phosphorylation may be necessary for an impact on biosynthesis. In PC12 cells, a two-fold increase in ser40 phosphorylation has no affect on L-DOPA biosynthesis, whereas a three-fold increase is associated with an increase (Salvatore et al, 2001). However, in the case of ser31, a two-fold increase may be sufficient to increase L-DOPA biosynthesis (Salvatore et al., 2001). These observations are highly relevant when applied to interpreting the impact of changes in ser31 and ser40 phosphorylation observed *in vivo*. Indeed, the results obtained in PC12 cells may have direct relevance to the *in vivo* situation because the basal phosphorylation of TH at ser31 and ser40 in the PC12 cell line versus that in the CNS are very similar, ranging from a phosphorylation stoichiometry of 0.02-0.05 for ser40 compared to 0.05 to 0.35 for ser31 (Salvatore et al., 2001; 2004; 2005; 2009a; 2009b) (Table 1). Therefore, in order to definitively answer whether any change in ser40 phosphorylation observed *in vivo* is of any consequence to L-DOPA biosynthesis capabilities, we must first define how much phosphorylation is necessary at ser40 and ser31 to affect L-DOPA biosynthesis capabilities *in vivo*.

Phosphorylation site	PC12 cells	striatum	Substantia nigra
Ser19	0.049	0.02 – 0.10	0.08 - 0.25
Ser31	0.088	0.15 – 0.35	0.05 - 0.10
Ser40	0.033	0.01 – 0.03	0.02 - 0.04

Table 1. **Tyrosine hydroxylase phosphorylation stoichiometry *in situ* and *in vivo*.** A comparison of TH phosphorylation in PC12 cells (Salvatore et al., 2001) versus the ranges reported in the nigrostriatal pathway *in vivo* (Salvatore et al., 2000; 2004; 2005; 2009a; 2009b). The *in vivo* TH phosphorylation ranges in striatum and substantia nigra represents results from mice (C57B1/6) and rats (Sprague-Dawley, Fischer 344, and Brown-Norway/Fischer 344 F_1 hybrid).

The first indication that increased ser40 phosphorylation might not necessary for activation of TH came from a study wherein depolarizing stimulation produced increased L-DOPA biosynthesis, even though the cells expressed TH with leucine substitution at ser40 (Harada et al., 1996). This study was the first to challenge the notion that only ser40 phosphorylation was important for regulation of TH activity. Yet, this conclusion was supported by earlier evidence to show that enhanced ser31 phosphorylation (or the peptide later found to correspond to ser31 in tryptic digest) alone was associated with enhanced TH activity (Tachikawa et al., 1987; Haycock et al., 1992). After the study by Harada and colleagues, it was shown in a cell line wherein PKA could not be activated (the A126 PC12 cell line) that a depolarization stimulated increase in ser31 phosphorylation could increase L-DOPA biosynthesis. Specifically, in both the wild-type PC12 and A126 cell line, the inhibition of mitogen-activated protein kinase produced a selective decrease in depolarization-stimulated ser31 phosphorylation accompanied by a reduction in depolarization-stimulated L-DOPA biosynthesis (Salvatore et al., 2001). This effect was later observed in striatal slices (Lindgren et al., 2002).

The finding that an increase in ser31 phosphorylation alone could enhance L-DOPA biosynthesis has significant impact for understanding how growth factors may improve locomotor activity (as to be discussed in the next section). Nearly two decades earlier, Greene and colleagues reported that the PC12 cell line was responsive to nerve growth factor (NGF) (Greene and Tischler, 1976). Furthermore, treatment with NGF increased TH activity for out to 1 hour (Greene et al., 1984). Subsequent studies indicated that the effect of NGF on TH phosphorylation is solely due to enhanced ser31 phosphorylation (Haycock 1990; Salvatore et al., 2001). There is also evidence that NGF-signaling can increase TH promoter activity (Suzuki et al., 2004). These findings are tremendously relevant for the evidence that growth factors can improve deficient locomotor activity in both PD and aging models. The synthesis of these three findings that 1) ser31 phosphorylation alone can increase L-DOPA biosynthesis in response to depolarizing stimulation, 2) a growth factor could accomplish the same end result, and 3) a growth factor like NGF can induce TH gene expression all make it plausible that the mechanism by which growth factors increase locomotor activity could be related to enhanced ser31 TH phosphorylation and regulation of TH protein expression, both of which would serve to regulate DA levels in a quantity sufficient to enhance locomotor capabilities.

While there is evidence for ser31 and ser40 phosphorylation in regulating TH activity, the role for ser19 phosphorylation *in vivo* is yet unknown. However, insights from cellular work indicate ser19 phosphorylation may be a sentinel for increased depolarizing activity, thus signaling that increased TH activity would be required to replenish DA lost from release.

Indeed, phosphorylation of ser19 requires Ca^{2+} (Waymire et al., 1988; Salvatore et al., 2001). Although ser19 does not directly influence TH activity (Sutherland et al.,1993; Haycock et al., 1998), it has been shown to facilitate ser40 phosphorylation *in situ* (Bevilaqua et al., 2001). To date, there are no reports on how ser19 phosphorylation may influence ser31 phosphorylation.

To date, there is evidence that ser31 may regulate basal DA biosynthesis capabilities *in vivo* (Salvatore et al., 2009b). We have recently shown that the differences in ser31 phosphorylation, but not ser40 phosphorylation, co-vary with differences in DA tissue content (Figure 1).

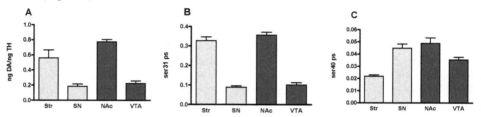

Fig. 1. Relationship of DA tissue content with tyrosine hydroxylase ser31 and ser40 phosphorylation stoichiometry *in vivo.* Four dopaminergic regions, striatum (Str), substantia nigra (SN), nucleus accumbens (NAc), and ventral tegmental area (VTA) were dissected from Brown-Norway/Fischer F344 F_1 hybrid rats and DA tissue content and TH protein inherent for each sample were analyzed from the same samples. **A)** The total recovered DA was normalized to total recovered TH protein to reveal differences in DA tissue content that could not be accounted for due to differences in TH protein recovery. To determine if phosphorylation at ser31 or ser40 could account for the differences in DA tissue content, we determined phosphorylation stoichiometry in each region. The differences in ser31 phosphorylation stoichiometry **(B)**, but not ser40 **(C)**, were similar to the differences in DA tissue content seen in **A**. *From Salvatore et al., 2009b*

In summary, there is no question that either increased ser31 or ser40 phosphorylation of TH can increase the biosynthesis of L-DOPA, leading to increased DA. There are still issues to be resolved. The first challenge lies in the acceptance of and practice of assessing ser31 phosphorylation in addition to ser40 phosphorylation in CNS studies of TH function or its role in behavioral paradigms. The second challenge is to ascertain how much phosphorylation at each site is necessary to produce an increase in L-DOPA biosynthesis.

4. Growth factors: dopamine & tyrosine hydroxylase

The objective in treating Parkinson's disease and aging-related Parkinsonism is to increase locomotor execution by increasing overall locomotor activity levels and the speed of execution. The discovery that glial cell line-derived neurotrophic factor (GDNF) delivery in CNS tissue can produce significant improvement in locomotor activity measures that are compromised in both aging and in PD models has revealed the critical importance of GDNF-signaling in maintenance of the nigrostriatal pathway (Hoffer et al., 1994; Gash et al., 1996; Gerhardt et al. 1999; Grondin et al 2003). There have also been successful outcomes to improve locomotor deficiencies from GDNF delivery via the use of viral-vectors. Delivery of GDNF using lentiviral vectors augments DA function in aged monkeys and reverses functional deficits caused by MPTP (Kordower et al., 2000). In fact, the precise delivery of specific quantities of the protein in the sub-nanogram quantities has shown promise for optimal outcomes in locomotor function and TH expression (Eslamboli et al., 2005). In the clinic, the outcomes from GDNF delivery on PD patients have been mixed (Gill et al., 2003; Slevin et al., 2005; Lang et al., 2006). There is evidence that the manner in which GDNF is infused into the brain may have significant impact on the clinical outcome due to the volume of distribution obtained following infusion (Hamilton et al., 2001; Ai et al., 2003; Gash et al., 2005; Salvatore et al., 2006). Notwithstanding the critical technical issues involved with GDNF delivery into the brain, there is substantial evidence that the neurobiological events triggered by GDNF delivery can have a positive influence on compromised locomotor function in PD and aging models, and possibly PD patients.

Recent work clearly indicates that maintaining GNDF signaling in the nigrostriatal pathway is critical for maintaining the DA phenotype into and beyond adulthood, as well as normal locomotor activity (Pascual et al., 2008; Nevalainen et al., 2010). Furthermore, there is definite evidence that GDNF-signaling regulates the DA phenotype through its impact on TH regulation. The mechanism by which GDNF signaling maintains or, in the case of treating PD, restores the DA phenotype involves its impact on TH expression and even TH phosphorylation. The partial depletion of the GDNF gene (GDNF +/- genotype) leads to a locomotor deficit at an earlier age during the course of aging (Boger et al., 2006). Not only is this deficit produced in the GDNF heterozygotes, but it is also observed in GDNF receptor (GFR α-1) heterozygote mice (Zaman et al., 2008). In both cases, there is significantly greater loss of TH protein with advancing age. These data suggest that there is a definite relationship between GDNF-signaling and locomotor activity, in which TH protein expression plays a vital mechanistic link. Other trophic factors can also enhance locomotor activity and DA signaling. Neurturin, an analog of GDNF, also enhances DA signaling and can protect against PD-like lesion (Gasmi et al., 2007; Cass and Peters, 2010). Most recently, there is evidence that another trophic factor, brain-derived neurotrophic factor (BDNF), also influences dopaminergic function and locomotor functions, as BDNF heterozygote mice exhibit declines in striatal DA release but, notably, without impact on TH protein expression (Boger et al., 2011). The possibility remains that diminished BDNF-signaling could affect TH phosphorylation, however, as GDNF has such effects, particularly on ser31 phosphorylation (Salvatore et al., 2004; 2009a).

Clearly the GDNF-related increase in DA tissue content or release capabilities seen in the nigrostriatal pathway has implications for involvement of enhanced tyrosine hydroxylase phosphorylation or TH protein biosynthesis. Indeed, in neuroblastoma and primary mesencephalic neurons it was shown that GDNF could increase TH phosphorylation (Kobori et al., 2003). The first in vivo study of the impact of GDNF on TH phosphorylation showed significant increases in TH phosphorylation in both striatum and substantia nigra, but the impact on specific phosphorylation sites showed a dichotomous result (Salvatore et al., 2004). In the substantia nigra, there was a profound increase in ser31, and only ser31 phosphorylation, the magnitude of which exceeded all other changes in TH phosphorylation examined (Salvatore et all, 2004). In striatum, all phosphorylation sites exhibited an increase in phosphorylation (Salvatore et al., 2004). Notably, this treatment also reduced TH protein levels in the nigrostriatal pathway, an effect which has also been reported in other studies in intact, but not lesioned, tissue (Georgievska et al., 2004). There is also evidence that the impact of GDNF on TH protein and phosphorylation is dose-dependent (Aoi et al., 2000; Salvatore et al., 2009a).

It is particularly notable that increased locomotor activity produced by GDNF is accompanied by increased DA tissue content in the SN, but not in striatum, regardless of the model of locomotor dysfunction, be it aging or a PD model (Hoffer et al., 1994; Gash et al., 1996; Hebert and Gerhardt, 1997; Gerhardt et al. 1999; Grondin et al 2003). However, the synaptic levels of striatal DA are affected following perburbations in GDNF-, BDNF-, or neurturin-related gene expression or delivery of these agents *in vivo* (Salvatore et al., 2004; Cass and Peters, 2010; Boger et al., 2011). These observations naturally raise the question of whether enhancement of locomotor activity by growth factors requires elevated DA-signaling in the striatum or SN. Furthermore, there is the question of how TH function in either region would ultimately affect DA signalling to affect locomotor activity. Bilateral improvement of locomotor activity after unilateral delivery of GDNF in striatum has been reported in clinical trials (Slevin et al., 2005) and bilateral effects on DA-regulating proteins like TH by unilateral GDNF have been shown to be limited to the SN (Salvatore et al., 2009a). Thus the increase in ser31 phosphorylation of TH, specifically in the SN, could be a critical molecular source to provide DA necessary for generating locomotor activity. This possibility leads to the necessity of asking how DA in striatum and the SN impact locomotor activity.

5. Tyrosine hydroxylase regulation in Parkinson's disease: role in dopaminergic compensation

It has been long noted that the pathological sequelae of PD include a major loss of TH protein in both the striatum and SN. There is evidence that TH activity may increase during PD progression, as increased DA release and TH activity occur in PD models (Snyder et al., 1990). TH activity may also be negatively affected by alpha-synuclein (to be discussed). Post-mortem analysis of PD brain tissue revealed the profound and yet unresolved finding that symptoms of PD were not apparent until the patient had at least 70% loss of the dopaminergic neuropil (Bernheimer et al., 1973). This observation led to formulating the concept of dopaminergic compensation, whereby locomotor functions continue normally in spite of loss of TH and other dopamine-regulating proteins until the 70-80% threshold is reached. One of the earliest observations to support dopaminergic compensation led to two hypotheses: one, that this mechanism was driving normal locomotion until the majority of the dopamine-regulating proteins were lost, but, two, at the same time could contribute to PD pathological progression (Agid et al., 1973). Other reports also suggest this compensatory mechanism may exacerbate toxicity to the nigrostriatal pathway (Zigmond et al, 2002). The human condition has been verified in MPTP-lesioned rhesus monkey in that the locomotor symptoms of PD are not present until there is nearly 80% loss of striatal DA (Bezard et al., 2001; Pifl et al., 2006). It is currently being debated as to whether or not increased striatal DA turnover can be observed during the asymptomatic stages of the disease or if, in fact, increased DA turnover is even a relevant index of dopaminergic compensation. There is support for dopaminergic compensation to maintain normal locomotion by evidence of enhanced striatal DA release (Perez et al., 2008). How TH activity is actually regulated by phosphorylation in a PD model is the subject of current investigation in this laboratory. Increased TH activity may be critical for ultimately maintaining normal locomotor activity during its progressive loss in PD. Infusion of the TH inhibitor AMPT hinders locomotor activity following nigrostriatal lesion (Leng et al, 2005), which argues that *de novo* DA biosynthesis is critical for dopaminergic compensation. As such, insights into which signaling pathway is more or less active could be made by determining how TH phosphorylation changes at each phosphorylation site in a PD model. This information, such as a decrease in ser31 phosphorylation for example, could be a guide to determining where deficiencies in signaling exist and reveal a therapeutic target. The regulation of TH during PD progression may also be affected by alpha-synuclein. Not only has this ubiquitous protein been well-studied in *in vitro, in situ,* and in animal models for potential involvement in PD pathogenesis, but there is evidence that it may control TH activity and expression. Indeed, perhaps the strongest evidence to date that implicates alpha-synuclein in PD vulnerability is a report that in both aged monkeys and humans, there is a strong correlation to nigral TH protein loss with aging-related accumulation of non-aggregated alpha-synuclein (Chu and Kordower, 2007). Under specific conditions, there is evidence that alpha-synuclein can act as a molecular chaperone to regulate TH activity through phosphorylation (Perez et al., 2002; Peng et al., 2005; Drolet et al., 2006). Therefore, the adverse impact of this protein on TH activity or its ability to be activated by phosphorylation may be considered when determining therapeutic options involving the targeting of TH.

These considerations must also include consideration of where TH could be best targeted, either in the terminal fields or somatodendritic region. As already mentioned in the discussion on growth factors, targeting TH may be best in the SN. There is evidence that the compensatory response is greater in the SN than in striatum, because extracellular DA levels in the SN are maintained despite 90% cell loss (Sarre et al., 2004). Furthermore, prevention of rotational behavior induced by L-DOPA can be blocked by intranigral infusion of a DA D_1 antagonist, and is more effective on blocking rotational behavior than striatal infusion (Robertson and Robertson, 1989). Thus, it may be possible that elevated TH activity in the SN could produce DA in quantities sufficient enough to sustain locomotion until a critical amount of TH protein is lost during PD progression.

6. Tyrosine hydroxylase regulation in aging-related Parkinsonism

Aging is a significant risk factor for developing Parkinson's disease. However, aging-related Parkinsonism is a much greater risk factor associated with aging, with up to 50% of the elderly developing bradykinesia after reaching age 80 (Bennet et al., 1996; Prettyman, 1998; Murray et al., 2004; Fleischman et al., 2007). However, unlike the loss of TH seen in PD, over the course of the lifespan the loss of striatal TH in humans is very minor and nowhere near the >70% loss seen in symptomatic PD (Haycock et al., 2003). It might be argued that there is a decrease in striatal TH phosphorylation during aging, which would support the evidence of striatal DA loss in human (Kish et al., 1992; Haycock et al., 2003), but the rodent models do not consistently support this possibility (Cruz-Muros et al., 2007; Salvatore et al., 2009b). Thus, the dominating hypothesis that >70% loss of striatal DA must be present for the emergence of locomotor symptoms associated with PD are challenged when viewed from the standpoint of striatal TH regulation during aging. In animal model studies of aging effects on DA regulation, no study has shown loss of DA or TH to reach that of the symptomatic threshold of striatal DA or TH loss. In fact, while some studies do show loss of DA or TH approaching that seen in PD, ~60% (Collier et al., 2007)), many studies report much less, if any, loss of striatal DA or TH (Ponzio et al., 1982; Marshall and Rosenstein, 1990; Emerich et al., 1993; Irwin et al, 1994; Hebert and Gerhardt, 1998; Yurek et al., 1998; Gerhardt et al., 2002; Haycock et al., 2003; Cruz-Muros et al., 2007; Salvatore et al., 2009). In fact, 60% striatal DA loss still does not produce bradykinesia in a PD model (Bezard et al., 2001).

Two fundamental observations should prompt us to pause and consider the prospect that nigral DA affects locomotor activity. First, GDNF enhances nigral DA tissue content in both aging and PD models in conjunction with increases locomotor activity. Second, aging work reveals that little or no striatal TH loss occurs with advanced age and there is a highly variable but consistently less than 60% DA loss in aging. A deficiency in nigral DA in either PD or in aging may contribute to decreased locomotor activity. Two aging studies have reported loss of both DA and ser31 TH phosphorylation of a 30-50%magnitude in the midbrain or SN (Cruz-Muros et al., 2007; Salvatore et al., 2009b). Loss of TH in the SN of aged non-human primates has been reported to be ~50% (Emborg et al., 1998). In a PD model, bradykinesia is present when nigral TH loss is at 50% (Bezard et al., 2001). Human data also indicate loss of DA neuropil of this magnitude in the SN in aging (Fearnley and Lees, 1991; Ross et al., 2004) or with PD (Marsden, 1990). Clinical studies of TH function in movement disorders is quite limited, but recent work in post-mortem tissue of Restless Leg Syndrome patients indicates that there is increased TH activity not only in putamen, but also in the SN (Connor et al., 2009). The possible importance of targeting the SN for treating PD has also been suggested for future work, as suggested in a recent report of a clinical trial involving the bilateral AAV-mediated gene delivery of neurturin in the putamen (Marks et al., 2010).

The abundance of GDNF-impact data has pointed to the possibility that DA regulation in the SN affects locomotor activity. In fact, a recent report has shown there is an aging-related decrease in the expression of the soluble isoform of the GDNF receptor, GFRα-1 only in the substantia nigra (Pruett and Salvatore, 2010). Taken together, these results all point to the possibility that TH regulation in the SN may be an important target for improving aging- or PD-related locomotor deficits, particularly bradykinesia. Thus, if deficits in nigral TH expression or phosphorylation in PD and aging are involved with locomotor dysfunction, an important question to ask is whether interference with DA signaling, specifically in the SN, could affect locomotor activity in otherwise normal rats.

7. Proposed role for nigral tyrosine hydroxylase function in locomotor activity

When it comes to defining how exactly DA modulates basal ganglia function, and hence locomotor activity, there is a wide consensus that DA function in the striatum is most critical. Yet, ever since somatodendritic DA release was reported (Cheramy et al., 1981), there have been reports from a variety of paradigms to suggest nigral DA alone can influence locomotor behavior. This possibility is a critical perspective to recognize if we are to understand how to successfully treat PD or aging-related bradykinesia. Specifically, from the perspective of striatal DA loss in PD and in aging, if striatal DA is most critical for bradykinesia arising from aging or PD, then there is a critical discrepancy at hand. That is, even though both conditions share a common symptom of bradykinesia, there is a starkly different magnitude of striatal DA loss in some cases and furthermore, no aging study has reported striatal DA to reach this critical threshold. Thus, if we are to accept that PD symptoms like bradykinesia are not present until there is 70% loss of TH or DA, which is supported by human PD pathology and PD models (Berheimer et al., 1973; Bezard et al., 2001), then how does bradykinesia come about in aging? Furthermore, do we dare ask if

70% striatal loss of TH or DA is really the threshold for symptom manifestation in PD, or is loss in another region like the SN more critical?

Observations in intact rats suggest that this question should be asked. Nigral application of DA modulates the output of the pars reticulata output (Waszczak and Walters, 1983; Kleim et al., 2007). Nigral infusion of a D_1 receptor antagonist suppresses operant behavior and open-field locomotion (Trevitt et al., 2001), and execution of motor performance (Bergquist et al., 2003). Depletion of nigral DA stores with tetrabenazine also hinders the ability to negotiate simple motor tasks (Andersson et al., 2006). We have most recently shown in longitudinally-characterized locomotor activity in rats that nigral DA correlates to lifetime locomotor activity initiation and maintenance, but not speed (Salvatore et al., 2009b).

These observations suggest that nigral TH function, as governed by TH protein expression and phosphorylation, may play a critical role in regulating the capacity for locomotor activity. The combination of phosphorylation at ser31 and the protein levels of TH may be a significant molecular source of producing DA that impacts the capacity for locomotor activity with regard to its initiation and frequency. Thus, the amount of local release of DA is proposed to be regulated by TH protein and phosphorylation. The released DA is proposed to act upon post-synaptic DA D_1 receptors. This local action in the SN increases GABA release from the striatonigral terminals, and disinhibits the inhibitory output neurons of the pars reticulata, thus facilitating locomotor activity. It is proposed that aging or PD-related deficits in locomotor activity may stem from deficiencies in either TH protein or TH phosphorylation at ser31 in the SN (Figure 2).

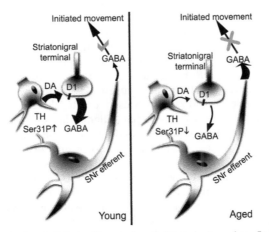

Fig. 2. **Proposed role of nigral DA leading to bradykinesia in aging**. It is proposed that inhibition of locomotion (bradykinesia) may occur by diminished local release of DA in the SN. Normally (as depicted in the young rat scenario on the left), released DA, acting upon post-synaptic D_1 receptors of the striatonigral terminals, promotes GABA release, which in turn reduces tonic release of GABA from the SNr efferent. This facilitates locomotor activity. When DA release capacity is deficient (as depicted in the aged rat scenario on the right), as proposed to be due to decreased TH protein or ser31 phosphorylation levels, the ability to promote GABA release from the striatonigral terminals is diminished, thereby removing an inhibition of GABA release from the SNr efferent, which promotes excess GABA release and inhibits locomotor activity.

8. Non-invasive approaches to target tyrosine hydroxylase function

The impact of exogenous sources of growth factors upon locomotor activity, DA tissue content and release, TH protein and phosphorylation is well-established. These observations allow us to question whether any non-invasive means exist to influence DA regulation *in vivo*. Increased production of growth factors from forced exercise, caloric restriction, and even components of the diet *in vivo* have been observed. Their impact on locomotor activity is an emerging and exciting topic as to the non-invasive measures we can take to improve locomotor deficits in PD or stave-off deficits produced by aging. Indeed, the enhancement of TH protein or its activity by phosphorylation may be a central mediator of the benefits to locomotor function realized by these non-invasive practices.

8.1 Exercise

Exercise is an activity that can be done at will with varying degrees of intensity, frequency, and longevity. Human and preclinical studies of exercise are revealing that these three variables associated with exercise have a significant impact upon our cognition and ability to move with advancing age and in the PD patient. For example in human studies, the volume of the hippocampus can increase and resist aging-related loss in volume as a result of aerobic exercise. Such changes are associated with improved memory function (Erickson et al., 2011). Exercise can prevent or reduce the risk of PD, as some longitudinal human studies support that regular exercise may lower the risk of PD (Chen et al., 2005). Other such studies do not support this hypothesis, with the caveat that study size was limited (Logroscino et al., 2006). The incidence of aging-related Parkinsonism and the disabilities arising from it may also be reduced from the quantity of physical activity that begins in midlife of healthy individuals (Savela et al., 2010). In the PD patient, there are definite benefits of exercise, and the frequency and intensity of it may be critical for its benefit. Exercise can improve motor performance and the physical activities of daily living in PD patients (Crizzle and Newhouse, 2006) and improve the efficacy of L-DOPA to improve motor performance (Muhlack et al., 2007). Most recently, the results of a forced exercise paradigm in human PD patients has shown that patients choosing to exercise on a bike with a trainer at a rate 30% greater than their preferred voluntary rate had a 35% improvement in their Unified Parkinson's Disease Rating Scale motor scores (Ridgel et al., 2009). Indeed, there is evidence from human studies that the intensity, frequency, and longevity of exercise may influence our innate capacity to move normally. The exciting aspect of this work is that exercise can be beneficial over short or long-term, even in a motorically-compromised state as seen in PD and may diminish the incidence of aging-related Parkinsonism.

The molecular events triggered in the CNS from exercise have been the subject of much study and appear to be related to growth factor production. An increase in mild cellular stress and angiogenesis are also thought to initiate signaling cascades that can be protective of DA neurons (rev. Zigmond et al., 2009). It is certainly believed that a relationship between innate DA function and physical activity exists (Knab and Lightfoot, 2010), and a number of studies examining this relationship supports this idea. Perhaps the single most compelling observation is that exercise does show a positive correlation to locomotor capabilities, which have a well-established relationship with DA regulation in the nigrostriatal pathway. Thus, the impact of exercise on TH regulation in aging and in PD models has been studied in several exercise paradigms. In animal studies, exercise paradigms are divided into voluntary or forced paradigms. In voluntary exercise, test subjects are given free access (within defined periods of time allowed for access) to an apparatus that permits and engages physical activity, most commonly a running wheel (Gerecke et al., 2010). In forced exercise, the test subjects are placed onto a treadmill on a near-daily basis and are coerced to run at a given rate of speed (12 – 20 meters/min) within a specific period of time that is typically much shorter that that used in voluntary (Tajari et al., 2010).

Regardless of the exercise paradigm used in animal studies, there is strong evidence of enhanced growth factor production, notably brain-derived neurotrophic factor (BDNF) and glial cell line-derived neurotrophic factor (GDNF) (Tajiri et al., 2010). In humans, there is a two- to three-fold increase in BDNF release from the human brain during exercise (Rasmussen et al., 2009) and endurance training also enhances the quantity of normal BDNF release compared to that seen at rest (Seifert et al., 2010). Given the well-established relationship of growth factors with TH and DA modulation, it would therefore be expected that exercise could affect TH and DA. Treadmill exercise in both PD and aging models does modulate DA tissue content and TH protein. In PD models, the impact of chemical lesions to the nigrostriatal pathway is lessened by treadmill exercise as evidenced by increased TH protein in the striatum and SN (Yoon et al., 2007). However, other reports show that despite locomotor activity improvements from exercise, no change in striatal DA or TH is observed (O'Dell et al., 2007; Petzinger et al., 2007), leaving open the possibility that enhancement of nigral TH function may be involved with locomotor activity effect. In fact, others have shown that extended periods of exercise (4-12 weeks), either treadmill (forced) or voluntary, increase nigral TH mRNA expression (Foley and Fleshner, 2008) or TH expression (Tumer et al., 2001; Gerecke et al., 2010; Tajiri et al., 2010). Thus, frequent exercise may enhance DA tone in the nigrostriatal pathway through enhancement of TH expression.

8.2 Diet: caloric restriction

The relationship of caloric intake with regulation of nigrostriatal DA function is becoming established. Seminal work showed aged rats that underwent calorie restriction (CR) had locomotor performances equal to that of younger adult rats. Furthermore, these CR aged rats had a 5-fold improvement in locomotor performance compared to age-matched controls, fed *ad libitum*. This work indicates that an innate molecular process associated with aging is hindered or diminished by CR. Calorie restriction increases striatal expression of GDNF in non-human primates (Maswood et al., 2004). Thus, if GDNF signaling is sufficiently active from CR, the impact of CR on locomotor activity could again, as in the case proposed in exercise, increase TH expression or activity enough to maintain DA signaling necessary for normal locomotor activity. Caloric restriction (CR) improves locomotor capabilities in PD models (Maswood et al., 2004) and preserves locomotor capabilities in aging models (Ingram et al., 1987; Weed et al., 1997; Kastman et al., 2010). Striatal DA loss from lesion is less severe in MPTP-treated monkeys on a 30% CR for about 6 months (Maswood et al., 2004) and amphetamine produces a marked enhancement locomotor activity in CR rats compared to rats fed *ab libitum* (Mamczarz et al., 2005; Marinkovic et al., 2007). An increase in DA release capacity from CR, as suggested by the Mamczarz study, strongly suggests an increase in DA biosynthesis capacity via increased TH protein or phosphorylation. The impact of CR on TH function has been studied sparingly. In fact, literature search yielded just one paper on the effect of 30 days CR on TH protein and ser40 phosphorylation (ser31 not studied). There was a trend toward increased TH protein in the SN. There was also an increase in striatal TH protein. There was no significant effect on ser40 phosphorylation of TH (Pan et al., 2006). However, through enhancement of GDNF expression, CR could increase TH activity via ser31 phosphorylation, which is increased by exogenous GDNF delivery *in vivo* (Salvatore et al., 2004). This would improve locomotor activity by enhancement of DA signaling, as already demonstrated in the Mamczarz and Marinkovic studies.

8.3 Diet: nutritive substances

There is an emerging literature on the relationship of fatty acid and cholesterol intake and the risk of PD (Liu et al., 2010; Miyake et al., 2010). Inhibition of cholesterol synthesis can reduce the severity of L-DOPA-induced dyskinesia in 6-OHDA lesioned rats (Schuster et al., 2008). A high-fat diet has been recently shown to promote greater DA depletion in both the striatum and SN following 6-OHDA (Morris et al., 2010). Cholesterol metabolites (oxysterols) do cross the blood-brain barrier and thus could interact with nigrostriatal neurons, possibly through liver X receptors (Sacchetti et al., 2009). Indeed, there is evidence that these oxysterols can modulate TH expression in neuroblastoma cells (Rantham Prabhakara et al., 2008). However, there is also evidence that a high dietary intake of omega-3 polyunsaturated fatty acids (PUFA), as found in fish oil extracts, is reported to be effective to sparing MPTP-induced loss of dopaminergic neuropil in the somatodendritic region of the nigrostriatal pathway (Bousquet et al., 2008). Furthermore, while the high PUFA was without effect on preventing MPTP-induced loss of TH protein in the striatum, there was a significant effect of the high PUFA diet on protecting against striatal DA loss (Bousquet et al., 2008). This exciting result may signify that high PUFA diet can activate signaling pathways to increase TH phosphorylation when loss of TH protein is occurring. The high-PUFA diet can increase BDNF expression in the striatum (Bouquet et al., 2009). Given that BDNF can increase ERK activity (Jovanovic et al., 2004), an increase in ERK activity would increase TH phosphorylation at ser31. Thus, a common denominator in enhancement or protection against nigrostriatal DA loss in a PD model, once again, appears to be an enhancement of ERK-signaling, via increased growth factor production, which could ultimately increase TH activity.

9. Future directions

Certainly there is evidence that the non-invasive lifestyle habits of exercise, caloric restriction, and diet could achieve a desirable end result of activating nigrostriatal TH to amounts sufficient to produce levels of DA necessary for normal locomotor activity. However, it is clear that the impact of these strategies upon striatal DA and TH have yielded ambiguous results and their relative impact on nigral DA and TH has yet to be fully revealed. Nonetheless, these lifestyle strategies can enhance growth factor expression. Growth factors also can enhance DA signaling and TH expression or phosphorylation *in vivo*, in conjunction with their locomotor benefits. Thus, it is an exciting prospect that TH function could be regulated from a non-invasive approach. Still, it is likely that some motorically-compromised individuals would be incapable of performing the rigorous demands of exercise required to yield an improvement in locomotor capabilities; certainly this would be the case for one afflicted with moderate-severe stage PD or one who has a physical impairment that prevents exercise. Thus the therapeutic options for such individuals, when removing the prospect of surgical approaches, are currently non-existent. Therefore, the ultimate challenge to maintain locomotor activity to conduct normal daily activities may be to take a pharmacological approach that targets TH and augments its expression and activity.

Clearly there is a critical battery of studies to support that augmenting nigral DA tissue content through enhancement of TH protein and phosphorylation could be the approach to improving the locomotor deficits seen in PD and aging. We have also known of the existence of somatodendritic DA release since the late 70s. There are handful of studies spanning nearly 30 years to support that nigral DA can influence aspects of locomotor activity. Clearly, there are still challenges in understanding the role of TH phosphorylation *in vivo*, notably, defining how much phosphorylation at TH is necessary at ser31 and ser40 to affect TH activity. Nonetheless, research efforts from a variety of angles that have been intended to improve locomotor impairment in PD and aging-related bradykinesia have shown, perhaps serendipitously, that targeting TH protein and its phosphorylation may be a promising molecular target to combat the locomotor deficits of PD and in aging.

10. References

Agid, Y, Javoy, F, & Glowinski, J. (1973). Hyperactivity of remaining dopaminergic neurones after partial destruction of the nigrostriatal dopaminergic system in the rat. *Nature New Biology* 245, 150-151. ISSN 0028-0836

Ai, Y, Markesbery, W, Zhang, Z, Grondin, R, Elseberry, D, Gerhardt, GA, & Gash, DM. (2003) Intraputamental infusion of GDNF in aged Rhesus monkeys: Distribution and dopaminergic effects. *J Comp Neurol* 461, 250-261. ISSN 0021-9967

Andersson, DR, Nissbrandt, H, & Bergquist, F. (2006). Partial depletion of dopamine in substantia nigra impairs motor performance without altering striatal dopamine neurotransmission. *Eur J Neurosci* 24, 617-624. ISSN 0953816X

Aoi, M, Date, I, Tomita, S, & Ohmoto, T. (2000). The effect of intrastriatal single injection of GDNF on the nigrostriatal dopaminergic system in hemiparkinsonian rats: behavioral and histological studies using two different dosages. *Neurosci Res* 36, 319-325. ISSN 1097-4547

Bennet, DA, Beckett, LA, Murray, AM, Shannon, KM, & Goetz, CG, Pilgrim, DM, & Evans, DA. (1996). Prevalence of Parkinsonian signs and associated mortality in a community population of older people. *New England J Med* 334, 71-76. ISSN 0028-4793

Bergquist, F, Shahabi, HN, & Nissbrandt, H. (2003). Somatodendritic dopamine release in rat substantia nigra influences motor performance on the accelerating rod. *Brain Res* 973, 81-91. ISSN 0006-8993

Bernheimer, H, Birkmayer, W, Hornykiewicz, O, Jellinger, K, & Seitelberger F, (1973). Brain dopamine and the syndromes of Parkinson and Huntington. Clinical, morphological and neurochemical correlations. *J. Neurological Sci.* 20, 415-455. ISSN 1302-1664

Bevilaqua, LRM, Graham, ME, Dunkley, PR, von Nagy-Felsobuki, EI, & Dickson, PW. (2001). Phosphorylation of Ser19 alters the conformation of tyrosine hydroxylase to increase the rate of phosphorylation of ser40. *J Biol Chem* 276, 40111-40116. ISSN 0021-9258

Bezard, E, Dovero, S, Prunier, C, Ravenscroft, P, Chalon, S, Guilloteau, D, Crossman, AR, Bioulac, B, Brotchie, JM, & Gross, CE. (2001). Relationship between the appearance of symptoms and the level of nigrostriatal degeneration in a progressive 1-methyl-

4-phenyl-1,2,3,6-tetrahydropyridine-lesioned Macaque model of Parkinson's disease. *J Neurosci* 21, 6853-6861. ISSN 0270-6474

Birkmayer, W, & Hornykiewicz, O. (1961). The L-3,4-dioxyphenylalanine (DOPA)-effect in Parkinson-akinesia. *Wien Klin Wochenschr* 73, 787-788. ISSN 0043-5325

Boger, HA, Middaugh, LD, Huang, P, Zaman, V, Smith, AC, Hoffer, BJ, Tomac, AC, & Granholm, AC. (2006). A partial GDNF depletion leads to earlier age-related deterioration of motor function and tyrosine hydroxylase expression in the substantia nigra. *Exp Neurol* 202, 336-347. ISSN 0014-4886

Boger, HA, Mannangatti, P, Samuvel, DJ, Saylor, AJ, Bender, TS, McGinty, JF, Fortress, AM, Zaman, V, Huang, P, Middaugh, LD, Randall, PK, Jayanthi, LD, Rohrer, B, Helke, KL, Granholm, AC, & Ramamoorthy, S. (2011). Effects of brain-derived neurotrophic factor on dopaminergic function and motor behavior during aging. *Genes, Brain, and Behavior* 10, 186-198. ISSN 1601-183X

Bousquet, M, Saint-Pierre, M, Julien, C, Salem, N, Cicchetti, F, & Calon, F. (2008). Beneficial effects of dietary omega-3 polyunsaturated fatty acid on toxin-induced neuronal degeneration in an animal model of Parkinson's disease. *FASEB J.* 22, 1213-1225. ISSN 1530-6860

Bousquet, M, Gibrat, C, Saint-Pierre, M, Julien, C, Calon, F, & Cicchetti, F. (2009). Modulation of brain-derived neurotrophic factor as a potential neuroprotective mechanism of action of omega-3 fatty acids in a parkinsonian animal model. *Prog Neuro-Psychopharm & Biol Psych* 33, 1401-1408. ISSN 0278-5846

Brown, VJ, & Robbins, TW. (1991). Simple and choice reaction time performance following unilateral striatal dopamine depletion in the rat. Impaired motor readiness but preserved response preparation. *Brain* 114, 513-525. ISSN 0006-8950

Calne, DB, & Sandler, M. (1970). L-DOPA and Parkinsonism. *Nature* 226, 21-24. ISSN 0028-0836

Cass, WA, & Peters, LE. (2010). Neurturin protects against 6-hydroxydopamine-induced reductions in evoked dopamine overflow in rat striatum. *Neurochem Int* 57, 540-546. ISSN 1872-9754

Chen, H, Zhang, SM, Schwarschild, MA, Hernan, MA, & Ascherio, A. (2005). Physical activity and the risk of Parkinson's disease. *Neurology* 64, 664-669. ISSN 0028-3878

Cheramy, A, Leviel, V, & Glowinski, J. (1981). Dendritic release of dopamine in the substantia nigra. *Nature* 289, 537-542. ISSN 0028-0836

Chu, Y, & Kordower, JH. (2007). Age-associated increases of a-synuclein in monkeys and humans are associated with nigrostriatal dopamine depletion: Is this the target for Parkinson's disease? *Neurobiol Aging* 25, 134-149. ISSN 0197-4580

Collier, TJ, Lipton, J, Daley, BF, Palfi, S, Chu, Y, Sortwell, C, Bakay, RA, Sladek, JR, & Kordower, JH. (2007). Aging-related changes in the nigrostriatal dopamine system and the response to MPTP in nonhuman primates: Diminished compensatory mechanisms as a prelude to parkinsonism. *Neurobiol Dis* 26, 56-65. ISSN 0969-9961

Connor, JR, Wang, X-S, Allen, RP, Beard, JL, Wiesinger, JA, Felt, BT, & Earley, CJ. (2009). Altered dopaminergic profile in the putamen and substantia nigra in restless leg syndrome. *Brain* 132, 2403-2412. ISSN 0006-8950

Crizzle, AM, & Newhouse, IJ. (2006). Is physical exercise beneficial for persons with Parkinson's disease? *Clin J Sport Med* 16, 422-425. ISSN 1050-642X

Cruz-Muros, I, Afonso-Oramas, D, Abreu, P, Barroso-Chinea, P, Rodríguez, M, Gonzalez, MC, & Hernandez, TG. (2007). Aging of the rat mesostriatal system: Differences between the nigrostriatal and the mesolimbic compartments. *Exp. Neurol.* 204, 147-161. ISSN 0014-4886

Drolet, RE, Behrouz, B, Lookingland, KJ, & Goudreau, JL. (2006). Substrate-mediated enhancement of phosphorylated tyrosine hydroxylase in nigrostriatal dopamine neurons: evidence for a role of alpha-synuclein. *J Neurochem* 96, 950-959. ISSN 0022-3042

Emborg, ME, Ma, SY, Mufson, EJ, Levey, AI, & Taylor, MD, Brown, WD, Holden, JE, & Kordower, JH. (1998). Age-related declines in nigral neuronal function correlate with motor impairments in rhesus monkeys. *J Comp Neurol* 401, 253-265. ISSN 0021-9967

Emerich, DF, McDermott, P, Krueger, P, Banks, M, Zhao, J, Marszalkowski, J, Frydel, B, Winn, SR, & Sanberg, PR. (1993). Locomotion of aged rats: Relationship to neurochemical but not morphological changes in nigrostriatal dopaminergic neurons. *Brain Res Bull* 32, 477-486. ISSN 0361-9230

Erickson, KI, Voss, MW, Prakash, RS, Basak, C, Szabo, A, Chaddock, L, Kim, JS, Heo, S, Alves, H, White, SM, Wojcicki, TR, Mailey, EL, Vieira, VJ, Martin, SA, Pence, BD, Woods, JA, McAuley, E, & Kramer, AF. (2011). Exercise training increases size of hippocampus and improves memory. *Proc Nat Acad Sci* 108, 3017-3022. ISSN 0027-8424

Eslamboli, A, Georgievska, B, Ridley, RM, Baker, HF, Muzyczka, N, Burger, C, Mandel, RJ, Annett, L, & Kirik, D. (2005). Continuous low-level glial cell line-derived neurotrophic factor delivery using recombinant adeno-associated viral vectors provides neuroprotection and induces behavioral recovery in a primate model of Parkinson's disease. *J Neurosci* 25, 769-777. ISSN 0270-6474

Fearnley, JM, & Lees, AJ. (1991). Ageing and Parkinson's disease: Substantia nigra regional selectivity. *Brain* 114, 2283-2301. ISSN 0006-8950

Fitzpatrick, PF. (1999). Tetrahydropterin-dependent amino acid hydroxylases. *Ann RevBiochem* 68, 355-381. ISSN 0066-4154

Fleischman, DA, Wilson, RS, Schneider, JA, Beinias, JL, & Bennet, DA. (2007). Parkinsonian signs and functional disability in old age. *Exp Aging Res,* 33, 59-76. ISSN 0361-073X

Foley, TE & Fleshner MR. (2008). Neuroplasticity of dopamine circuits after exercise: implications for central fatigue. *Neuromolec Med* 10: 67-80, 2008. ISSN 1535-1084

Gash, DM, Zhang, Z, Ai, Y, Grondin, R, Coffey, R, & Gerhardt, GA. (2005). Trophic factor distribution predicts functional recovery in Parkinsonian monkeys. *Ann Neurol* 58, 224-233. ISSN 0364-5134

Gash, DM, Zhang, Z, Ovadia, A, Cass, WA, Ai, Y Simmerman, L, Russell D, Martin, D, Lapchak, PA, Collins, F, Hoffer, BJ, & Gerhardt, GA. (1996). Functional recovery in parkinsonian monkeys treated with GDNF. Nature 380: 252-255. ISSN 0028-0836

Gasmi, M, Brandon, EP, Herzog, CD, Wilson, A, Bishop, KM, Hofer, EK, Cunningham, JJ, Printz, MA, Kordower, JH, & Bartus, RT. (2007). AAV2-mediated delivery of human neurturin to the rat nigrostriatal system: long-term efficacy and tolerability of CERE-120 for Parkinson's disease. *Neurobiol Dis* 27, 67-76. ISSN 0969-9961

Georgievska, B, Kirik, D, & Bjorklund, A. (2004). Overexpression of glial cell line-derived neurotrophic factor using a lentiviral vector induces time- and dose-dependent downregulation of tyrosine hydroxylase in the intact nigrostriatal dopamine system. *J Neurosci* 24, 6437-6445. ISSN 0270-6474

Gerecke, KM, Jiao, Y, Pani, A, Pagala, V, & Smeyne, RJ. (2010). Exercise protects against MPTP-induced neurotoxicity in mice. *Brain Res* 1341, 72-83. ISSN 0006-8993

Gerhardt, GA, Cass WA, Huettl P, Brock S, Zhang Z, & Gash,D.M. (1999).GDNF improves dopamine function in the substantia nigra but not the putamen of unilateral MPTP-lesioned rhesus monkeys. *Brain Res* 817, 163-171. ISSN 0006-8993

Gerhardt, GA, Cass, WA, Yi, A, Zhang, Z, & Gash, DM. (2002). Changes in somatodendritic but not terminal dopamine regulation in aged rhesus monkeys. *J Neurochem* 80, 168-177. ISSN 0022-3042

Gill, SS, Patel, NK, Hotton, GR, O'Sullivan, K, McCarter, R, Bunnage, M, Brooks, DJ, Svendsen, CN, & Heywood, P. (2003). Direct brain infusion of glial cell line-derived neurotrophic factor in Parkinson disease. *Nature Med* 9, 589-595. ISSN 1078-8956

Greene LA, & Tischler AS. (1976). Establishment of a noradrenergic clonal line of rat adrenal pheochromocytoma cells which respond to nerve growth factor. *Proc Nat Acad Sci* 73, 2424-2428. ISSN 0027-8424

Greene, LA, Seeley, PJ, Rukenstein, A, DiPiazza, M, & Howard, A. (1984). Rapid activation of tyrosine hydroxylase in response to nerve growth factor. *J Neurochem* 42, 1728-1734. ISSN 0022-3042

Grondin, R, Cass, WA, Zhang, Z, Stanford, JA, Gash, DM, & Gerhardt, GA. (2003). Glial Cell Line-Derived Neurotrophic Factor Increases Stimulus-Evoked Dopamine Release and Motor Speed in Aged Rhesus Monkeys. *J Neurosci* 23, 1974-1980. ISSN 0270-6474

Hamilton, JF, Morrison, PF, Chen, MY, Harvey-White, J, Pernaute, RS, Phillips, H, Oldfield, E, & Bankiewicz, KS. (2001). Heparin coinfusion during convection-enhanced delivery (CED) increases the distribution of the glial-derived neurotrophic factor (GDNF) ligand family in rat striatum and enhances the pharmacological activity of neurturin. *Exp Neurol* 168, 155-161. ISSN 0014-4886

Harada, K, Wu, J, Haycock, JW, & Goldstein, M. (1996). Regulation of L-DOPA biosynthesis by site-specific phosphorylation of tyrosine hydroxylase in AtT-20 cells expressing wild-type and serine 40-substituted enzyme. *J Neurochem* 67, 629-635. ISSN 0022-3042

Haycock, JW. (1990). Phosphorylation of tyrosine hydroxylase *in situ* at serine 8, 19, 31, and 40. *J Biol Chem* 265, 11682-11691. ISSN 0021-9258

Haycock, JW, & Haycock, DA. (1991). Tyrosine hydroxylase in rat brain dopaminergic nerve terminals: Multiple-site phosphorylation *in vivo* and in synaptosomes. *J Biol Chem* 266, 5650-5657. ISSN 0021-9258

Haycock, JW, Ahn, NG, Cobb, MH, & Krebs, EG. (1992) ERK1 and ERK2, two microtubule-associated protein 2 kinases, mediate the phosphorylation of tyrosine hydroxylase at serine-31 in situ. *Proc Natl Acad Sci* 89, 2365-2369. ISSN 0027-8424

Haycock, JW, Lew, JY, Garcia-Espana, A, Lee, KY, Harada, K, Meller, E, & Goldstein, M. (1998). Role of Serine-19 phosphorylation in regulating tyrosine hydroxylase studied with site- and phosphospecific antibodies and site-directed mutagenesis. *J Neurochem* 71, 1670-1675. ISSN 0022-3042

Haycock, JW, Becker, L, Ang, L, Furukawa, Y, Hornykiewicz, O, & Kish, SJ. (2003). Marked disparity between age-related changes in dopamine and other presynaptic dopaminergic markers in human striatum. *J Neurochem* 87, 574-585. ISSN 0022-3042

Hebert, MA, & Gerhardt, GA. (1998). Normal and drug-induced locomotor behavior in aging: comparison to evoked DA release and tissue content in Fischer 344 rats. *Brain Res* 797, 42-54. ISSN 0006-8993

Hoffer, BJ, Hoffman, AF, Bowenkamp, KE, Huettl, P, Hudson, J, Martin, D, Lin, LF, & Gerhardt, GA (1994). Glial cell line-derived neurotrophic factor reverses toxin-induced injury to midbrain dopaminergic neurons in vivo. *Neurosci Lett* 182:107-111. ISSN 0304-3940

Ingram, DK, Weindruch, RH, Spangler, EL, Freeman, JR, & Walford, RL. (1987). Dietary restriction benefits learning and motor performance of aged mice. *J Gerontol* 42, 78-81. ISSN 0022-1422

Irwin, I, DeLanney, LE, McNeill, T, Chan, P, Forno, LS, Murphy, GM, DiMonte, DA, Sandy, MS, Langston, JW. (1994). Aging and the nigrostriatal dopamine system: a non-human primate study. *Neurodegeneration* 3, 251-265. ISSN 1522-9661

Jovanovic, JN, Czernik, AJ, Fienberg, AA, Greengard, P, & Sihra, TS. (2004). Synapsins as mediators of BDNF-enhanced neurotransmitter release. *Nat Neurosci* 3, 323-329. ISSN 1097-6256

Kastman, EK, Willette, AA, Coe, CL, Bendlin, BB, Kosmatka, KJ, McLaren, DG, Xu, G, Canu, E, Field, AS, Alexander, AL, Voytko, ML, Beasley, TM, Colman, RJ, Weindruch, RH, & Johnson, SC. (2010). A calorie-restricted diet decreases brain iron accumulation and preserves motor performance in old rhesus monkeys. *J Neurosci* 30, 7940-7947. ISSN 0270-6474

Kish, SJ, Shannak, K, Rajput, A, Deck, JH, & Hornykiewicz, O. (1992). Aging produces a specific pattern of striatal dopamine loss: Implications for the etiology of idiopathic Parkinson's disease. J *Neurochem* 58, 642-648. ISSN 0022-3042

Kliem, MA, Maidment, NT, Ackerson, LC, Chen, S, Smith, Y, & Wichmann, T. (2007). Activation of nigral and pallidal dopamine D1-like receptors modulates basal ganglia outflow in monkeys. *J Neurophysiol* 98, 1489-1500. ISSN 0022-3077

Kobori, N, Waymire, JC, Haycock, JW, Clifton, GL, & Dash, PK. (2003). Modulation of tyrosine hydroxylase phosphorylation and activity by glial cell line-derived neurotrophic factor. *J Biol Chem* 279, 2182-2191. ISSN 0021-9258

Kordower, JH, Emborg, ME, Bloch, J, Ma, SY, Chu, Y, Leventhal, L, McBride, J, Chen, E-Y, Palfi, S, Roitberg, BZ, Brown, WD, Holden, JE, Pyzalski, R, Taylor, MD, Carvey, P, Ling, Z, Trono, D, Hantraye, P, Deglon, N, & Aebischer, P. (2000). Neurodegeneration prevented by lentiviral vector delivery of GDNF in primate models of Parkinson's disease. *Science* 290, 767-773. ISSN 0036-8075

Knab, AM, & Lightfoot, JT. (2010). Does the difference between physically active and couch potato lie in the dopamine system? *Int J Biol Sci* 6, 133-150. ISSN 1449-2288

Lang, AE, Gill, SS, Patel, NK, Lozano, A, Nutt, JG, Penn, R, Brooks, DJ, Hotton, G, Moro, E, Heywood P, Brodsky MA, Burchiel K, Kelly P, Dalvi A, Scott B, Stacy M, Turner D, Wooten, GF, Elias, WJ, Laws, ER, Dhawan, V, Stoessl, AJ, Matcham, J, Coffey, RJ, & Traub, M. (2006). Randomized controlled trial of intraputamenal glial cell line-derived neurotrophic factor infusion in Parkinson's disease. *Ann Neurol* 59, 459-466. ISSN 0364-5134

Leng, A, Mura, A, Hengerer, B, Feldon, J, & Ferger, B. (2005). Effects of blocking the dopamine biosynthesis and of neurotoxic dopamine depletion with 1-methyl-4-phenyl-1,2,3,6-tetrahydropyridine (MPTP) on voluntary wheel running in mice. *Behav Brain Res* 154, 375-383.

Leviel, V, Guibert, B, Mallet, J, & Faucon-Biguet, N. (1991). Induction of Tyrosine Hydroxylase in the Rat Substantia Nigra by Local Injection of Forskolin. *J Neurosci Res* 30, 427-432. ISSN 0360-4012

Lim, S-Y, & Lang, AE. (2010). The nonmotor symptoms of Parkinson's disease-an overview. *Movt Disord* 25, S123-S130. ISSN 1531-8257

Lindgren, N, Goiny, M, Herrera-Marschitz, M, Haycock ,JW, Hokfelt, T, Fisone, G (2002) Activation of extracellular signal-regulated kinases 1 and 2 by depolarization stimulates tyrosine hydroxylase phosphorylation and dopamine synthesis in rat brain. *Eur J Neurosci* 15, 769-773. ISSN 0953-816X

Liu, JP, Tang, Y, Zhou, S, Toh, BH, McLean, C, &Li, H. (2010). Cholesterol involvement in the pathogenesis of neurodegenerative diseases. *Mol Cell Neurosci* 43, 33-42. ISSN 1095-9327

Logroscino, G, Sesso, HD, Paffenbarger, RS, & Lee, I-M. (2006). Physical activity and risk of Parkinson's disease: a prospective cohort study. *J Neural Neurosurg Psychiatry* 77, 1318-1322.

Mamczarz, J, Bowker, JL, Duffy, K, Zhu, M, Hagepanos, A, & Ingram, DK. (2005). Enhancement of amphetamine-induced locomotor response in rats on different regimens of diet restriction and 2-deoxy-D-glucose treatment. *Neuroscience* 131, 451-464. ISSN 1873-7544

Marinkovic, P, Pesic, V, Loncarevic, N, Smiljanic, K, Kanazir, S, & Ruzdijic, S. (2007). Behavioral and biochemical effects of various food-restriction regimens in the rats. *Physiol Behav* 92, 492-499. ISSN 0031-9384

Marks, WJ, Bartus, RT, Siffert, J, Savis, CS, Lozano, A, Boulis, N, Vitek, J, Stacy, M, Turner, D, Verhagen, L, Bakay, R, Watts, R, Guthrie, B, Jankovic, J, Simpson, R, Tagliati, M, Alterman, R, Stern, M, Baltuch, G, Starr, PA, Larson, PS, Ostrem, JL, Nutt, J, Kieburtz, K, Kordower, JH, & Olanow, CW. (2010). Gene delivery of AAV2-neurturin for Parkinson's disease: a double-blind, randomised, controlled trial. *Lancet Neurology* 9, 1164-1172. ISSN 1474-4422

Marsden, CD. (1990). Parkinson's disease. *The Lancet* 335, 948-952. ISSN 0099-5355

Marshall, JF, & Rosenstein, AJ. (1990). Age-related decline in rat striatal dopamine metabolism is regionally homogeneous. *Neurobiol Aging* 11, 131-137. ISSN 0197-4580

Maswood, N, Young, J, Tilmont, E, Zhang, Z, Gash, DM, Gerhardt, GA, Grondin, R, Roth, GS, Mattison, JA, Lane, MA, Carson, RE, Cohen, RM, Mouton, PR, Quigley, C, Mattson, MP, & Ingram, DK. (2004). Caloric restriction increases neurotrophic factor levels and attenuates neurochemical and behavioral deficits in a primate model of Parkinson's disease. *Proc Natl Acd Sci* 100, 18171-18176. ISSN 0027-8424

Mitchell JP, Hardie DG, Vulliet PR (1990) Site-specific phosphorylation of tyrosine hydroxylase after KCl depolarization and nerve growth factor treatment of PC12 cells. *J Biol Chem* 265, 22358-22364. ISSN 0021-9258

Miyake, Y, Sasaki, S, Tanaka, K, Fukushima, W, Kiyohara, C, Tsuboi, Y, Yamada, T, Oeda, T, Miki, T, Kawamura, N, Sakae, N, Fukuyama, H, Hirota, Y, &Nagai, M. (2010).

Dietary fat intake and risk of Parkinson's disease: a case-control study in Japan. *J Neurol Sci* 288(1-2), 117-122. ISSN 1302-1664

Miyamoto, E, Kuo, JF, & Greengard, P. (1969). Adenosine 3',5'-monophosphate-dependent protein kinase from brain. *Science* 165, 63-65. ISSN 0036-8075

Morgenroth, VH, Hegstrand, LR, Roth, RH, & Greengard, P. (1975). Evidence for involvement of protein kinase in the activation by adenosine 3':5'-monophosphate of brain tyrosine 3-monooxygenase. *J Biol Chem.* 250, 1946-1948. ISSN 0021-9258

Morris, JK, Bomhoff, GL, Stanford, JA, & Gieger, PC. (2010). Neurodegeneration in an animal model of Parkinson's disease is exacerbated by a high-fat diet. *Am J Physiol Integr Comp Physiol* 299, R1082-1090. ISSN 0363-6119

Muhlack, S, Welnic, J, Woitalla, D, & Muller, T. (2007). Exercise improves the efficacy of levodopa in patients with Parkinson's disease. *Movement Disord* 22,427-430. ISSN 1531-8257

Murray, AM, Bennet, DA, Mendes, de Leon CF, Beckett, LA, & Evans, DA. (2004). A longitudinal study of Parkinsonism and disability in a community population of older people. *J Gerontol Medical Sciences* 59A, 864-870. ISSN 1079-5006

Nevalainen, N, Chermenina, M, Rehnmark, A, Berglof, E, Marschinke, F, & Stromberg, I. (2010). Glial cell line-derived neurotrophic factor is crucial for long-term maintenance of the nigrostriatal system. *Neuroscience* 171, 1357-1366. ISSN 1873-7544

Obeso, JA, Rodriguez-Oroz, MC, Goetz, CG, Marin, C, Kordower, JH, Rodriguez, M, Hirsch, EC, Farrer, M, Schapira, AHV, & Halliday, G. (2010). Missing pieces in the Parkinson's disease puzzle. *Nat Medicine* 16, 653-661. ISSN 1078-8956

O'Dell, SJ, Gross, NB, Fricks, AN, Casiano, BD, Nguyen, TB, & Marshall JF. (2007). Running wheel exercise enhances recovery from nigrostriatal dopamine injury without inducing neuroprotection. *Neuroscience* 144, 1141-1151. 1873-7544

Pan, Y, Berman, Y, Haberny, S, Meller, E, & Carr, KD. (2006). Synthesis, protein levels, activity, and phosphorylation state of tyrosine hydroxylase in mesoaccumbens and nigrostriatal dopamine pathways of chronically food-restricted rats. *Brain Res* 1122, 135-142. ISSN 0006-8993

Pascual, A, Hidalgo-Figueroa, M, Piruat, JI, Pintaldo, CO, Gomez-Diaz, R, & Lopez-Barneo, J. (2008). Absolute requirement of GDNF for adult catecholaminergic neuron survival. *Nat Neurosci* 11, 755-761. ISSN 1097-6256

Peng, XM, Tehranian, R, Dietrich, P, Stefanis, L, & Perez, RG. (2005). alpha-synuclein activation of protein phosphatase 2A reduces tyrosine hydroxylase phosphorylation in dopaminergic cells. *J Cell Sci* 118, 3523-3530. ISSN 0021-9533

Perez, RG, Waymire, JC, Lin, E, Liu, JJ, Guo, F, & Zigmond, MJ. (2002). A Role for alpha - Synuclein in the Regulation of Dopamine Biosynthesis. *J Neurosci* 22,3090-3099. ISSN 0270-6474

Perez, XA, Parameswaran, N, Huang, L, O'Leary, KT, & Quik, M. (2008). Pre-synaptic dopaminergic compensation after moderate nigrostriatal damage in non-human primates. *J Neurochem* 105, 1861-1872. ISSN 0022-3042

Petzinger, GM, Walsh, JP, Akopian, G, Hogg, E, Abernathy, A, Arevalo, P, Turnquist, P, Vuckovic, M, Fisher, BE, Togasaki, DM, Jakowec, MW. (2007). Effects of treadmill exercise on dopaminergic transmission in the 1-methyl-4-phenyl-1,2,3,6-tetrahydropyridine-lesioned mouse model of basal ganglia injury. *J Neurosci* 27, 5291-5300. ISSN 0270-6474

Pifl, C, & Hornykiewicz, O. (2006). Dopamine turnover is upregulated in the caudate putamen of asymptomatic MPTP-lesioned rhesus monkeys. *Neurochem Int* 49, 519-524. ISSN 0197-0186

Ponzio, F, Calderini, G, Lomuscio, G, Vantini, G, Toffano, G, & Algeri, S. (1982). Changes in monoamines and their metabolite levels in some brain regions of aged rats. *Neurobiol Aging* 3, 23-29. ISSN 0197-4580

Prasanthi, JR, Huls, A, Thomasson, S, Thompson, A, Schommer, E, & Ghribi, O. (2008). Differential effects of 24-hydroxycholesterol and 27-hydroxycholesterol on beta-amyloid precursor protein levels and processing in human neuroblastoma SH-SY5Y cells. *J Neurochem* 107, 1722-1729. ISSN 0022-3042

Prettyman, R. (1998). Extrapyramidal signs in cognitively intact elderly people. *Age and Ageing* 27, 557-560. ISSN 0002-0729

Pruett, BS, & Salvatore, MF. (2010). GFRα-1 receptor expression in the aging nigrostriatal and mesoaccumbens pathways. *J Neurochem*, 115, 707-715. ISSN 0022-3042

Rantham Prabhakara, JP, Feist, G, Thomasson, S, Thompson, A, Schommer, E, & Ghribi, O. (2008). Differential effects of 24-hydroxycholesterol and 27-hydroxycholesterol on tyrosine hydroxylase and alpha-synuclein in human neuroblastoma SH-SY5Y cells. *J Neurochem* 107, 1722-1729. ISSN 0022-3042

Rasmussen, P, Brassard, P, Adser, H, Pedersen, MV, Leick, L, Hart, E, Secher, NH, Pedersen, BK, & Pilegaard, H. (2009). Evidence for a release of brain-derived neurotrophic factor from the brain during exercise. *Exp Physiol* 94, 1062-1069. ISSN 0958-0670

Rech, RH, Borys, HK, & Moore, KE. (1966). Alterations in behavior and brain catecholamine levels in rats treated with alpha-methyltyrosine. *J Pharmacol Exp Ther*, 153, 412-419. ISSN 0022-3565

Ridgel, AL, Vitek, JL, & Alberts, JL. (2009). Forced, not voluntary, exercise improves motor function in Parkinson's disease patients. *Neurorehabil Neural Repair* 23, 600-608. ISSN 1545-9683

Robertson, GS, & Robertson, HA. (1989). Evidence that L-DOPA-induced rotational behavior is dependent on both striatal and nigral mechanisms. *J Neurosci* 9, 3326-3331. ISSN 0270-6474

Ross, GW, Petrovich, H, Abbott, RD, Nelson, J, Markesbery, W, Davis, D, Hardman, J, Launer, L, Masaki, K, Tanner, CM, & White, LR. (2004). Parkinsonian signs and substantia nigra neuron density in decendents elders without PD. *Ann Neurol* 56, 532-539. ISSN 0364-5134

Sacchetti, P, Sousa, KM, Hall, AC, Liste, I, Steffensen, KR, Theofilopoulos, S, Parish, CL, Hazenberg, C, Richter, LA, Hovatta, O, Gustafsson, J-A, & Arenas, E. (2009). Liver X receptors and oxysterols promote ventral midbrain neurogenesis in vivo and in human embryonic stem cells. *Cell Stem Cell* 5, 409-419. ISSN 1934-5909

Salvatore, MF, Garcia-Espana, A, Goldstein, M, Deutch, AY, & Haycock, JW. (2000). Stoichiometry of tyrosine hydroxylase phosphorylation in the nigrostriatal and mesolimbic systems *in vivo*: Effects of acute haloperidol and related compounds. *J Neurochem* 75, 225-232. ISSN 0022-3042

Salvatore, MF, Waymire, JC, & Haycock, JW. (2001). Depolarization-stimulated catecholamine biosynthesis: involvement of protein kinases and tyrosine hydroxylase phosphorylation sites *in situ*. *J Neurochem* 79, 349-360. ISSN 0022-3042

Salvatore, MF, Zhang, JL, Large, DM, Wilson, PE, Gash, CR, Thomas, TC, Haycock, JW, Bing, G, Stanford, JA, Gash, D, & Gerhardt, GA. (2004). Striatal GDNF administration increases tyrosine hydroxylase phosphorylation in the rat striatum and substantia nigra. *J Neurochem* 90, 245-254. ISSN 0022-3042

Salvatore, MF, Fisher, B, Surgener, SP, Gerhardt, GA, & Rouault, TA. (2005). Neurochemical investigations of dopamine neuronal systems in iron-regulatory protein 2 (IRP-2) knockout mice. *Mol Brain Res* 139, 341-347. ISSN 0169-328X

Salvatore, MF, Ai, Y, Fischer, B, Zhang, A, Grondin, RC, Zhang, Z, Gerhardt, GA, & Gash, DM. (2006). Point source concentration of GDNF may explain failure of phase II clinical trial. *Exp Neurol* 202, 497-505. ISSN 0014-4886

Salvatore, MF, Gerhardt, GA, Dayton, RD, Klein, RL, & Stanford, JA. (2009a). Unilateral striatal GDNF bilaterally affects nigrostriatal dopamine-regulating proteins in substantia nigra and GABA-regulating proteins in striatum. *Exp Neurol*, 219, 197-207. ISSN 0014-4886

Salvatore, MF, Pruett, BS, Spann, SL, & Dempsey, C. (2009b). Aging reveals a role for nigral tyrosine hydroxylase ser31 phosphorylation in locomotor activity generation. *PLoS ONE*, 4 (12), e8466. ISSN 1932-6203

Sarre, S, Yuan, H, Jonkers, N, Van Hemelrijck, A, Ebinger, G, & Michotte, Y. (2004). *In vivo* characterization of somatodendritic dopamine release in the substantia nigra of 6-hydroxydopamine-lesioned rats. *J Neurochem* 90, 29-39. ISSN 0022-3042

Savela, SL, Koistinen, P, Tilvis, RS, Strandberg, AY, Pitkala, KH, Salomaa, VV, Miettinen, TA, & Strandberg, TE. (2010). Physical activity at midlife and health-related quality of life in older men. *Arch Intern Med* 170, 1171-1172. ISSN 0003-9926

Schuster, S, Nadjar, A, Guo, JT, Li, Q, Ittrich, C, Hengerer, B, &Bezard, E. (2008). The 3-hydroxy-3-methylglutaryl-CoA reductase inhibitor lovastatin reduces severity of L-DOPA-induced abnormal involuntary movements in experimental Parkinson's disease. *J Neurosci* 28, 4311-4316. ISSN 0270-6474

Seifert, T, Brassard, P, Wissenberg, M, Rasmussen, P, Nordby, P, Stallknecht, B, Adser, H, Jakobsen, AH, Pilegaard, H, Nielsen, HB, & Secher, NH. (2010). Endurance training enhances BDNF release from the human brain. *Am J Physiol Regul Integr Comp Physiol* 298, R372-R377. ISSN 0363-6119

Slevin, JT, Gerhardt, GA, Smith, CD, Gash, DM, Kryscio, R, & Young,B. (2005). Improvement of bilateral motor functions in patients with Parkinson disease through the unilateral intraputamenal infusion of glial cell line-derived neurotrophic factor. *J Neurosurg* 102, 216-222. ISSN 0022-3085

Snyder, GL, Keller, RW, & Zigmond, MJ. (1990). Dopamine efflux from striatal slices after intracerebral 6-hydroxydopamine: evidence for compensatory hyperactivity of residual terminals. *J Pharm Exp Ther* 253, 867-876. ISSN 0022-3565

Sutherland, C, Alterio, J, Campbell, DG, LeBourdelles, B, Mallet, J, Haavik, J, & Cohen, P. (1993). Phosphorylation and activation of human tyrosine hydroxylase in vitro by mitogen-activated protein (MAP) kinase and MAP-kinase-activated kinases 1 and 2. *Eur J Biochem* 217, 715-722. ISSN 0014-2956

Suzuki, T, Kurahashi, H, & Ichinose, H. (2004). Ras/MEK pathway is required for NGF-induced expression of tyrosine hydroxylase gene. *Biochem Biophys Res Comm.* 315, 389-396. ISSN 0006-291X

Tachikawa, E, Tank, AW, Weiner, DH, Mosimann, WF, Yanagihara, N, & Weiner, N. (1987). Tyrosine hydroxylase is activated and phosphorylated on different sites in rat pheochromocytoma PC12 cells treated with phorbol ester and forskolin. *J Neurochem* 48, 1366-1376. ISSN 0022-3042

Tajari, N, Yasuhara, T Shingo, T, Kondo, A, Yuan, W, Kadota, T, Wang, F, Baba, T, Tayra, JT, Morimoto, T, Jing, M, Kikuchi, Y, Kuramoto, S, Agari, T, Miyoshi, Y, Fujino, H, Obata, F, Takeda, I, Furuta, T, & Date, I. (2010). Exercise exerts neuroprotective effects on Parkinson's disease model of rats. *Brain Res* 1310, 200-207. ISSN 0006-8993

Trevitt, JT, Carlson, BB, Nowend, K, & Salamone, JD. (2001). Substantia nigra pars reticulate is a highly potent site of action for the behavioral effects of the D1 antagonist SCH23390 in rat. *Psychopharmacol* 156, 32-41. ISSN 1432-2072

Tümer, N, Demirel, HA, Serova, L, Sabban, EL, Broxson, CS, & Powers, SK. (2001) Gene expression of catecholamine biosynthetic enzymes following exercise: modulation by age. *Neuroscience* 103: 703-711, 2001. ISSN 0306-4522

Waszczak, BL & Walters,J.R. (1983). Dopamine modulation of the effects of gamma-aminobutyric acid on substantia nigra pars reticulata neurons. *Science* 220, 218-221. ISSN 0036-8075

Waymire, JC, Johnston, JP, Hummer-Lickteig, K, Lloyd, A, Vigny, A, & Craviso, GL. (1988). Phosphorylation of bovine adrenal chromaffin cell tyrosine hydroxylase. Temporal correlation of acetylcholine's effect on site phosphorylation, enzyme activation, and catecholamine synthesis. *J Biol Chem* 263, 12439-12447. ISSN 0021-9258

Waymire, JC, Craviso, GL, Lichteig, K, Johnston, JP, Baldwin, C, Zigmond, RE. (1991). Vasoactive intestinal peptide stimulates catecholamine biosynthesis in isolated adrenal chromaffin cells: Evidence for a cyclic AMP-dependent phosphorylation and activation of tyrosine hydroxylase. J Neurochem 57, 1313-1324. ISSN 0022-3042

Weed, JL, Lane, MA, Roth, GS, Speer, DL, & Ingram, DK. (1997). Activity Measures in Rhesus Monkeys on Long-Term Calorie Restriction. *Physiology and Behavior* 62, 97-103. ISSN 0031-9384

Yoon, MC, Shin, MS, Kim, TS, Kim, BK, Ko, IG, Sung, YH, Kim, SE, Lee, HH, Kim, YP, & Kim, CJ. (2007). Treadmill exercise suppresses nigrostriatal dopaminergic neuronal loss in 6-hydroxydopamine-induced Parkinson's rats. *Neurosci Lett* 423, 12-17. ISSN 0304-3940

Yurek, M, Hipkens, SB, Hebert, MA, Gash, DM, & Gerhardt, GA. (1998). Age-related decline in striatal dopamine release and motoric function in Brown Norway/Fischer 344 hybrid rats. *Brain Res* 791, 246-256. ISSN 0006-8993

Zaman, V, Boger, HA, Granholm, AC, Rohrer, B, Moore, A, Buhusi, M, Gerhardt, GA, Hoffer, BJ, & Middaugh, LD. (2008). The nigrostriatal dopamine system of aging GFRalpha-1 heterozygous mice: neurochemistry, morphology and behavior. *Eur J Neurosci* 28, 1557-1568. ISSN 0953-816X

Zigmond, MJ, Hastings, TG, & Perez, RG. (2002). Increased dopamine turnover after partial loss of dopaminergic neurons: compensation or toxicity? *Parkinsonism & Related Dis* 8, 389-393. ISSN 1353-8020

Zigmond, MJ, Cameron, JL, Leak, RK, Mirnics, K, Russell, VA, Smeyne, RJ, & Smith, AD. (2009). Triggering endogenous neuroprotective processes through exercise in models of dopamine deficiency. *Parkinsonism & Related Dis* 15S3, S42-S45. ISSN 1353-8020

2

Successes of Modelling Parkinson Disease in Drosophila

Brian E. Staveley
Memorial University of Newfoundland
Canada

1. Introduction

Over one hundred years of innovative experimentation with the "common fruit fly" or *Drosophila melanogaster* has placed this remarkable organism at the forefront of contemporary biological research. Whether we consider the implications of modern genetic technologies and comprehensive genomic research, or we are interested in leading-edge aspects of molecular and cellular biology or complex developmental biology systems, or our studies range from the pin-point accuracy of proteomics to the large-scale questions of population biology, research with fruit flies has made very significant contributions to our understanding of the basic and complex functions of life. Although research into a wide range of biological questions has benefited greatly from experimentation with Drosophila, it never fails to surprise how often an approach that uses this model organism is undervalued or ignored. Any experimental system can be and should be criticized; however the opportunity to explore the biological basis of disease should never be missed. One shining example of this point is our understanding of Parkinson disease which has expanded through and continues to benefit from basic research into the biology of Drosophila, a model organism whose genome has been so thoroughly understood as to make it indispensable for medical research. These recent advances provide significant support for the use of *Drosophila melanogaster* models in the study of the biological basis of many human diseases and disorders.

Parkinson disease is the most common movement disorder and the second most common neurodegenerative disorder. Most apparent to even the most casual of observers is the fact that patients with Parkinson disease present with symptoms that are related to locomotion and motor control. These symptoms include resting tremor, slowness of movement, rigidity and postural instability. As the common underlying source that gives rise to these movement difficulties, Parkinson disease is most often associated with and distinguished by the degeneration of neurons, especially the dopamine-producing, or dopaminergic, neurons in the *substantia nigra* of the midbrain and the subsequent loss of dopamine (Dauer & Przedborski, 2003). Associated with these degenerating neurons is the appearance in many cases of the disease of large aggregates of proteins that are often referred to as the Lewy bodies. Often ignored are the additional non-motor symptoms, where non-dopaminergic neurons including olfactory and brain stem neurons, can frequently deteriorate before the dopaminergic neurons show signs of loss (Braak et al., 2003). Additional Parkinson disease symptoms are common and comprise a number of behavioural symptoms that include dementia, depression, anxiety and difficulties with sleep, plus non-behavioural symptoms such as the development of muscular and skeletal anomalies and skin lesions (Simuni & Sethi, 2008). Given the importance and the complexity of this disease, the application of a multifaceted, interdisciplinary approach to understanding the biological basis of Parkinson disease, including the modelling of the disease in well-known genetically versatile organisms, cannot be stressed enough.

The inherited or familial forms of Parkinson disease are, for the most part, indistinguishable in nature and severity from the sporadic forms of the disease (Hardy et al., 2009). As of only a few years ago, Parkinson disease was believed to be completely sporadic in nature, yet the identification of the inherited forms of the disease along with subsequent characterization of the causative genetic defects has revolutionized this area of research. It is now known that the familial cases comprise approximately 10 to 15% of the cases and arise from mutations in several identified genes with new loci associated with Parkinson disease being routinely discovered. Of the loci identified early in this process, mutations in the *alpha-synuclein* gene (designated as both *PARK1/PARK4*) (Polymeropoulos et al., 1997; Singleton et al., 2003) and *Leucine-rich repeat kinase 2* or *LRRK2* (identified as *PARK8*) (Paisan-Ruiz et al., 2004; Zimprich et al., 2004) cause autosomal dominant or "gain-of-function" forms of the disease. Mutations in the *parkin* gene (designated as *PARK2*)(Kitada et al., 1998), *PTEN-induced kinase 1* or *Pink1* (*PARK6*)(Valente et al., 2004), and *Dj-1* (*PARK7*) (Bonifati et al., 2003) are associated with autosomal recessive or "loss-of-function" forms of Parkinson disease. With the identification of the underlying genetic contributions to, at the very least, a sizable proportion of the incidents of Parkinson disease, it has become possible to apply the principles of disease modelling in genetically tractable animal systems to the study of this disease.

To demonstrate the great utility of the application of research into *Drosophila melanogaster* in the modelling of Parkinson disease, I will describe some of the most exciting recent advances in this field. To begin, a brief description of the wealth of genetic and transgenic approaches that are most commonly used to model aspects of human disease in Drosophila will be provided as an introduction to the organism. The first model of Parkinson disease, one based upon the toxic expression of the human *alpha-synuclein* gene, the first gene identified as a genetic cause of Parkinson disease, will be discussed. This model offered the opportunities to study a wide range of biological contributions to Parkinson disease including aspects of protein structural stability, oxidative stresses and other disease genes. Investigation of *Lrrk/LRRK2* in flies has revealed roles in dopamine distribution, protein synthesis and cell death in another model of a dominant form of Parkinson disease. Then, the processes of modelling Parkinson disease through examination of the loss-of–function of the Drosophila homologues of the *parkin* and *Pink1* genes, both responsible for recessive forms of Parkinson disease will be detailed. Of a very significant nature, this area of research has lead to the fundamental understanding the activity of these gene products at the mitochondria. Furthermore, recent studies have lead to the proposal of a mechanism that outlines the normal role of *parkin* and *Pink1* in mitochondrial dynamics. It is very likely that the loss of this mechanism leads to failure of the cell's ability to clear damaged mitochondria and ultimately results in the degeneration of these cells and, subsequently, the disease state. Finally, continued study of Drosophila models of Parkinson disease is clearly well positioned to contribute a great deal to the future of research into the basis of this disease.

2. The Drosophila approach to model human disease

Drosophila melanogaster has been extensively studied and a wealth of genetic, genomic, cellular and developmental knowledge and reagents are readily available. Drosophila are inexpensive to propagate and can produce a large number of genetically homogenous progeny. Flies display surprisingly intricate behaviours and have complicated brain and nervous systems. For many purposes, the fly provides a well-characterized system that is relatively easy to manipulate but complex enough to be relevant to the development of human disease models.

Often, once a gene has been implicated in a given disease, a bioinformatic search of genomic sequences can readily identify a potential homologue or orthologue from among the genes that comprise the well-characterized genome of *Drosophila melanogaster* as well as the genomes of a number of other Drosophila species for comparison. Application of reverse genetics can lead the production of both loss-of-function and gain-of-function phenotypes that may recapitulate symptoms of a given disease. Loss-of-function can be achieved either through the creation of mutations that lower or abolish gene activity or through the directed expression of an interfering RNAi transgene. A gain of function phenotype can be generated by the directed expression of a gene to where there is normally low or no expression or by inducing elevated levels of expression far above the norm. As a very well studied system, the Drosophila's pre-existing loss-of-function mutations, as well as transposon-bearing lines that can be employed to direct the expression, are available through stock centres and individual research laboratories from around the world. Due to the genomics projects, it is easy to access cDNA and genomic clones along with various vectors for generation of a variety of transgenic animals.

2.1 Drosophila genetics: genes, mutants and transgenics

In most cases, genes that have been identified as playing a role in human disease have counterparts in the genome of *Drosophila melanogaster*. Through the analysis of pre-existing mutants, the application of genetic screens to generate novel loss-of-function mutants and the implementation of "interfering RNA" or RNAi technology to reduce or eliminate gene activity can mimic the effect of recessively inherited diseases. For dominantly inherited disease, some pre-existing dominantly inherited alleles may exist in the stock centre collections. However, hypermorphic gain-of-function phenotypes can be generated by the directed overexpression of a transgene introduced into the fly genome through germ-line transformation. In addition, neomorphic and antimorphic gain-of-function phenotypes may be produced by *in vitro* construction and transformation of Drosophila transgenes that replicate molecular defects that have been determined to cause disease in people. Alternatively, a transgene that can express a variant form of a human gene can be fashioned and transformed. This approach has been applied to study the function and the potential contribution of genes to a number of diseases, including Parkinson disease. This approach can be instrumental in providing insight into the function of an identified gene involved in a human disease when the function is difficult to determine.

To produce the gain-of-function or the RNAi loss-of-function phenotypes described above, the Gal4/UAS system has been widely employed for the ectopic expression of specific genes in Drosophila (Brand & Perrimon 1993). For the most part, a gene of interest is cloned within a P element transposon-bearing plasmid containing several copies of the DNA-binding target of the yeast transcription factor GAL4 designated as the 'Upstream Activating

Sequence' (UAS) along with a selectable marker to readily track the presence of the transgene. As there is no Drosophila transcription factor that acts though binding of this sequence, in the absence of GAL4 these fusion transgenes are mostly inactive. Once established, individuals bearing a responsive transgene can be mated to specific lines that express Gal4 in any one or combination of expression patterns. Many choices of expression are available including ubiquitous, pan-neural, dopaminergic neuron-specific, early or late in eye development, inducible by heat shock, and many more. When the Gal4 transgene and the UAS target gene are combined in the offspring of the controlled breeding experiments, the gene of interest is subject to control of expression with regard to level, timing and tissue specificity. Analyses of these progeny provide the opportunity to approach a wide range of fundamental biological investigations including the detailed modelling of human disease.

When dealing with living systems, and in particular when carrying out complex manipulation of a model organism, careful evaluation and consideration of the techniques employed are necessary. With this in mind, it is important to note that a very limited number of Gal4 transgenes had been demonstrated to lead to cell death: first in the neuron-rich compound eye (Kramer & Staveley, 2003) and later in the nervous system (Rezaval et al., 2007). This suggests that the use of the Gal4/UAS system requires some caution because there may be a compounding Gal4-effect in some experiments when interpreting experimental observations. As always, control experiments must be subjected to proper evaluation and scrutiny. Nevertheless, the Gal4/UAS ectopic gene expression system in Drosophila is an extremely powerful tool and is one of the reasons that modelling human disease in flies is such an attractive pursuit.

2.2 Drosophila dopaminergic neurons

For a model system to functionally approach a condition as complex as Parkinson disease, changes to specific tissues that result in recapitulation of phenotypes that resemble symptoms of the disease are key. The Drosophila adult brain has been characterized to contain clusters of dopaminergic neurons (Nassel & Elekes, 1992). The feeding of rotenone, the complex I inhibitor that initiates degeneration of dopaminergic neurons in mammals, can cause the loss of these clusters of dopaminergic neurons in flies (Coulom & Birman, 2004). This demonstrates that there is a susceptibility of dopamine-producing neurons to toxins that is conserved between mammals and flies. As described below, altering the expression of selected genes in these dopaminergic neurons has resulted in loss of the neurons coupled with an age-dependent loss of locomotor abilities. The basic similarities between the genetically manipulated Drosophila models and Parkinson disease patients, given that the loss of the dopamine-producing neurons and the subsequent change in behaviour occurs over time, suggests that significant aspects of the disease may be well modelled in flies.

3. The alpha-synuclein-dependent Drosophila model of Parkinson disease

Once the genetic basis of a familial form of Parkinson disease was identified (the *alpha-synuclein* gene or *PARK1* and, later, *PARK4* as well) and the molecular basis of the defect determined (as specific changes to the protein), exploring the function or dysfunction of this gene was greatly aided by study in the Drosophila system.

3.1 The alpha-synuclein gene (PARK1) models Parkinson disease in Drosophila

Although instances are rare, mutations that result in substitution of amino acid residues within the human alpha-synuclein protein, specifically A30P, A53T and E46K, produce a dominant autosomally inherited version of Parkinson disease (PARK1; Polymeropoulos et al. 1997; Kruger et al. 1998; Zarranz et al. 2004). An early onset familial version of Parkinson disease results when a duplication of the region bearing this gene produces an increase in gene copy number (PARK4; Singleton et al. 2003). Although abundant in Lewy bodies, the precise physiological function of alpha-synuclein is uncertain. Because two of the original designated PARK loci (PARK1 and PARK4) have mapped to the *alpha-synuclein* gene, the native role and consequences of dysfunction appear complex and deserve to undergo extensive evaluation.

It is of extreme importance to the modelling of Parkinson disease in Drosophila that the first and most exploited Drosophila model of Parkinson disease depends upon the Gal4/UAS system for the ectopic expression of various forms of the human alpha-synuclein gene (Feany & Bender, 2000). Expression of human wild-type and Parkinson disease-causing mutant forms of *alpha-synuclein* in Drosophila results in the loss of the dopamine-producing neurons. The loss of neurons is coupled with the loss of the ability to climb over time in adult flies. As well, the development of Lewy body-like cytoplasmic inclusions and degeneration of the retina occurs with the expression of A30P, A53T and wild-type versions of *alpha-synuclein* using different Gal4 drivers. The observed phenotypic end-points produced by the disease-associated forms of the alpha-synuclein protein appear to display some differences and may mirror aspects of the toxicity that lead to various sub-types of Parkinson disease. To be clear, bioinformatic analysis of the genome of *Drosophila melanogaster* has not identified genes that encode any member of the synuclein family of proteins, including alpha synuclein. However, the recapitulation of phenotypes in Drosophila caused by the toxicity of *alpha-synuclein* gene product that somewhat mimic the consequences of Parkinson disease certainly seems to validate such study in this model organism. As with Parkinson disease patients, Drosophila models of Parkinson disease involve multiple defects, the cellular basis that provides insight into the pathogenesis of Parkinson disease.

3.2 Controversial detection of neurodegeneration in the model

Briefly, visualization of the dopaminergic neurons in Drosophila brains or brain sections has been accomplished through two main methods: detection of the tyrosine hydroxylase enzyme via immunohistochemistry, or detection of a *green fluorescent protein* or *GFP* reporter gene placed under the control of the *tyrosine hydroxylase-Gal4* transcription factor. For the most part, the determination of the specific death of dopaminergic neurons over time in response to the expression of *alpha-synuclein* has been demonstrated reproducibly since development of the alpha-synuclein-induced Drosophila model of Parkinson disease (Feany & Bender, 2000; Auluck et al., 2002; Cooper et al., 2006; Wassef et al., 2007; Botella et al., 2008; Trinh et al., 2008). Not all studies could detect dopaminergic neurodegeneration using anti-tyrosine hydroxylase immunostaining (Pesah et al., 2005) or detection of transgenic GFP (Whitworth et al. 2006). Clearly differences in the approach or methodology used to measure loss of dopaminergic neurons can influence the sensitivity of the assay (Auluck et al., 2005). In addition, as a definite decrease in the strength of the nuclear GFP signal has been observed the dopaminergic neurons of ageing flies that express *alpha-synuclein*, (Botella et al. 2008) a significant proportion of the differences could have easily been overlooked. In primary cultures of neurons cultivated from Drosophila that express *alpha-synuclein*, an *in vitro* model for Parkinson disease that shows great potential, the observed decrease in detection of GFP in these cultured neurons has been strongly associated with the early stages of apoptosis and signs of neurodegeneration (Park et al., 2007). Although this has been a contentious issue, the loss of immunological staining of the tyrosine hydroxylase enzyme, or detection of the tyrosine hydroxylase-responsive GFP reporter, seems to be very well correlated to neuronal dysfunction and degeneration.

This controversy highlights one great advantage of the study of Parkinson disease in an organism that presents complex phenotypes that reflect the consequences of the disease in humans. Of great importance, experiments where the loss of neurons is correlated to the loss of locomotor ability over time have provided sufficient comparison. For example, when oxidative stress is prevented, the loss of locomotor activity and the loss of dopaminergic neurons are diminished together in flies expressing alpha-synuclein (Pendleton et al., 2002, Yang et al., 2003, Wassef et al., 2007, Botella et al., 2008). As such, the loss of climbing ability seems to be a meaningful and modifiable phenotype that allows for the detection and validation of subtle influences.

3.3 Mechanisms to prevent alpha-synuclein-dependent toxicity

To address the possibility that chaperone activity may actively counteract protein toxicity, elevated expression of Heat Shock Protein 70 (HSP70) was demonstrated to toxicity of a-synuclein expression although aggregates were found (Auluck et al., 2002). Reduced chaperone activity contributed to increased loss of neurons resulting from expression of alpha-synuclein. Providing transgenic flies with geldanamycin, an inducer of chaperone activity, added to the food source contributed to survival of *alpha-synuclein*-expressing neurons (Auluck et al., 2005). The phosphorylation of alpha-synuclein at residue Serine residue-129, a modification often found in brains from Parkinson disease patients, apparently leads to toxicity (Fujiwara et al., 2002). In *Drosophila melanogaster*, study of the consequences of *in vivo* alteration of this site of phosphorylation suggests that this amino-acid residue is responsible for keeping the alpha-synuclein protein in a soluble form instead of in a state of aggregation (Chen & Feany, 2005). Prevention of phosphorylation at this site results in aggregation and reduced toxicity. This observation supports the hypothesis that the soluble form of the protein has a much greater potential for toxicity than does the non-phosphorylated form. Taken all together, this suggests that the process of aggregation acts as a protective cellular mechanism that works to neutralize the toxic forms of the alpha-synuclein protein.

While oxidative stress seems to contribute to Parkinson disease, a relationship to the mechanism behind alpha-synuclein toxicity is unclear. The degeneration of neuronal phenotypes induced by expression of mutant forms of *alpha-synuclein* is enhanced growth under conditions of hyperoxia while the elevated expression of the oxygen free radial scavenger superoxide dismutase suppresses the neuronal degeneration and the loss of locomotor activity over the lifespan of alpha-synuclein-expressing flies (Botella et al., 2008). To support the role of oxidative insult in the disease process, the alpha-synuclein-induced phenotypes are suppressed by other known antioxidants. These include the overexpression of methionine sulfoxide reductase and the supplementation of the Drosophila growth medium with S-methyl-L-cysteine (Wassef et al., 2007), and the induction of glutathione synthesis or glutathione conjugation activity (Trinh et al., 2008). As the toxicity of alpha-synuclein is sensitive to oxidative stress, manipulation of antioxidants may make a significant contribution to modify these effects.

One of the great advantages of employing the Drosophila model is the ability to combine and evaluate various components identified to contribute to Parkinson disease in an animal model organism. The first example of combining gene products that are known to cause inherited forms of Parkinson disease was the demonstration that the overexpression of *parkin* can act to counteract the toxic effects of both wild type and mutant forms of alpha-synuclein to restore climbing ability and to prevent degeneration of the retina when co-expressed in the eye (Haywood & Staveley, 2004; 2006). Similarly, the directed expression of *Pink1*, an upstream activator of *parkin*, acts to restore locomotor abilities and prevent subtle developmental defects in the eye (Todd & Staveley, 2008). This approach demonstrates that the directed expression of some of the recessive Parkinson genes can act to balance defects caused by a dominantly inherited Parkinson disease gene.

4. The LRRK2/Lrrk (PARK8) models of Parkinson disease in Drosophila

Leucine-rich repeat kinase 2 or *LRRK2* (first identified as *PARK8*) causes an autosomal dominant or "gain-of-function" form of Parkinson disease (Paisan-Ruiz et al., 2004; Zimprich et al., 2004). Dysfunction of LRRK2 has been mapped to several amino-acid substitutions in the protein and is very prominent among sporadic and inherited forms of Parkinson disease. The *LRRK2* gene encodes a very large protein with a leucine-rich repeat (LRR) domain, a kinase domain, a RAS-like GTPase domain and WD-40 domain and is very similar to an orthologous gene *LRRK1*.

There is a single homologue, *Lrrk*, in *Drosophila melanogaster*. Perhaps due to difficulties in the detection of neurodegeneration, as discussed above, there has been some confusion with studies of *Lrrk/LRRK2* in flies. In one case, Lrrk mutant flies display impaired locomotive activity and a reduction in the immunostaining of tyrosine hydroxylase in dopaminergic neurons (Lee et al., 2007). While the dopaminergic neurons display abnormal morphologies, the absolute number of the neurons appears to be unchanged although they may be degenerating slowly. Under other circumstances, *Lrrk* mutants seemed relatively normal which lead to the claim that *Lrrk* is not required for the survival of dopaminergic neurons (Wang et al., 2008). Directed expression of wild type of *Lrrk* did not lead to detectable degeneration of dopaminergic neurons (Lee et al., 2007). However, expression of mutant forms of both human (G2019S) and Drosophila (I2020T) did lead to documented loss of dopaminergic neurons (Imai et al., 2008; Liu et al., 2008). Nevertheless, the few studies of Lrrk/LRRK2 in flies have revealed a great deal that may influence our understanding of Parkinson disease.

The *Lrrk* mutants undergo lipid peroxidation and mutant flies containing the carboxy-terminal kinase domain truncated Lrrk transgene are sensitive to hydrogen peroxide (Wang et al., 2008). However, *Lrrk* mutants seem to be reasonably resistant to the oxidative stresses presented by paraquat and hydrogen peroxide (Imai et al., 2008). The relationship between Lrrk/LRRK2 and oxidative stress is unclear for now.

Lrrk/LRRK2 has been demonstrated to be involved in the negative regulation of normal levels of dopamine. The over expression of select mutants of Lrrk, but not wild-type Lrrk, causes a severe reduction in the dopamine levels of the brain (Imai et al., 2008). Treatment with I –DOPA causes improvement in movement not survival of dopaminergic neurons (Liu et al., 2008). Conversely, dopamine content is highly elevated in *Lrrk* mutants, as changes in dopamine levels must not be due to survival neurons but due to either defects in metabolism or processing and handling.

The eukaryotic initiation factor 4E (eIF4E)-binding protein, a major controller of protein synthesis and as such a key regulator of responses to cellular stress is phosphorylated by the Lrrk/LRRK2 kinase (Imai et al., 2008). This strongly suggests that the survival of dopaminergic neurons is compromised by pathogenic forms of Lrrk/LRRK2 through the deregulation or mis-regulation of protein translation. The Lrrk and LRRK2 proteins have been shown to phosphorylate and activate the transcription factor foxo (Kanao et al., 2010). This suggests that downstream targets of foxo, such as *hid* in flies (and *Bim* in humans), act to activate the apoptotic machinery to cause the neurodegeneration in Lrrk/LRRK2 models of PD. These research findings demonstrate a very meaningful connection between the control of protein synthesis, activation of cell death programs and the development of Parkinson disease.

5. The parkin/Pink1-dependent Drosophila models of Parkinson disease

5.1 The consequences of parkin and Pink1 loss in Drosophila

The loss-of-function in the *parkin* gene (PARK2), which encodes a highly conserved ubiquitin E3 ligase, is responsible for a rare autosomal recessive subtype of Parkinson disease. The Drosophila *parkin* gene is highly expressed in the Drosophila central nervous system (Horowitz et al. 2001; Bae et al. 2003). In *parkin* mutants, the dopaminergic neurons degenerate (Greene et al., 2003; Cha et al., 2005; Whitworth et al., 2005; Wang et al., 2007). In flies that that overexpress some mutant forms of *parkin*, dopaminergic neurons degeneration occurs (Sang et al., 2007). Although viable, *parkin* mutants present with a reduction in life-span, locomotor defects and extensive degeneration of muscle fibres, the latter is clearly associated with mitochondrial deterioration (Greene et al., 2005). The male *parkin* mutants are sterile due to failure of mitochondrial activities during spermatogenesis (Riparbelli and Callaini, 2007). Reduction of neuronal-specific staining (either GFP or TH) and/or cell death has been reported in these *parkin* mutants (Greene et al., 2003; Cha et al., 2005; Whitworth et al., 2005; Wang et al. 2007). The localization of this protein to the mitochondria (Darios et al., 2003) coupled with the consequences of *parkin* loss is a strong indication that it protects this organelle.

Mutations in the *PTEN-induced kinase 1* (*Pink1* or PARK6) gene are a common cause of autosomal recessive Parkinson disease (Valente et al., 2004). In flies, the *Pink1* gene, like *parkin*, is highly expressed in adult heads and testes (Park et al. 2006). The Pink1 serine-threonine kinase, along with a kinase domain, contains a mitochondrial-targeting signal (Clark et al., 2006). A decrease in the levels of dopamine with age plus a somewhat limited loss of dopaminergic neurons was found in the *Pink1* mutants along with the presence of abnormal mitochondria in the surviving dopaminergic neurons. When the function of *Pink1* was inhibited through the directed expression of an RNAi transgene, loss of dopaminergic neurons as well as the age-dependent degeneration of ommatidia was observed (Wang et al. 2006; Yang et al. 2006). The potential for a functional association with the mitochondria and the similarity in the consequences of dysfunction clearly suggest a shared role for these two proteins.

5.2 The parkin and Pink1 proteins act in one pathway

Although not identical, the flies that have lost *Pink1* function share a number of defects found in the *parkin* mutants including shortened lifespan, apoptotic muscle degeneration, male sterility, defects in mitochondrial morphology and disruption of locomotor abilities. These mitochondria are lost with age from the dopaminergic neurons of Pink1 mutants. While, for the most part, double *Pink1-parkin* mutants show the same phenotypes as either of the single mutants, the overexpression of *parkin* is able to rescue the mitochondrial defects found in *Pink1*, whereas *Pink1* overexpression does not rescue the *parkin* phenotypes. The parkin and Pink1 proteins have been reported to interact physically in at least some contexts (Kim et al., 2008; Xiong et al., 2009). This, at least in part, indicates that the Pink1 and parkin proteins function in the same pathway with Pink1 functioning upstream of parkin activity. This Pink1/parkin pathway is necessary for the integrity of dopaminergic neurons, because the loss of neurons due to loss of *Pink1* function could be rescued by additional expression of parkin (Clark et al., 2006; Park et al., 2006). The contribution of the study of the relationship between *parkin* and *Pink1* to our understanding of mitochondrial pathology in Parkinson disease highlights the utility of Drosophila to model Parkinson disease.

Similar to *parkin* and *Pink1*, mutations in the *Dj-1* gene cause autosomal recessive forms of Parkinson disease (Bonifati et al., 2003) and it has been suggested that they will become another potential component of this pathway. *Drosophila melanogaster* has two homologues of Dj-1 and is viable when both are deleted or silenced by RNAi transgenes (Menzies et al., 2005; Meulener et al., 2005; 2006). The loss of *Dj-1* activities leads to increased sensitivity to oxidative stress when exposed to paraquat or rotenone. However, the overexpression of *Dj-1* does not rescue the *Pink1* mutant phenotypes (Yang et al., 2006). The possibility exists that *Dj-1* may act much further upstream or through a parallel mechanism. However, at this time the relationship in unclear and *Dj-1* may or may not influence the Pink1/parkin pathway.

5.3 The parkin and Pink1 proteins co-operate at the mitochondria

Mitochondria undergo fission and fusion to change shape and share components (Chen & Chan, 2009). The fusion of mitochondria requires fusion of both the inner and outer mitochondrial membranes. The control of outer membrane fusion requires the activity of the protein mitofusin, and the inner membrane fusion requires the product of the *Optic atrophy-1* gene. Mitochondrial fission is promoted by the recruitment of dynamin-related protein 1 (Drp1) to the mitochondria, and this recruitment requires the activity of Fis1, a mitochondrial outer membrane protein. The regulation of this process is essential to the maintenance of a healthy cell.

To focus upon the mitochondria, in the dopaminergic neurons and the adult flight muscles of *parkin* mutants, the mitochondria are swollen with fragmented cristae (Greene et al., 2003; Pesah et al., 2004). A similar phenomenon is observed in flies that have lost the function of *Pink1* (Clark et al., 2006; Park et al., 2006; Yang et al., 2006). During Drosophila spermatogenesis, the spermatid's mitochondria aggregate and fuse to produce the nebenkern, a structure composed of two entangled strings of fused mitochondria. During subsequent elongation, the nebenkern disentangles to yield two fused structures that are maintained throughout the process of spermatogenesis. Whether due to reduced mitochondrial fission or excess fusion, in *parkin* and *Pink1* mutants only one mitochondrial fusion product has been detected (Deng et al., 2008). These mitochondrial defects, along with locomotion defects, flight muscle degeneration, cell death and diminishment of dopamine levels in heads, are suppressed both by the directed expression of the pro-fission genes *drp1* or *fis1* and by decreasing levels of the pro-fusion genes *mitofusin* or *opa1* (Deng et al., 2008; Park et al., 2009; Poole et al., 2008; Yang et al., 2008). In a *Pink1* mutant background, a reduction in the gene copy number of *drp1*, as seen with mutant heterozygotes, causes lethality (Deng et al., 2008; Poole et al., 2008). This clearly suggests that *parkin* and *Pink1* must act to promote mitochondrial fission. It is extremely important to point out that the phenotypes that arise from the loss of *parkin* or *Pink1* are very different from the loss of *drp1* (Deng et al., 2008). This is a strong indication that the Pink1-parkin pathway acts to regulate mitochondrial fission machinery.

5.4 The regulation of Mitophagy by parkin and Pink1 proteins

The process of mitophagy is a recently described specialized mitochondrial-specific version of autophagy (Goldman et al., 2010). In this procedure, the mitochondria undergo engulfment by autophagosomes and are degraded. This essential mechanism is absolutely dependent upon the dynamics of the continual fission and fusion of the mitochondria that alter the size and shape of the organelle and allow the exchange of components. With the failure of mitophagy, the quality of cellular respiration is severely diminished as is illustrated through the accumulation of oxidized proteins. Through the regulation of the fission/fusion dynamics of the cellular mitochondria, the Pink1 and parkin collaborate to contribute to this process.

First of all, although the parkin E3 ubiquitin ligase can target toxic proteins for proteasomal degradation, as the loss of *parkin* results in the accumulation of toxic proteins and overexpression can suppress toxicity of potential targets, other cellular processes can be regulated by ubiquitination by parkin (Geisler et al., 2009). With this in mind, a mechanism has been proposed that outlines the potential roles of the parkin and Pink1 proteins in the regulation of mitochondrial dynamics, changes in which can lead to alterations in the process of mitophagy (Geisler et al., 2009; Narendra et al., 2009; Vives-Bauza et al., 2010; Ziviani et al., 2010). The recruitment of parkin from the cytoplasm to the mitochondria depends on the activity of the Pink1 kinase. Pink1 is localized to the outer mitochondrial membrane through a well-conserved mitochondrial targeting signal peptide located near the amino-terminus of the protein (Zhou et al., 2008). This arrangement leaves the carboxy-terminal kinase-containing remainder of the protein exposed to the cytoplasm. It is proposed that under normal conditions, the tethered Pink1 protein is cleaved in a constitutive way to release the portion of Pink1 that contains the kinase activity into the cytoplasm (Narendra et al., 2009; Vives-Bauza et al., 2010; Ziviani et al., 2010). As a result, under standard conditions, Pink1 activity at the mitochondrial membrane is maintained at a steady but low level.

However, when stressed mitochondria undergo a critical amount of damage, the routine degradation of the Pink1 kinase is discontinued (Narendra et al., 2009; Vives-Bauza et al., 2010; Ziviani et al., 2010). This leaves intact and active versions of Pink1 to accumulate at the mitochondrial membrane in response to the termination of Pink1 inactivation. The initiation and maintenance of the accumulation of Pink1 may depend upon a signal generated when the mitochondria are not able to maintain membrane potential. Although the Rhomboid-7 protease is a candidate enzyme that can cleave Pink1 (Whitworth et al., 2008), this protease may not be the one responsible for this activity in response to mitochondria signalling for destruction. In the first major step of this process, the result is the differential identification of damaged mitochondria through the build up of active Pink1 activity bound and secured to the outer mitochondrial membrane. According to this mechanism, the next step in the regulation of mitophagy depends upon the recruitment of the parkin E3 ubiquitin ligase though Pink1 activity to the outer mitochondrial membrane (Narendra et al., 2009; Vives-Bauza et al., 2010; Ziviani et al., 2010). Recruitment of parkin to the mitochondrial membrane depends upon the localization of the Pink1 kinase to the mitochondria. An alternative method of mitochondrial targeting of Pink1 also recruits parkin (Narendra et al., 2009). Finally, the presence of the parkin ligase at the mitochondria results in the ubiquitination and subsequent degradation of the fusion-promoting outer mitochondrial membrane protein mitofusin (Ziviani et al., 2010). The mitofusin protein has been shown to accumulate with the loss of *Pink1* and *parkin* gene functions. If this proposal holds true, the initiation of mitophagy may very well depend upon signaling through the ubiquitination of mitofusin. In turn, whether mitofusin is targeted for degradation or modified to a form that no longer contributes to the process, this situation leads to the prevention of the fusion of the outer mitochondrial membrane. Although there is no evidence that fission is directly influenced, the subsequent failure of damaged mitochondria to be isolated would likely result from their loss of the ability to undergo proper segregation.

In summary, when mitochondria accumulate sufficient damage, the Pink1 protein becomes stabilized at the mitochondria. This acts to recruit parkin to the damaged mitochondria that in turn causes degradation or modification of mitofusin to promote mitochondrial fission and mitophagy to remove these damaged mitochondria. In Pink1/parkin mediated Parkinson disease, the damaged mitochondria are not cleared as efficiently to result in cellular damage.

6. The future of drosophila models of Parkinson disease

Drosophila is proving to have great advantages in the genetic and cell biological study of Parkinson disease. As more genes are found to be associated with Parkinson disease, further applications of reverse genetics should lead to greater understanding of the disease. The Drosophila phenotypes offer many diverse clues that may benefit from greater scrutiny. As well as future screens that modify the more obvious phenotypes such as male sterility, muscle degeneration, abnormal wing positioning, locomotion defects as well as mitochondrial defects in multiple tissues in young adults, these can be examined/scored for suppression or enhancement without having to carry out aging studies that can span months. Studies of candidate genes that may modify the activities of genes that mediate familial Parkinson disease are rigorous, but allow for rapid and straightforward means to deduce mechanisms. Given that mitochondria defects accumulate during normal aging, identification of multiple means to activate mitophagy may have applications to many aspects of aging. Drosophila provides an indispensable and unique opportunity to contribute to the Parkinson disease field.

7. Conclusion

To summarize, the recent expansion of research interest in the well understood laboratory organism *Drosophila melanogaster* to provide highly informative models of Parkinson disease demonstrates some of the great advantages that this system has to offer. The first model of Parkinson disease, one based on the toxic expression of the human *alpha-synuclein* gene, has allowed a great deal of investigation into various biological factors, such as protein folding, oxidative stress and protein detoxification, that may contribute to the disease. Studies of

Lrrk/LRRK2 have revealed roles for the management of dopamine handling, the control of protein synthesis and the initiation of programmed cell death in models of Parkinson disease. Further modelling of Parkinson disease through careful evaluation of *parkin* and *Pink1* loss-of-function in Drosophila has revealed that these two genes contribute to a pathway where the parkin E3 ubiquitin ligase is under the regulatory control of the Pink1 protein kinase. In flies, the relationship between *parkin* and *Pink1* has been extended from the neurons to other tissues including the mitochondrial-rich flight muscle and the male gametes. This has led to investigation of the products of these highly conserved genes in the processes that promote mitochondrial survival. The routine participation of *parkin* and *Pink1* in mitochondrial activities reveals that the loss of the fusion/fission dynamic can result in the failure of the cells to adequately deal with mitochondria that present a burden to the health of the cell. Future study of Parkinson disease in Drosophila models will continue to reveal much about the basis of this disease. As the past century has made clear, over and over again, investigations that apply our collective knowledge of the genetics and biology of *Drosophila melanogaster* to explore the fundamentals of disease, such as Parkinson disease, are very difficult to ignore.

8. Acknowledgments

I wish to thank the Natural Sciences and Engineering Research Council of Canada (NSERC) Discovery Grants, NSERC Research Tool Instruments Grants, and Parkinson Society Canada Friedman Pilot Project Grants for funding my research programs. In a special acknowledgement, I wish to thank the family of Jerry Friedman for supporting Parkinson disease research in Canada. I wish to thank the School of Graduate Studies at Memorial University of Newfoundland and the NSERC post-graduate scholarship and NSERC undergraduate scholarship programs for funding the students that have studied aspects of Parkinson disease in Drosophila in my laboratory. I thank the talented technical and the patient administrative support staff within the Department of Biology, the Faculty of Science and the Office of Research at Memorial University of Newfoundland. I thank Annika F.M. Haywood, Amy M. Todd, Githure (Peter) M'Angale, Lisa Baker (Saunders), Gillian Sheppard, Sharleen Hoffe, Michael Nightingale, Jo-Anna Clark, Kevin Mitchell, Greg Dale, Meghan O'Leary, Kate Bassett, Heather Stone, Kimberley Chafe, David Lipsett and Jamie M. Kramer for participation in modelling Parkinson disease in *Drosophila melanogaster* in my laboratory.

Finally, as the recent progress in this field has been extensive, I must offer my sincere apologies to those colleagues whom I have failed to include in this discussion. There are many research groups that have made and continue to make extremely significant contributions to the study of Parkinson disease through the study of the Drosophila model system.

9. References

Auluck, P.K.; Chan, H.Y., Trojanowski, J.Q., Lee, V.M. & Bonini, N.M. (2002). Chaperone suppression of alpha-synuclein toxicity in a Drosophila model for Parkinson's disease. *Science*, 295, pp. 865-8.

Auluck, P.K.; Meulener, M.C. & Bonini, N.M. (2005). Mechanisms of suppression of {alpha}-synuclein neurotoxicity by geldanamycin in Drosophila. *J Biol Chem*, 280, pp. 2873-8.

Bae, Y.J.; Park, K.S. & Kang, S.J. (2003). Genomic organization and expression of parkin in Drosophila melanogaster. *Exp Mol Med*, 35, pp. 393-402.

Bonifati, V.; Rizzu, P., van Baren, M.J., Schaap, O., Breedveld, G.J., Krieger, E., Dekker, M.C., Squitieri, F., Ibanez, P., Joosse, M., van Dongen, J.W., Vanacore, N., van Swieten, J.C., Brice, A., Meco, G., van Duijn, C.M., Oostra, B.A. & Heutink, P. (2003). Mutations in the DJ-1 gene associated with autosomal recessive early-onset parkinsonism. *Science*, 299, pp. 256-9.

Botella, J.A.; Bayersdorfer, F. & Schneuwly, S. (2008). Superoxide dismutase overexpression protects dopaminergic neurons in a Drosophila model of Parkinson's disease. *Neurobiol Dis*, 30, pp. 65-73.

Braak, H.; Del Tredici, K., Rüb, U., de Vos, R.A., Jansen Steur, E.N. & Braak, E. (2003). Staging of brain pathology related to sporadic Parkinson's disease. *Neurobiol Aging*, 24, pp. 197-211.

Brand, A.H.; & Perrimon, N. (1993). Targeted gene expression as a means of altering cell fates and generating dominant phenotypes. *Development*, 118, pp. 401-15.

Cha G.H.; Kim, S., Park, J., Lee, E., Kim, M., Lee, S.B., Kim, J.M., Chung, J. & Cho K. S. (2005), Parkin negatively regulates JNK pathway in the dopaminergic neurons of Drosophila. *Proc Natl Acad Sci U S A*, 102, pp. 10345-50.

Chen, H.; & Chan, D.C. (2009), Mitochondrial dynamics--fusion, fission, movement, and mitophagy-in neurodegenerative diseases. *Hum Mol Genet*, 18, pp. R169-76.

Chen, L.; & Feany, M.B. (2005). Alpha-synuclein phosphorylation controls neurotoxicity and inclusion formation in a Drosophila model of Parkinson disease. *Nat Neurosci*, 8, pp. 657-63.

Clark, I.E.; Dodson, M.W., Jiang, C., Cao, J.H., Huh, J.R., Seol, J.H., Yoo, S.J., Hay, B.A. & Guo, M. (2006). Drosophila pink1 is required for mitochondrial function and interacts genetically with parkin. *Nature*, 441, pp. 1162-6.

Cooper, A.A.; Gitler, A.D., Cashikar, A., Haynes, C.M., Hill, K.J., Bhullar, B., Liu, K., Xu, K., Strathearn, K.E., Liu, F., Cao, S., Caldwell, K.A., Caldwell, G.A., Marsischky, G., Kolodner, R.D., Labaer, J., Rochet, J.C., Bonini, N.M. & Lindquist, S. (2006). Alpha-synuclein blocks ER-Golgi traffic and Rab1 rescues neuron loss in Parkinson's models. *Science*, 313, pp. 324-8.

Coulom H.; & Birman S. (2004). Chronic exposure to rotenone models sporadic Parkinson's disease in Drosophila melanogaster. *J Neurosci*, 24, pp. 10993-8.

Darios, F.; Corti, O., Lücking, C.B., Hampe, C., Muriel, M.P., Abbas, N., Gu, W.J., Hirsch, E.C., Rooney, T., Ruberg, M., & Brice, A. (2003). Parkin prevents mitochondrial swelling and cytochrome c release in mitochondria-dependent cell death. *Hum Mol Genet*, 12, pp. 517-26.

Dauer, W.; & Przedborski, S. (2003). Parkinson's disease: mechanisms and models. Neuron, 39, pp. 889-909.

Deng, H.; Dodson, M.W., Huang, H. & Guo, M. (2008). The Parkinson's disease genes pink1 and parkin promote mitochondrial fission and/or inhibit fusion in Drosophila. *Proc Natl Acad Sci U S A*, 105, pp. 14503-8.

Feany, M.B.; & Bender, W.W. (2000). A Drosophila model of Parkinson's disease. *Nature*, 404, pp. 394-8.

Fujiwara, H.; Hasegawa, M., Dohmae, N., Kawashima, A., Masliah, E., Goldberg, M.S., Shen, J., Takio, K. & Iwatsubo, T. (2002). alpha-Synuclein is phosphorylated in synucleinopathy lesions. *Nat Cell Biol*, 4, pp. 160-4.

Geisler, S.; Holmström, K.M., Skujat, D., Fiesel, F.C., Rothfuss, O.C., Kahle, P.J. & Springer W. (2010). PINK1/Parkin-mediated mitophagy is dependent on VDAC1 and p62/SQSTM1. *Nat Cell Biol*, 12, pp. 119-31.

Goldman, S.J.; Taylor, R., Zhang, Y. & Jin, S. (2010). Autophagy and the degradation of mitochondria. *Mitochondrion*, 10, pp. 309-15.

Greene, J.C.; Whitworth, A.J., Kuo, I., Andrews, L.A., Feany, M.B. & Pallanck, L.J. (2003). Mitochondrial pathology and apoptotic muscle degeneration in Drosophila parkin mutants. *Proc Natl Acad Sci U S A*, 100, pp. 4078-83.

Greene, J.C.; Whitworth, A.J., Andrews, L.A., Parker, T.J. & Pallanck, L.J. (2005). Genetic and genomic studies of Drosophila parkin mutants implicate oxidative stress and innate immune responses in pathogenesis. *Hum Mol Genet*, 14, pp. 799-811.

Hardy, J.; Lewis, P., Revesz, T., Lees, A. & Paisan-Ruiz, C. (2009). The genetics of Parkinson's syndromes: a critical review. *Curr Opin Genet Dev*, 19, pp. 254-65.

Haywood, A.F.; & Staveley, B.E. (2004). Parkin counteracts symptoms in a Drosophila model of Parkinson's disease. *BMC Neurosci*, 5:14.

Haywood, A.F.; & Staveley, B.E. (2006). Mutant alpha-synuclein-induced degeneration is reduced by parkin in a fly model of Parkinson's disease. *Genome*, 49, pp. 505-10.

Horowitz, J.M.; Vernace, V.A., Myers, J., Stachowiak, M.K., Hanlon, D.W., Fraley, G.S. & Torres, G. (2001). Immunodetection of Parkin protein in vertebrate and invertebrate brains: a comparative study using specific antibodies. *J Chem Neuroanat*, 21, pp. 75-93.

Imai, Y.; Gehrke, S., Wang, H.Q., Takahashi, R., Hasegawa, K., Oota, E. & Lu B. (2008). Phosphorylation of 4E-BP by LRRK2 affects the maintenance of dopaminergic neurons in Drosophila. *EMBO J*, 27, pp. 2432-43.

Kanao, T.; Venderova, K., Park, D.S., Unterman, T., Lu, B. & Imai Y. (2010). Activation of FoxO by LRRK2 induces expression of proapoptotic proteins and alters survival of postmitotic dopaminergic neuron in Drosophila. *Hum Mol Genet*, 19, pp. 3747-58.

Kim, Y.; Park, J., Kim, S., Song, S., Kwon, S.K., Lee, S.H., Kitada, T., Kim, J.M. & Chung, J. (2008). PINK1 controls mitochondrial localization of Parkin through direct phosphorylation. *Biochem Biophys Res Commun*, 377, pp. 975-80.

Kitada, T.; Asakawa, S., Hattori, N., Matsumine, H., Yamamura, Y., Minoshima, S., Yokochi, M., Mizuno, Y. & Shimizu N. (1998). Mutations in the parkin gene cause autosomal recessive juvenile parkinsonism. *Nature*, 392, pp. 605-8.

Kramer, J.M.; & Staveley, B.E. (2003). GAL4 causes developmental defects and apoptosis when expressed in the developing eye of Drosophila melanogaster. *Genet Mol Res*, 2, pp. 43-7.

Krüger R.; Kuhn, W., Müller, T., Woitalla, D., Graeber, M., Kösel, S., Przuntek, H., Epplen, J.T., Schöls, L. & Riess, O. (1998). Ala30Pro mutation in the gene encoding alpha-synuclein in Parkinson's disease. *Nat Genet*, 18, pp. 106-8.

Lee, S.B.; Kim, W., Lee, S. & Chung J. (2007). Loss of LRRK2/PARK8 induces degeneration of dopaminergic neurons in Drosophila. *Biochem Biophys Res Commun*, 358, pp. 534-9.

Liu, Z.; Wang, X., Yu, Y., Li, X., Wang, T., Jiang, H., Ren, Q., Jiao, Y., Sawa, A., Moran, T., Ross, C.A., Montell, C. & Smith, W.W. (2008). A Drosophila model for LRRK2-linked parkinsonism. *Proc Natl Acad Sci U S A*, 105, pp. 2693-8.

Menzies, F.M.; Yenisetti, S.C. & Min, K.T. (2005). Roles of Drosophila DJ-1 in survival of dopaminergic neurons and oxidative stress. *Curr Biol*, 15, 1578-82.

Meulener, M.; Whitworth, A.J., Armstrong-Gold, C.E., Rizzu, P., Heutink, P., Wes, P.D., Pallanck, L.J. & Bonini, N.M. (2005). Drosophila DJ-1 mutants are selectively sensitive to environmental toxins associated with Parkinson's disease. *Curr Biol*, 15, pp. 1572-7.

Meulener, M.C.; Xu, K., Thomson. L., Ischiropoulos, H. & Bonini, N.M. (2006). Mutational analysis of DJ-1 in Drosophila implicates functional inactivation by oxidative damage and aging. *Proc Natl Acad Sci U S A*, 103, pp. 12517-22.

Narendra, D.P.; Jin, S.M., Tanaka, A., Suen, D.F., Gautier, C.A., Shen, J., Cookson, M.R. & Youle, R.J. (2010). PINK1 is selectively stabilized on impaired mitochondria to activate Parkin. *PLoS Biol*, 8, pp. e1000298.

Nässel, D.R.; & Elekes, K. (1992). Aminergic neurons in the brain of blowflies and Drosophila: dopamine- and tyrosine hydroxylase-immunoreactive neurons and their relationship with putative histaminergic neurons. *Cell Tissue Res*, 267, pp. 147-67.

Paisán-Ruíz, C.; Jain, S., Evans, E.W., Gilks, W.P., Simón, J., van der Brug, M., López de Munain, A., Aparicio, S., Gil, A.M., Khan, N., Johnson, J., Martinez, J.R., Nicholl, D., Carrera, I.M., Pena, A.S., de Silva, R., Lees, A., Martí-Massó, J.F., Pérez-Tur, J. & Wood, N.W. & Singleton, A.B. (2004). Cloning of the gene containing mutations that cause PARK8-linked Parkinson's disease. *Neuron*, 44, pp. 595-600.

Park, J.; Lee, S.B., Lee, S., Kim, Y., Song, S., Kim, S., Bae, E., Kim, J., Shong, M., Kim, J.M. & Chung, J. (2006). Mitochondrial dysfunction in Drosophila PINK1 mutants is complemented by parkin. *Nature*, 441, pp. 1157-61.

Park, J.; Lee, G. & Chung, J. (2009). The PINK1-Parkin pathway is involved in the regulation of mitochondrial remodeling process. *Biochem Biophys Res Commun*, 378, pp. 518-23.

Park, S.S.; Schulz, E.M. & Lee, D. (2007). Disruption of dopamine homeostasis underlies selective neurodegeneration mediated by alpha-synuclein. *Eur J Neurosci*, 26, pp. 3104-12.

Pendleton, R.G.; Parvez, F., Sayed, M. & Hillman R. (2002). Effects of pharmacological agents upon a transgenic model of Parkinson's disease in Drosophila melanogaster. *J Pharmacol Exp Ther*, 300, pp. 91-6.

Pesah, Y.; Pham, T., Burgess, H., Middlebrooks, B., Verstreken, P., Zhou, Y., Harding, M., Bellen, H. & Mardon G. (2004). Drosophila parkin mutants have decreased mass and cell size and increased sensitivity to oxygen radical stress. *Development*, 131, pp. 2183-94.

Polymeropoulos, M.H.; Lavedan, C., Leroy, E., Ide, S.E., Dehejia, A., Dutra, A., Pike, B., Root, H., Rubenstein, J., Boyer, R., Stenroos, E.S., Chandrasekharappa, S., Athanassiadou, A., Papapetropoulos, T., Johnson, W.G., Lazzarini, A.M., Duvoisin, R.C., Di Iorio, G., Golbe, L.I. & Nussbaum, R.L. (1997). Mutation in the alpha-synuclein gene identified in families with Parkinson's disease. *Science*, 276, pp. 2045-7.

Poole, A.C.; Thomas, R.E., Andrews, L.A., McBride, H.M., Whitworth, A.J. & Pallanck, L.J. (2008). The PINK1/Parkin pathway regulates mitochondrial morphology. *Proc Natl Acad Sci U S A*, 105, pp. 1638-43.

Rezával, C.; Werbajh, S. & Ceriani, M.F. (2007). Neuronal death in Drosophila triggered by GAL4 accumulation. *Eur J Neurosci*, 25, pp. 683-94.

Riparbelli, M.G.; & Callaini, G. (2007). The Drosophila parkin homologue is required for normal mitochondrial dynamics during spermiogenesis. *Dev Biol*, 303, pp. 108-20.

Sang, T.K.; Chang, H.Y., Lawless, G.M., Ratnaparkhi, A., Mee, L., Ackerson, L.C., Maidment, N.T., Krantz, D.E. & Jackson, G.R. (2007). A Drosophila model of mutant human parkin-induced toxicity demonstrates selective loss of dopaminergic neurons and dependence on cellular dopamine. *J Neurosci*, 27, pp. 981-92.

Simuni, T.; & Sethi, K. (2008). Nonmotor manifestations of Parkinson's disease. *Ann Neurol*, 64, pp. S65-80.

Singleton, A.B.; Farrer, M., Johnson, J., Singleton, A., Hague, S., Kachergus, J., Hulihan, M., Peuralinna, T., Dutra, A., Nussbaum, R., Lincoln, S., Crawley, A., Hanson, M., Maraganore, D., Adler, C., Cookson, M.R., Muenter, M., Baptista, M., Miller, D., Blancato, J., Hardy, J., & Gwinn-Hardy, K. (2003). alpha-Synuclein locus triplication causes Parkinson's disease. *Science*, 302, pp. 841.

Todd, A.M.; & Staveley, B.E. (2008). Pink1 suppresses alpha-synuclein-induced phenotypes in a Drosophila model of Parkinson's disease. *Genome*, 51, pp. 1040-6.

Trinh, K.; Moore, K., Wes, P.D., Muchowski, P.J., Dey, J., Andrews, L. & Pallanck LJ. (2008). Induction of the phase II detoxification pathway suppresses neuron loss in Drosophila models of Parkinson's disease. *J Neurosci,* 28, pp. 465-72.

Valente, E.M.; Abou-Sleiman, P.M., Caputo, V., Muqit, M.M., Harvey, K., Gispert, S., Ali, Z., Del Turco, D., Bentivoglio, A.R., Healy, D.G., Albanese, A., Nussbaum, R., González-Maldonado, R., Deller, T., Salvi, S., Cortelli, P., Gilks, W.P., Latchman, D.S., Harvey, R.J., Dallapiccola, B., Auburger, G. & Wood N.W. (2004). Hereditary early-onset Parkinson's disease caused by mutations in PINK1. *Science*, 304, pp. 1158-60.

Vives-Bauza, C.; Zhou, C., Huang, Y., Cui, M., de Vries, R.L., Kim, J., May, J., Tocilescu, M.A., Liu, W., Ko, H.S., Magrané, J., Moore, D.J., Dawson, V.L., Grailhe, R., Dawson, T.M., Li, C., Tieu, K. & Przedborski, S. (2010). PINK1-dependent recruitment of Parkin to mitochondria in mitophagy. *Proc Natl Acad Sci U S A*, 107, pp. 378-83.

Wang, D.; Qian, L., Xiong, H., Liu, J., Neckameyer, W.S., Oldham, S., Xia, K., Wang, J., Bodmer, R.& Zhang, Z. (2006). Antioxidants protect PINK1-dependent dopaminergic neurons in Drosophila. *Proc Natl Acad Sci U S A*, 103, pp. 13520-5.

Wang, C.; Lu, R., Ouyang, X., Ho, M.W., Chia, W., Yu, F. & Lim, K.L. (2007). Drosophila overexpressing parkin R275W mutant exhibits dopaminergic neuron degeneration and mitochondrial abnormalities. *J Neurosci*, 27,pp. 8563-70.

Wassef, R.; Haenold, R., Hansel, A., Brot, N., Heinemann, S.H. & Hoshi, T. (2007). Methionine sulfoxide reductase A and a dietary supplement S-methyl-L-cysteine prevent Parkinson's-like symptoms. *J Neurosci*, 27, pp. 12808-16.

Whitworth, A.J.; Theodore, D.A., Greene, J.C., Benes, H., Wes, P.D. & Pallanck, L.J. (2005). Increased glutathione S-transferase activity rescues dopaminergic neuron loss in a Drosophila model of Parkinson's disease. *Proc Natl Acad Sci U S A*, 102, pp. 8024-9.

Whitworth, A.J.; Wes, P.D. & Pallanck, L.J. (2006). Drosophila models pioneer a new approach to drug discovery for Parkinson's disease. *Drug Discov Today*, 11, pp. 119-26.

Whitworth, A.J.; Lee, J.R., Ho, V.M., Flick, R., Chowdhury, R. & McQuibban, G.A. (2008). Rhomboid-7 and HtrA2/Omi act in a common pathway with the Parkinson's disease factors Pink1 and Parkin. *Dis Model Mech*, 1, pp. 168-74.

Xiong, H.; Wang, D., Chen, L., Choo, Y.S., Ma, H., Tang, C., Xia, K., Jiang, W., Ronai, Z., Zhuang, X. & Zhang, Z. (2009). Parkin, PINK1, and DJ-1 form a ubiquitin E3 ligase complex promoting unfolded protein degradation. *J Clin Invest*, 119, pp. 650-60.

Yang, Y.; Nishimura, I., Imai, Y., Takahashi, R. & Lu, B. (2003). Parkin suppresses dopaminergic neuron-selective neurotoxicity induced by Pael-R in Drosophila. *Neuron*, 37, pp. 911-24.

Yang, Y.; Gehrke, S., Imai, Y., Huang, Z., Ouyang, Y., Wang, J.W., Yang, L., Beal, M.F., Vogel, H. & Lu, B. (2006). Mitochondrial pathology and muscle and dopaminergic neuron degeneration caused by inactivation of Drosophila Pink1 is rescued by Parkin. *Proc Natl Acad Sci U S A*, 103, pp. 10793-8.

Yang, Y.; Ouyang, Y., Yang, L., Beal, M.F., McQuibban, A., Vogel, H. & Lu, B. (2008). Pink1 regulates mitochondrial dynamics through interaction with the fission/fusion machinery. *Proc Natl Acad Sci U S A*, 105, pp. 7070-5.

Zarranz, J.J.; Alegre, J., Gómez-Esteban, J.C., Lezcano, E., Ros, R., Ampuero, I., Vidal, L., Hoenicka, J., Rodriguez, O., Atarés, B., Llorens, V., Gomez Tortosa, E., del Ser, T., Muñoz, D.G. & de Yebenes, J.G. (2004). The new mutation, E46K, of alpha-synuclein causes Parkinson and Lewy body dementia. *Ann Neurol*, 55, pp. 164-73.

Zhou, C.; Huang, Y., Shao, Y., May, J., Prou, D., Perier, C., Dauer, W., Schon, E.A. & Przedborski, S. (2008). The kinase domain of mitochondrial PINK1 faces the cytoplasm. *Proc Natl Acad Sci U S A*, 105, pp. 12022-7.

Zimprich, A.; Biskup, S., Leitner, P., Lichtner, P., Farrer, M., Lincoln, S., Kachergus, J., Hulihan, M., Uitti, R.J., Calne, D.B., Stoessl, A.J., Pfeiffer, R.F., Patenge, N., Carbajal, I.C., Vieregge, P., Asmus, F., Müller-Myhsok, B., Dickson, D.W., Meitinger, T., Strom, T.M., Wszolek, Z.K. & Gasser, T. (2004). Mutations in LRRK2 cause autosomal-dominant parkinsonism with pleomorphic pathology. *Neuron*, 44, pp. 601-7.

Ziviani, E; Tao, R.N. & Whitworth, A.J. (2010). Drosophila parkin requires PINK1 for mitochondrial translocation and ubiquitinates mitofusin. *Proc Natl Acad Sci U S A*, 107, pp. 5018-23.

3

Wading into a Theoretical Model for Parkinson's Disease

Diana W. Verzi
San Diego State University-Imperial Valley Campus
USA

1. Introduction

While a lot of work has been done on theoretical models for learning and memory, with implications for Alzheimer's disease, little mathematical modeling has been offered for Parkinson's disease, a neurodegenerative disorder of the basal ganglia. The disease is characterized by progressive loss of dopaminergic neurons in the substantia nigra pars compacta, and movement disorders are associated with abnormalities in electrical activity within the substantia nigra pars reticulata. (Brown et al., 1982; Guatteo et al., 2005)
An early study implicated a thermoregulatory role for dopamine receptors in the substantia nigra, but the functional significance of this location in temperature regulation remained to be elucidated (Brown et al., 1982). More recently, changes in temperature of up to several degrees have been reported in different brain regions during various behaviors or in response to environmental stimuli. This lead to the conclusion that temperature-gated TRPV3 and TRPV4 cationic channels are expressed in nigral dopaminergic neurons, and they are active in brain slices at near physiological temperatures, affecting neuronal excitability and calcium homeostasis (Guatteo et al., 2005).
A reduction in the frequency of neuron firing within the striata nigra has been linked to a loss of dopaminergic neurons. A study of spontaneous neuron firing, cell membrane potential and currents, and intracellular calcium levels in dopaminergic neurons of the rat substantia nigra was conducted under varying temperature controls (Guatteo et al., 2005). Cooling evoked slowing of firing, cell membrane hyperpolarization, increase in cell input resistance, and outward current under voltage clamp, along with a decrease in intracellular Ca2+. Warming induced an increase in firing frequency, a decrease in input resistance, an inward current and a rise in Ca2+. Neurons within the globus pallidus and substantia nigra form a functional network that ideally resonates around *70Hz* for normal voluntary movement. However, this network has been observed to oscillate at frequencies below *30Hz* in Parkinson patients, and these oscillations are believed to disrupt normal motor function (Basu et al., 2010).
Post-morten cortices from Parkinson patients exhibit biochemical and physical alterations within dendritic arbors (Patt et al., 1991; Stephens et al., 2005), and it has been suggested that activity-dependent intraspine calcium may regulate dendritic morphology, affecting the synaptic connection between neurons (Stephens et al., 2005). One theory holds that sporadic Parkinson's involves a breakdown of the mitochondria (Surmeier et al., 2010), and recent experimental work implicates mitochondrial Ca2+ dysregulation (Celsi et al., 2009). In particular, the Cav1.3 calcium channel on striatopallidal neurons expressing the D2

dopamine receptor has been linked to the degeneration of dendritic spines on striatal projection neurons. Particular to this chapter, the density of spines within the striata nigra have been found to be greatly reduced for Parkinson's patients, along with a reduction in their dendritic arbors (Gerfen, 2006).

Earlier theoretical models have studied how activity-dependent calcium release from mitochondria may alter dendritic spine morphology (Verzi et al., 2004; Verzi & Baer, 2005), and how activity may directly affect the density and distribution of spines along the dendrite (Verzi et al., 2004). Models have demonstrated that in dendrites with excitable spines, generation and propagation of action potentials depend on the morphology and spatial distribution of spines (Verzi et al., 2004; Verzi & Baer, 2005). A wave can propagate if localized excitatory synaptic input into spine heads causes a few excitable spines to fire, initiating a chain reaction of spine firings along the dendrite. Baer and Rinzel (1991) found that a sustained wavelike response is possible for a certain range of spine densities and electrical parameters. They found that propagation is precluded when spine stem resistance is either too small or too large and that success or failure of local excitation to spread as a chain reaction depends on the spatial distribution of spines (Baer and Rinzel, 1991).

It is painfully obvious that Parkinson's is a complex disorder, involving alterations in brain chemistry, morphology and activity, and an enhanced understanding of the interdependence of these processes will increase our understanding of this devastating disease. This chapter will offer several models to consider these relationships within the striata nigra.

2. Methods

This section develops variations on models for activity-dependent and calcium-regulated spine density and morphology, with age-, temperature- and disease-related changes in the dendritic arbor of the Parkinsonian striata nigra. Dopamine has been implicated as a thermoregulator for dopaminergic neurons (Brown et al., 1982), along with the observation of localized variations in neuronal temperature (Guatteo et al, 2005). Since ionic activity is the driving force in the following models, a study of how temperature may affect the magnitude and frequency of activity is an implicit model for dopamine-dependent levels of neuronal activity.

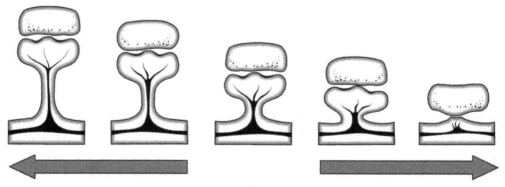

Fig. 1. **Spine loss as a contributor in neuronal death.** Spines may be reabsorbed into the dendrite, or stretch to a point where resistance from the spine stem hinders signal transduction, contributing to neuronal isolation.

2.1 Activity-dependent spine densities

Spines are mushroom shaped protrusions from the soma or dendritic arbor of a neuron, and the loci of 90% of excitatory synaptic connections. Spine loss is observed in normal aging, with an accelerated loss for patients with Parkinson's disease. A dendrite may be populated with thousands of spines of different sizes, shapes and configurations. The basic model for a dynamic distribution of spines is based on Baer and Rinzel's cable theory (1991), where the membrane potentials vary continuously in space and time. Spines interact indirectly by voltage spread along the dendritic cable.

Consider a dendrite with passive membrane properties of a prescribed (dimensionless) electrotonic length (el), studded with a population of spines. The spine density $\bar{n}(X,t)$ represents the average number of spines per unit el. At each location X, the spines deliver current $\bar{n}I_{ss}$, where I_{ss} represents the current flowing through an individual spine stem. The spine stem is modeled as a lumped Ohmic resistor, (Segev & Rall, 1988), so that the stem current is expressed as a voltage drop across the resistor, $R_{ss}(M\Omega)$:

$$I_{ss}(X,t) = \frac{V_{sh}(X,t) - V_d(X,t)}{R_{ss}}. \tag{1}$$

The variables V_{sh} (mV) and V_d (mV) are, respectively, the membrane potential in the head and dendritic base. If potential in the spine head is larger than in the dendrite, $I_{ss} > 0.0$, then the current is flowing from spine head to base. Conversely, if the potential in the base is larger than in the spine head, $I_{ss} < 0.0$, then current flow is from base to head. The spine stem resistance (R_{ss}) represents the ratio of specific cytoplasmic resistance to cross-sectional area, integrated over the length of the stem. A constriction at any location along the stem would decrease the cross sectional area, significantly increasing R_{ss}. Likewise, a stem occlusion could significantly increase internal cytoplasmic resistance, and increase R_{ss}.

The electrical potential in a passive dendrite, studded with $\bar{n}$ spines per unit length, satisfies the cable equation

$$\tau_m \frac{\partial V_d}{\partial t}(X,t) = \frac{\partial^2 V_d}{\partial X^2} - V_d + R_\infty \bar{n} I_{ss}, \tag{2}$$

where τ_m is the membrane time constant, R_∞ is the cable input resistance, and $\bar{n}$ is the average density of spines at each location $X = x/\lambda$, with $\lambda(\mu m)$ the physical length. The model assumes that the dendrite has sealed-end boundary conditions and that both the dendrite and spines have zero resting potentials.

An equation for the membrane potential in each spine head is obtained from a current-balance relation for the capacitive, ionic, synaptic and spine stem currents:

$$C_{sh} \frac{\partial V_{sh}}{\partial t}(X,t) = -I_{syn} - I_{ion} - I_{ss}. \tag{3}$$

The term I_{ion} represents ionic currents passing through the spine head membrane and I_{syn} the synaptically applied current. In a simulation involving spines with passive membrane properties, the ionic current is modeled simply as the ratio of head potential to resistance:

$$I_{ion}(X,t) = \frac{V_{sh}(X,t)}{R_{sh}} . \tag{4}$$

If the spines are considered to have excitable membrane properties, Hodgkin-Huxley kinetics model temperature- and voltage-dependent ion channel currents (Hodgkin & Huxley, 1952), and

$$I_{ion}(X,t) = \gamma A_{sh}\left[g_{NA}m^3h(V_{sh} - V_{NA}) + g_K n^4(V_{sh} - V_K) + g_L(V_{sh} - V_L) \right]. \tag{5}$$

The parameters γ and A_{sh} represent channel density and spine head area, and the gate activation/inactivation variables m, n and h satisfy first-order rate equations with voltage-dependent time constants and steady-state functions (Hodgkin & Huxley, 1952). The parameters V_{Na}, V_K and V_L are synaptic reversal potentials for sodium, potassium and leakage currents, with maximal conductances of g_{Na}, g_K and g_L, respectively .
Synapses over a small interval are activated by applying a brief synaptic conductance to the spines in that interval

$$I_{syn} = g_p \frac{t}{t_p} \exp\left(1 - \frac{t}{t_p} \right)\left(V_{sh} - V_{syn}\right), \tag{6}$$

where V_{syn} is the synaptic reversal potential. The synaptic current is applied periodically, maximizing to g_p, when $t = t_p$ in each period.
Let I_{ss} , the spine stem current from Eq. (1), be a measure for local activity. Then, the density of spines at any location X along the dendrite is assumed to be a dynamic variable that changes slowly over time and depends on electrical interactions between the spine head and dendritic shaft, as measured by the spine stem current. Let $\overline{n}(X,t)$ the average density of spines per unit el be a dynamic variable that changes slowly over time and space, and depends on electrical interactions between the spine head and the dendritic base. In general, the change in $\overline{n}$ is assumed to be bounded and proportional to I_{ss} . Then,

$$\frac{\partial \overline{n}}{\partial t}(X,t) = \varepsilon_n K_n I_{ss}\left(1 - \frac{\overline{n}}{n_{max}} \right)\left(\overline{n} - n_{min}\right), \tag{7}$$

describes this change, where $\varepsilon_n \ll 1$ is dimensionless, and K_n is a positive parameter scaled to cable input resistance. Density increases in response to local synaptic activity, decreases in response to centripedal flow, and remains unchanged in regions experiencing no measurable level of activity. Changes in spine density depend on changes in I_{ss} , which in turn depend on the integrative properties of the surrounding membrane and synaptic activity. A more detailed derivation of this model may be found in Verzi et al. (2004).

2.2 A model of dendritic spine loss with age and Parkinsonism
An early model for idiopathic Parkinsonism considered the temporal profile for neurodegeneration in dopaminergic neurons, assuming a linear loss for normal aging, and a quadratic or exponential loss consistent with the duration of symptoms (Schulzer et al., 1994). Since ten percent of these neurons seem to survive, a lower bound was placed on the

temporal function. A reduction in dendritic spines may be considered as a reduction in axo-dendritic synapses, and a total loss of synaptic contact may be considered as neuronal isolation or cell death.

To consider the implications of activity-dependent spine densities in the substantia nigra, consistent with age-related linear and Parkinson-related quadratic loss of dopaminergic neurons, one could remove the upper bound for spine density, and append linear and quadratic terms to Eq. (7), replacing it with

$$\frac{\partial \overline{n}}{\partial t}(X,t) = \varepsilon_n K_n I_{ss}\left(\overline{n} - n_{min}\right) - \delta\left(\overline{n} - n_{min}\right) - \theta\left(\overline{n} - n_{min}\right)^2. \tag{8}$$

2.3 A model for the interdependence of activity, calcium and dendritic spine morphology

While activity affects, and is affected by the distribution and density of spines along the dendrite, so also are the structures of individual spines. Earlier theoretical models (Verzi et al., 2004; Verzi & Baer, 2005) have considered how activity-dependent calcium-regulated dendritic morphology could alter neuronal firing patterns to enhance or impede the efficacy of a neuronal network. This was based on experimental observations that a moderate amount of neuronal activity may release Ca2+ from mitochondria, reshaping dendritic spines to increase synaptic efficacy, but that too much activity may raise Ca2+ within the cytosol to a caustic level and cause the spines to pull away from the synaptic connection, thereby contributing to isolation of the neuron (Harris, 1999) .

This section considers how activity-dependent free intraspine calcium may function as a second messenger in regulating continuous changes in dendritic spine morphology. For a fixed distribution of spines along the dendrite, let the spine stem resistance R_{ss} (reciprocal of conductance) be a measure for dynamic spine stem morphology. Spines with longer and thinner stems, or those deformed by organelle occlusions, such as mitochondria or endoplasmic reticula, generally have higher measures of stem resistance and are more isolated from the dendrite, while those with shorter and wider stems generally have lower input resistance, and may be more electrically connected to the dendrite. A continuum model consistent with the above assumptions utilizes Eqs. (1-6), replacing Eq. (7) in the model for activity-dependent dendritic spine densities with the following slow subsystem for calcium-regulated dendritic spine morphology:

$$\frac{\partial C_a}{\partial t}(X,t) = -\varepsilon_C\left(C_a - C_{min}\right) + |I_{ss}| / K_C \tag{9}$$

$$\frac{\partial R_{ss}}{\partial t}(X,t) = -\varepsilon_R\left(\frac{C_a}{C_{crit}} - 1\right)\left(\frac{C_a}{C_{min}} - 1\right)\left(1 - \frac{R_{ss}}{R_{max}}\right)\left(R_{ss} - R_{min}\right) \tag{10}$$

In this model, local activity is measured by the magnitude, or absolute value, of the spine stem current, regardless of direction. Local calcium levels increase, so long as $|I_{ss}|$ is large enough, with respect to the current saturation of calcium, relative to a minimum amount. The parameter K_C scales this relationship. The model prescribes a critical intraspine calcium level (C_{crit}), consistent with Harris (1999), as threshold for whether or not local spines become long and thin or short and stubby. The stem resistance increases for $C_a < C_{crit}$

(subcritical), modeling spine stem elongation, and decreases for $C_a > C_{crit}$ (supercritical), modeling spine stem shortening.

Now the spine density ($\bar{n}$) is no longer dynamic, but the spine stem resistance ($R_{ss}(X,t)$) is a bounded, dynamic function of activity and free intraspine calcium, relative to some minimal level. When synaptic activity is present, stem resistance approaches steady-state if R_{ss} approaches the bounds of R_{max} or R_{min}, or if I_{ss} drives C_a to C_{crit}.

For ε_C and $\varepsilon_R \ll 1$, the slow subsystem described in Eqs. (9-10) connects to the fast equations for activity (Eq. 1-6) by I_{ss} in Eqs. 2, 3 and 9, and by R_{ss} in Eqs. 1 and 10. In the absence of activity, the system approaches equilibrium, since C_a approaches C_{min} when $I_{ss} = 0$, and $\partial R_{ss} / \partial t = 0$ when $C_a = C_{min}$. In the model, the cable input resistance (R_∞) is fixed, while R_{ss} varies over time and space. The difference between spine head and base potentials in Eq. (1) becomes negligible since $V_{sh} \to V_d$ in Eq. (1) as $R_{ss} \to R_{min}$, imposing a kinetic upper bound on calcium (i.e. $|I_{ss}| = |V_{sh} - V_d| / R_{ss}$ becomes small enough that Eq. (9) is negative).

2.4 A discussion of temperature-dependent neuronal firing patterns

Hodgkin & Huxley (1952) hypothesized in their famous study of the squid giant axon that sodium movement depends on the distribution of charged particles that allow sodium to pass through the membrane, so that changes in membrane permeability are a function of membrane potential, rather than current. They supposed that the rate of movement of the activating particles determined the rate at which the sodium conductance approached its maximum, concluding that temperature had a large effect on this rate, and the frequency for repetitive firing and recovery. While of opposite charge, similar statements were made about changes in sodium permeability.

Many theoretical models utilize Hodgkin-Huxley kinetics for excitable (or active) membrane response, with an implicit adjustment for temperature. The gating variables m, n and h in Eq. (5) consider the voltage-dependent probability that the sodium and potassium channels are open as

$$\frac{dm}{dt} = \alpha_m(V_{sh})(1-m) - \beta_m m$$
$$\frac{dh}{dt} = \alpha_h(V_{sh})(1-h) - \beta_h h \qquad (11)$$
$$\frac{dn}{dt} = \alpha_n(V_{sh})(1-n) - \beta_n n$$

where the voltage-dependent, gating functions $\alpha_i(V_{sh})$ and $\beta_i(V_{sh})$ for i=m, n and h

$$\alpha_m(T,V_{sh}) = \Phi(T)\frac{0.1(25-V_{sh})}{\exp(0.1(25-V_{sh})-1)}$$
$$\beta_m(T,V_{sh}) = \Phi(T)\exp(-V_{sh}/18)$$
$$\alpha_h(T,V_{sh}) = \Phi(T)0.07\exp(-V_{sh}/20)$$
$$\beta_h(T,V_{sh}) = \Phi(T)\frac{1}{\exp(0.1(30-V_{sh})+1)} \qquad (12)$$
$$\alpha_n(T,V_{sh}) = \Phi(T)\frac{0.01(10-V_{sh})}{\exp(0.1(10-V_{sh})-1)}$$
$$\beta_n(T,V_{sh}) = \Phi(T)0.125\exp(-V_{sh}/80)$$

are adjusted for variation from Hodgkin & Huxley (1952) results obtained at $T = 6.3$ Celsius (C), by the factor:

$$\Phi(T) = 3^{\left(\frac{T-6.3}{10}\right)}. \tag{13}$$

Modeling an increase in temperature in Eq. (13) decreases the time-duration for an action potential, with a decrease in maximal amplitude (see Fig. 2 below). Conversely, a decrease in temperature stretches out the action potential over time and increases the maximum membrane potential. Increasing temperature also raises the voltage threshold for action potential generation, and decreasing temperature lowers this threshold (Fitzhugh, 1966).

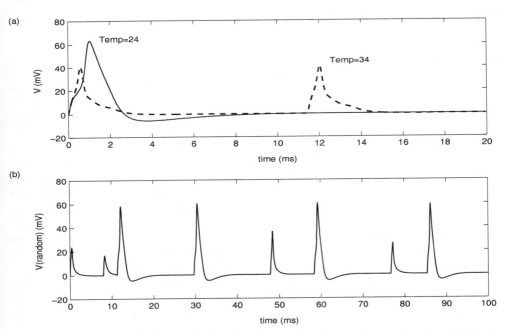

Fig. 2. **Temperature-dependent variations in neuronal activity.** The magnitude and shape of neuronal response depends on localized membrane temperature. Periodic synaptic activation is temperature-dependent.

Earlier theoretical studies demonstrated the interdependence of dendritic activity, morphology and chemistry for fixed temperature and activation periods (Verzi et al., 2004; Verzi & Baer, 2005). This chapter considers how slow changes in morphology and chemistry affect and are affected by temperature-dependent changes in ionic activity. In most of the simulations, temperature is defined iteratively for each activation cycle, remaining constant for the duration of a cycle k as

$$T(1) = \omega \text{ , and } T(k+1) = T(k) + \sigma \text{ .} \tag{14}$$

For $|\sigma| \ll 1$, continuous changes in temperature describe a simulation for warming if $\sigma > 0$ and cooling for $\sigma < 0$. Since studies have observed a decrease in temperature and firing frequency in Parkinsonism (Guatteo et al., 2005), simulations will, likewise, consider the effect of temperature-dependent continuous changes in activation frequency, describing the period between synaptic firings from Eq. (6) as

$$P = \upsilon - \rho T .$$
(15)

For $\rho > 0$, the length of an activation cycle is inversely proportional to temperature for an increasing period during gradual cooling, and decreasing period for warming. Figure 2a displays two temperature-dependent magnitudes for excitable membrane response (Eq. 5). Note the slower rise in sodium to a greater maximum for cooler temperatures (Fitzhugh, 1966). In Fig. 2b, temperature is random on T in [24,39] to display the range of magnitudes and frequencies from Eq. (15).

3. Results

In the simulations that follow, the models are numerically integrated using a semi-implicit Crank-Nicholson/Adams-Bashforth finite differencing method. The spatial step is set to $\Delta X = 0.4$, with a corresponding time step of $\Delta t = .005$ for simulations with R_{ss} of higher values, and $\Delta X = 0.1$, with $\Delta t = .0005$ to maintain stability for R_{ss} of lower values. Computations are performed in Fortran double-precision on a *Sun-Solaris 9* computer. Since, in reality, a significant increase in spine density takes place on a time scale of hours to days and individual action-potentials are on a time scale of milliseconds, the computation time for a simulation could be on the order of hours. For most simulations, the synaptic input is repeated at greater than or equal to 8 *ms*, long enough to allow potentials in the head and dendrite to return to resting values. For each of the time scaling values that define slowly changing variables, one must identify a value that preserves the basic dynamics of the system as $\varepsilon_i \to 0$. Using a computer animation program with uniform activation periods, an initial value is chosen to animate the time course at three spatial locations over 60 synaptic events for a typical run involving the development of a propagating wave. Then each ε_i is halved, and simulations are repeated for 120 activation cycles. The results are superimposed, using every-other cycle of the 120-cycle simulation. The process is repeated several times, successively halving ε_i and doubling superimposed cycles, until the animations converge at ε_i^*. Then ε_i is set to ε_i^* for each i, sufficiently small and computationally efficient, without compromising the integrity of the dynamics for smaller values that define chemical and morphological changes over hours to days.

3.1 Dendritic spine loss with age and Parkinsonism

Equations (1-3) and (8) are used in four separate simulations, with initially 23 spines/unit *el*, uniformly distributed over a dendrite of length 3. Spines over X in [0, 0.2] are activated every 10 *ms* with Eq. (6). In two of the simulations, the spines are considered to have passive membrane properties, merely passing the signal along the dendrite, so that the ionic membrane current is modeled with Eq. (4). In the other two simulations, the spines are considered to have excitable, or active membrane properties to modulate a signal on its way

Cable and Spine Model	τ_m	Membrane time constant	$2.5ms$
	R_∞	Cable input resistance	$1233M\Omega$
	λ	Physical length	$180\mu m$
	C_{sh}	Spine head capacitance	$C_m A_{sh}$
	C_m	Membrane capacitance	$1mF/cm^2$
	A_{sh}	Spine head surface area	$1.31/\mu m^2$
	R_{sh}	Spine head membrane resistance	$10.02 \cdot 10^{11}\Omega$
	R_{ss}	Spine stem resistance	See simulations
Spine Density Models	ε_n	Density time constant	$8.02 \cdot 10^{-6}$
	K_n	Scaling parameter	10^9
	n_{max}	Upper bound	$50/e.l.$
	n_{min}	Lower bound	$0/e.l.$
	δ	Linear rate of loss	10^{-3}
	θ	Quadratic rate of loss	10^{-4} or 0
Calcium-Morphology	ε_C	Calcium time constant	$3 \cdot 10^{-3}$
	ε_R	Resistance time constant	$7.5 \cdot 10^{-5}$
	K_C	Scaling parameter	$3.3 \cdot 10^{-10}$
	C_{min}	Calcium lower bound	$5nM$
	C_{crit}	Calcium critical level	$300nM$
	R_{min}	Stem resistance lower bound	$90M\Omega$
	R_{max}	Stem resistance upper bound	$2000M\Omega$
Kinetics	γ	Channel density scale factor	2.5
	g_{NA}	Maximal sodium conductance	$120mS/cm^2$
	g_K	Maximal potassium conductance	$36mS/cm^2$
	g_L	Maximal leakage conductance	$0.3mS/cm^2$
	V_{NA}	Sodium reversal potential	$115mV$
	V_K	Potassium reversal potential	$-12mV$
	V_L	Leakage reversal potential	$10.5989mV$
Synaptic activation	g_p	Peak synaptic conductance	$0.074nS$
	t_p	Time to peak synaptic conductance	$0.2ms$
	V_{syn}	Synaptic reversal potential	$100mV$
Temperature and Period	ω	Initial temperature	See simulations
	σ	Rate of change in temperature	See simulations
	υ	Period scaling constant	40
	ρ	Rate of change in period	0.8

Table 1. Table of model parameters

to the soma, modeled here with kinetics from Eq. (5). Figure 3 graphs results for two passive simulations (left) and two active simulations (right), reporting results for spines "downstream" of the synaptic activation at X=0.5, to observe local response without input current from the axon.

In Eq. (8), spine density may increase for sufficiently high levels of activity to offset linear and/or quadratic loss due to age or the onset of Parkinson's disease, respectively. The spine density over time is graphed in Fig. 3a for two passive (left) and two active (right) simulations, superimposing results for linear assumptions for aging only (NL) over linear and quadratic assumptions for both aging and Parkinsonism (NQ).

Simulations with passive or active membrane in dendritic spines shows a linear decrease when θ = 0, to model only age-related loss of spines in Eq. (8), and a quadratic decrease in spine density when θ is positive, modeling the effect of both aging and Parkinson's disease on the loss of synaptic connections. Parameter values chosen here are set to emphasize qualitative differences for age- and Parkinson-related spine loss, and results are observed over a relatively short period of time. Since the action potential is rapidly shut down by spine loss, the rate of spine loss is similar from passive to active simulation.

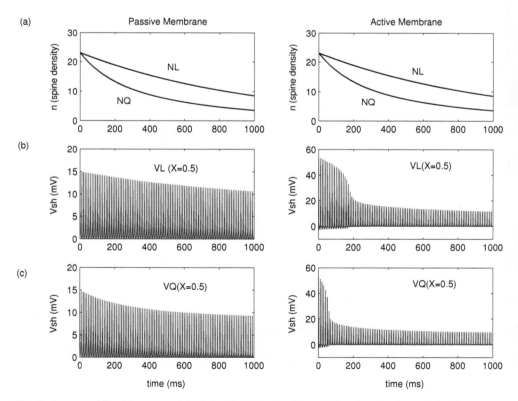

Fig. 3. **Age- and Parkinson- related dendritic spine loss.** Spine density is modeled to decrease linearly with age, and quadratically after the onset of Parkinson's disease.

Figure 3b graphs the time course for spine head potential in the linear simulation (VL). In the passive simulation (left) peak potential in each 10-*ms* activation cycle decreases linearly with NL (above). Spine density is initially large enough to cause an action potential in the active spine simulation (right), but quickly decreases below threshold NL=20, so that maximum potentials decrease linearly for the duration of the simulation. In Fig. 3c, potential in the spine heads is graphed over time for the quadratic simulation (VQ). Peak potentials decrease quadratically with NQ in Fig. 3a for the passive simulation (left). In the active simulation (right), VQ loses its nonlinear response much earlier, when NQ falls below threshold to generate an action potential for spines with stem resistance uniformly set to $R_{ss} = 1240 M\Omega$. Spine density decreases at each time step linearly or quadratically, with a decrease in the rate of change as $\bar{n} \to n_{min} = 0$. The strength of the signal passed to the dendrite decreases proportional to the density of spines.

3.2 Temperature-regulated dendritic spine density

To model how cooling temperatures due to dopamine depletion affect the density of spines and resultant efficacy of signal transduction in the dendrite, Equations (1-3) and Eq. (7) are used in a single simulation for spines with excitable membrane properties. The initial spine density is set to 23 spines/unit *el*, uniformly distributed over a dendrite of length 3. Since the spines are assumed active, I_{ion} from Eq. (5) models voltage-dependent membrane kinetics. Spines are stimulated over X in [0, 0.2] with I_{syn} from Eq. (6) that peaks at $t_p = 0.2ms$ in each activation cycle. Different in this simulation, the period between activations is temperature-dependent from Eq. (15) with υ and ρ chosen to vary the period from 8 to 20 *ms* over a temperature range of 39 to 24° C. The temperature decreases from $\omega = 39$ in Eq. (14) at a rate of $\alpha = -0.05$.

In Fig. 4a (left) temperature changes with each cycle, with the rate of change decreasing as cycles grow longer for cooler temperatures. On the right side of Fig. 4a, spine density is graphed in a spatial profile over the entire dendrite at three frozen moments in time: The initial condition is indicated by the top dashed line at $\bar{n} = 23$, with a slight rise in density over the activation site at t=1000 *ms*, with a decrease in densities downstream. After 5000 *ms*, density has significantly decreased over the entire length of the dendrite.

In Fig. 4b, spine head potential is graphed over time within the activation site (left) and downstream (right). Downstream, $I_{ss} \leq 0$ until the spines initiate their own action potential to propagate the signal. At t=1000 *ms*, action potential generation begins at X=1.0, but spine densities continue to decrease across the dendrite (4a right), even in the presence of a propagating wave, due to the increasingly longer periods with little or no activity. Shorter cycles for higher temperatures may be observed in the dark shading (t<800ms), compared to the shading for longer periods (t>3000).

Spine density is an important parameter for action potential generation and propagation, since more spines increase membrane potential per location X. While the initial density of 23 would be sufficient for an action potential under normal temperatures, the higher voltgage-threshold for T=39 degrees prevents generation at the beginning of the simulation. The voltage-dependent gating functions α_i and β_i from Eq. (12) contain a temperature-dependent factor from Eq. (13) that increases the magnitude and decreases the voltage-threshold for action potential response under cooler temperatures (Fitzhugh, 1966). Figure

4c graphs the change in density over time within the activation site (left) and downstream (right). Note the rate of decrease is constant in the activation site (left), but greater downstream (right) in the absence of local action potential generation.

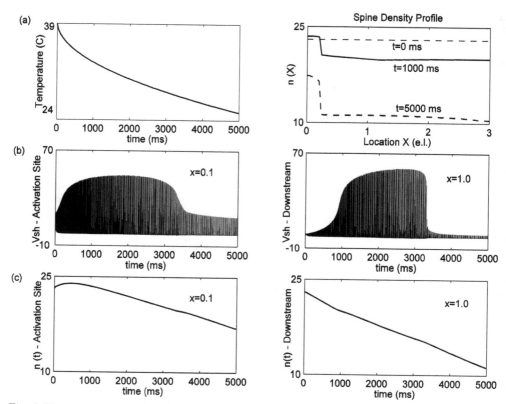

Fig. 4. **Temperature regulated excitable dendritic spine densities.** Spine densities decrease for cooler temperatures and longer activation cycles, even in the presence of action potential generation and propagation.

3.3 Steady-state calcium regulated spine morphology

The model for calcium-regulated spine morphology demonstrates how variations in the frequency of synaptic activation may affect the shape and efficacy of dendritic spines (Verzi et al., 2004; Verzi & Baer, 2005). Eqs. (1-3) and (9-10) model the interdependence of activity, chemistry and morphology for a fixed population of spines along the dendrite. Using the stem resistance as a measure for morphology, the model identifies a variation in steady-states for calcium and spine shape, based on the frequency of activation.

Figure 5 illustrates two such steady-states. A uniform density of 23 spines/unit *el* are distributed along a dendrite of length 3. They are assumed passive, so that Eq. (4) describes the ionic current. Now the spine density is fixed, but the morphology of each spine is a dynamic variable, measured by the spine stem resistance, $R_{ss}(X,t)$. The morphology depends on the local level of calcium $C_a(X,t)$ (Eq. 10), which, in turn, is regulated by the magnitude of local activity, as measured by $|I_{ss}|$ (Eq. 9). Initially, stem resistance and calcium are uniformly set to $R_{ss} = 750 M\Omega$, and $C_a = 15nM$. Spines are activated over X in [0, 0.2] with Eq. (6) every 20 ms or 50 Hz (left), and every 8 ms or 125 Hz (right), and results are shown for spines under synaptic activation. The parameter $C_{crit} = 300nM$ for Eq. (10), so that R_{ss} increases when C_a is below the dashed line in Fig. 5a, and decreases when C_a is above the dashed line.

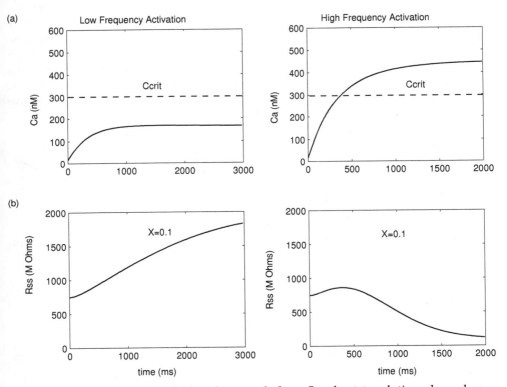

Fig. 5. **Calcium-regulated dendritic spine morphology.** Steady-state solutions depend on the frequency of synaptic activation. If calcium is supercritical/subcritical, the spines display higher/lower input resistance.

The upper bound for free intraspine calcium settles to a sub-critical steady-state for low-frequency activation (Fig. 5a left) and a super-critical steady-state for high-frequency activation (Fig. 5a right). In Fig. 5b (left), stem resistance rises rapidly as calcium increases, but reaches an inflection point to slow its ascent toward R_{max} as calcium approaches steady-state, for low-frequency synaptic activation. In Fig. 5b (right), stem resistance increases while calcium is below C_{crit}, and begins to decrease toward R_{min} when calcium becomes super-critical for high-frequency stimulation.

3.4 Frequency-dependent calcium regulation for spines with passive membrane properties

It has been observed in Parkinson's disease that a decrease in temperature causes a reduction in the frequency of neuronal firing in the striata nigra, along with a decrease in the amount of free interstitial calcium. Likewise, an increase in temperature has been shown to cause an increase in the frequency of firing, with an increase in free calcium, citing temperatures ranging from -10 to +5 degrees from 34 C (Guatteo et al., 2005). While temperature is not explicit in the model for spines with passive membrane properties, it may be inferred from the positive correlation between temperature and firing frequency.

Figure 6 illustrates two simulations to study the effect of a continuous change in temperature-dependent frequency variations from Eq. (15) for the calcium-regulated spine morphology model, using Eqs. (1-3) to model rapid changes in activity and Eqs. (9-10) for the slow subsystem of calcium and spine stem resistance, as in the steady-state simulations from Fig. 5 above. Once again, a dendrite of length 3 is assumed to have a fixed density of 23 uniformly distributed passive spines/unit el, with initial uniform morphology $R_{ss} = 750 M\Omega$. This time, initial free calcium is uniformly set to $C_a = 150 nM$. Since the spines are assumed to have passive membrane properties, the ionic current is modeled with Eq. (4).

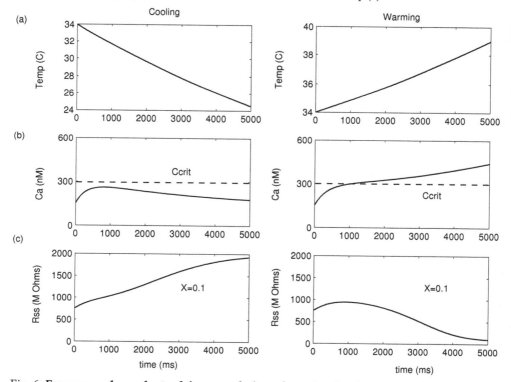

Fig. 6. **Frequency-dependent calcium regulation of passive dendritic spine shape.**
Longer/shorter periods between activations cause calcium to decrease/increase and spine length to increase/decrease.

The period between activations is modeled to be temperature-dependent from Eq. (15), with υ and ρ chosen to, again, vary the period from 8 to 20 ms over a temperature range of 39 to 24 degrees. Figure 6a graphs temperature over 5000 ms for cooling (left) and warming (right). The initial temperature is set to change from $\omega = 34$ in Eq. (14) at a rate of $\alpha = -0.03$ in each activation period for the simulation over 10 degrees of cooling in Fig. 6 (left), and $\alpha = 0.01$ for the simulation over 5 degrees of warming in Fig. 6 (right), since activation cycles are much shorter over time for warmer temperatures.

In Fig. 6b, calcium does not approach equilibrium, but remains subcritical during cooling (left), and climbs steadily beyond C_{crit} as both the temperature and frequency of activation increase during warming (right). In response, Fig. 6c displays an increase in stem resistance toward maximum as the temperature cools (longer activation period) and decreases toward its minimum under warming conditions (shorter activation period), consistent with experimental observations (Guatteo et al., 2005). It is interesting to note that the balance between local activity and free intraspine calcium from Eq. (9) changes sign so that calcium begins to decrease (6b left) when the length of each activation period equals 13.6 ms ($T=32$ C). It is also interesting to observe that calcium increases almost linearly with warming (6b right) after stem resistance begins to decrease.

3.5 Temperature-dependent calcium regulation for spines with active membrane properties

Different from the previous simulation for calcium regulated passive spine morphology, a simulation of the same model for spines with active membrane properties has a direct link to temperature. Recall that the gating functions in the Hodgkin-Huxley kinetics are adjusted for temperature by Eq. (13). Once again, Eqs. (1-3) and (9-10) model activity-dependent calcium, and calcium-regulated spine morphology, under the assumption that the period between synaptic activations is a function of temperature from Eq. (15). Twenty-five spines/unit el with excitable membrane properties are uniformly distributed across a dendrite of length 3. Spines over X in [0, 0.2] are activated with I_{syn} from Eq. (6), and the active ionic membrane currents are modeled by Eq. (5).

Figure 7 illustrates results from a simulation for temperatures cooling (Eq. 14) from $\omega = 34$ to 24 degrees at a rate of $\sigma = -0.03$ degrees/activation cycle. Initial values for calcium and spine stem resistance are uniformly 15 nM and 900 $M\Omega$, respectively. While the rate of cooling is constant between cycles, Fig. 7a (left) again shows a reduction in the rate of cooling over time, since the length of activation cycles lengthens as the temperature cools. In Fig. 7a (right) calcium rises quickly to supercritical, since voltage is above threshold to generate an action potential for the current values of stem resistance and temperature. Voltage in the spine heads under synaptic activation rises in the presence of an action potential briefly in Fig. 7b (left) until the temperature drops below. It is interesting that the magnitude of an action potential may be higher for cooler temperatures, but the voltage threshold for generation decreases as temperatures cool (Fitzhugh, 1966).

Stem resistance rises when calcium is below the dashed line for C_{crit} and falls when calcium is above it in Fig. 7 (right). When action potential generation ceases, $|I_{ss}| / K_c < \varepsilon_c (C_a - C_{min})$ in Eq. (9), so that the change in calcium is negative and calcium falls below subcritical to a steady-state balance between these two terms. However, since the steady-state is subcritical, as in Fig. 5 for low frequency activation, R_{ss} continues to rise for the duration of the simulation. After

6500 ms, stem resistance has returned to its initial value of 900 $M\Omega$ (7b right), but the maximum spine head potential has fallen from 28 mV to 13 mV for the same number of spines with the same morphology. The temperature has fallen from 34 to 24, affecting voltage threshold to generate an action potential. Note also the hyperpolarization of head potential in the presence an action potential at the beginning of the simulation, and after 2500 ms, when the temperature has fallen below 30. Compare this result with Figs. 3 and 4 for dynamic spine density where there is no hyperpolarization for passive membrane simulations, and only in the presence of an action potential for active simulations.

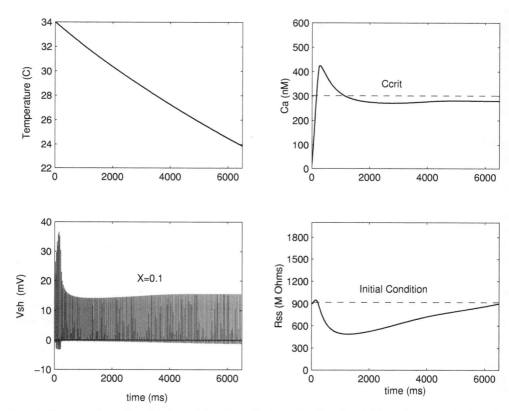

Fig. 7. **Temperature-dependent calcium regulation of active dendritic spine morphology.** Cooler temperatures lengthen the period between synaptic activations, decreasing the amount of local activity and free intraspine calcium levels, which increases spine stem length and input resistance.

4. Conclusions

It is challenging to consider the long-term effect over months to years of activity that scales on the order of milliseconds. The length of time for density and structural transition in the models presented depends on the magnitude of ε_i, for $i=n$, C, R, selected here for computational efficiency. To achieve the results shown in this paper over several months, one would need to set the rate of change in spine structure on the order of 10^{-25}. An alternative to speed up computation time in systems with periodic activation would be to exploit the fact that the slow variables are piecewise continuous over time and relatively constant within each activation cycle. One might then use the average measure of local activity (such as I_{ss}) in each cycle to compute changes in the slow system at the end of each cycle of length P, rather than integrating the entire system at each time step. While simulations in this paper consider repetitive input to a fixed site along the dendrite, an interesting question for future work is to observe long term effects for simulations where the activation site is randomly selected in each cycle.

The results in this chapter agree with earlier generalized neuronal studies for spine density (Annis et al., 1994) and morphology (Harris, 1999), and specifically to recent studies within the striata nigra for Parkinsonism (Guatteo et al., 2005; Patt et al., 1991; Schulzer et al., 1994). Earlier studies (Verzi et al., 2004; Verzi & Baer, 2005) identified both analytic and numeric equilibria, centers and limit cycles for calcium and stem resistance that coincide with healthy or ailing spine morphologies illustrated in this chapter, and suggested in the literature (Guatteo et al., 2005; Harris, 1999). There are numerous observations about spine loss in the literature (Gerfen, 2006, Patt et al., 1991, and Schulzer et al., 1994), and studies that involve the thermoregulatory role of dopamine within the striata nigra suggest cooling, a reduction in firing frequency, and a decrease in cell input resistance (Brown et al., 1982, Guatteo et al., 2005). The model for calcium and spine morphology uses stem resistance as a measure for cell shape, suggesting long, thin spines under warming conditions and short stubby spines under cooling conditions. One cannot help but wonder what is the morphological precursor to the loss of a dendritic spine? Do spines die as a result of stretching out their stems and increasing input resistance (under cooling and low frequency activation) to the point that the synaptic connection is isolated from the dendrite? Or do they die as a result of being driven down into the dendrite, decreasing input resistance (under warming and high frequency activation) to the point that they can no longer boost or modulate a signal? These are interesting questions that beg more study.

With evidence that ion channel proteins within the dendritic arbor play an important role in thermoregulation (Geffen et al., 1976; Simon, 2006), experimentalists will need to work closely with theoretical biologists to include components within ionic membrane modeling to include dopamine uptake and release, as well as TRPV3 and TRPV4 channel function. Likewise, mathematical modelers need to include components to more accurately capture important dynamics within the striata nigra. A recent Ranvier node model (Smit et al., 2009), based on a modification of the Hodgkin-Huxley model accurately captures excitable membrane properties within the range for human temperatures for large-diameter nerve fibres. Likewise, a model by Moore (1958, as cited in Fitzhugh, 1966) suggests that sodium and potassium conductances (g_{NA} and g_K) in Eq. (5) increase linearly with temperature, where the Hodgkin-Huxley model (1952) assumes they are independent of temperature. Since temperature has been shown to be a significant variable in the study of Parkinson's disease, it may be prudent to multiply these conductances by

$$\eta = A\left[1 + B(T - 6.3)\right], \tag{16}$$

where A is the ratio between ionic conductions of the axon at 6.3 C and the values used by Hodgkin & Huxley (1952), and B is the rate of change in conductance with temperature, (Fitzhugh, 1966). Measurement data within the striata nigra will be required to accurately fit the parameters A and B. Moreover, with the recent identification of variations in intracellular calcium levels as a contributor to mitochondrial damage (Celci et al, 2009), it is important to include calcium as a component of activity, as well as a consequence. Calcium currents should be included in further theoretical studies to consider the effect of calcium influx to localized cell deterioration.

Patients not adequately controlled with medication may be treated with deep brain stimulation, a current that is thought to block abnormal nerve signals (Benabid, 2003). Other work has demonstrated that high frequency electro-acupucture stimulation could enhance survival of dopamineric neurons and interfere with abnormal signaling (Jia et al., 2010). These studies suggest that high-frequency stimulation may result in changes in neuronal activity within the basal ganglia, by correcting signal rather than chemical abnormalities. Deep brain stimulation or high frequency electro-acupuncture may induce an inhibitory current, blocking abnormal synaptic activation and excitation (Benabid, 2003, Ascoli et al., 2010). Synaptic inhibition may be thought of as increased membrane permeability to negatively charged ions such as potassium and chloride, which tend to extinguish excitation. Inhibitory conductance in the spine head creates a current path to ground, shunting local currents. For an inhibitory reversal potential, it produces a hyperpolarizing inhibitory postsynaptic potential in the spines. In the presence of synaptic excitation, it reduces the net depolarizing current produced by both the excitatory input and the active channels (Segev & Rall, 1988). Theoretical biologists need to address the connection between deep brain stimulation and Parkinson's disease.

Because a neuron may have as many as ten or twenty thousand spines, small changes in one or more spine parameters could affect the relative weighting of several different synaptic inputs. Nonlinear dynamics in thousands of these compartments along a dynamic geometry within the dendritic arbor may change a single neuron's response to varying input patterns, as well as the dynamic behavior of the entire neuronal subsystem (Segev & Rall, 1988). Severe pathological changes, such as decrease of dendritic length, loss of dendritic spines, and several types of dendritic varicosities have been found in the melanin-containing neurons of substantia nigra pars compacta for Parkinson's patients (Patt et al., 1991). Continuing theoretical studies of action potential generation and propagation under geometric and chemical fluctuations will give insight to the pathology of this complex and devastating disease.

5. Acknowledgments

The author gratefully acknowledges Frank Perez of Frank's Graffik Graffiti in Brawley, California, for illustrations; SM Baer of Arizona State University for inspiration; and Oliver Velarde of San Diego State University-Imperial Valley Campus for technical assistance. This work was supported by National Institutes of Mental Health Grant MH1065515 to Terry Cronan of SDSU.

6. References

Annis, C. M.; O'Dowd, D. K. & Robertson, R. T. (1994). Activity-dependent regulation of dendritic spine density on cortical pyramidal neurons in organotypic slice cultures. *Journal of Neurobiology*, 25(12), (December, 1994), pp. 1483-1493.

Ascoli, G. A.; Gasparini, S., Medinilla, V.; & Migliore, M. (2010). Local control of postinhibitory rebound spiking in CA1 pyramidal neuron dendrites. *Journal of Neuroscience*, 30(18), (May, 2010), pp. 6434-6442.

Basu I., Graupe, D; Tuninetti, D. & Slavin, K. V. (2010). Stochastic modeling of the neuronal activity in the subthalamic nucleus and model parameter identification from Parkinson patient data. *Biological Cybernetics*, 103(6), (June, 2010) pp. 273-283.

Benabid, A. L. (2003). Deep brain stimulation for Parkinson's disease. *Current Opinion in Neurobiology*, 13(6), (December, 2003), pp. 696-706.

Brown, S. J.; Gisolfi, C. V. & Mora, F. (1982). Temperature regulation and dopaminergic systems in the brain: does the substatia nigra play a role? *Brain Research*, 234(2), (February, 1982), pp. 275-286.

Celsi, F.; Pizzo, P.; Brini, M.; Leo, S.; Fotino, C.; Pinton, P. & Rizzuto, R. (2009). Mitochondria, calcium and cell death: a deadly triad in neurodegeneration. *Biochimica, Biophysica Acta.* 1787(5), (May, 2009), pp. 335-344.

Fitzhugh, R. (1966). Theoretical effect of temperature on threshold in the Hodgkin-Huxley nerve model. *General Physiology*, 49(5), (May, 1966), pp. 989-1005.

Geffen, L. B.; Jessell, T. M.; Cuello, A. C.; & Iversen, L. L. (1976). Release of dopamine from dendrites in rat substantia nigra. *Nature*, (March, 1976), 260(3), pp. 258-260.

Gerfen, C. R. (2006). Indirect-pathway neurons lose their spines in Parkinson disease. *Nature Neuroscience*, 9(2), (February, 2006), pp. 157-158.

Guatteo, E.; Chung, K. K.; Bowala, T. K.; Bernardi, G.; Mercuri, N.B. & Lipski, J. J. (2005). Temperature sensitivity of dopaminergic neurons of the substantia nigra pars compacta: involvement of transient receptor potential channels. *Journal of Neurophysiology*, 94(5), (May, 2005), pp. 3069-80.

Harris, K. M. (1999). Calcium from internal stores modifies dendritic spine shape. *Proceedings of the National Academy of Sciences, USA*, 96(22), (October, 1999), pp. 12213-12215.

Hodgkin, A. L. & Huxley, A. F. (1952). A quantitative description of membrane current and its application to conduction and excitation in nerves. *Journal of Physiology*, 117, (March, 1952), pp. 500-544

Jia, J.; Li, B.; Sun, Z. L.; Yu, F.; Wang, X.; & Wang, X. M. (2010). Electro-acupuncture stimulation acts on the basal ganglia output pathway to ameliorate motor impairment in Parkinsonian model rats. *Behavioral Neuroscience*, 124(2), (February, 2010), pp. 305-310.

Patt, S.; Gertz, H. J.; Gerhard, L. & Cervos-Navarro, J. (1991). Pathological changes in dendrites of substantia nigra neurons in Parkinson's diseases: a Golgi study. *Journal of Histology and Histopathology*, 6(3), (July, 1991), pp. 373-380.

Schulzer, M.; Lee, C. S.; Mak, E. K.; Vingerhoets, F. J. G.; & Calne, D. B. (1994). A mathematical model of pathogenesis in idopathic parkinsonism. *Brain*, 117(3), (March, 1994), pp. 509-516.

Segev, I & Rall, W. J. (1988). Computational study of an excitable dendritic spine. *Journal of Neurophysiology*, 60(2), (February, 1988), pp. 499-523.

Simon, E . (2006). Ion channel proteins in neuronal temperature transduction: from inferences to testable theories of deep body thermosensitivity. *American Journal of Physiology: Regulatory, Integraative and Comparative Physiology* , 291(4), (April, 2006), pp. 273-283.

Smit , J. E.; Hanekom, T.; & Hanekom, J. J. (2009). Modelled temperature-dependent excitability behavior of a generalised human peripheral sensory nerve fibre. *Biological Cybernetics*, 101(7), (July, 2009), pp. 115-`30.

Stephens, B; Mueller, A. J.; Shering, A. F.; Hood, S. H.; Taggart, P.; Arbuthnott, G. W.; Bell, J. E.; Kilford, L; Kingsbury, A. E.; Daniel, S. E.; & Ingham, C. A. (2005). Evidence of a breakdown of corticostriatal connections in Parkinson's disease. *Neuroscience*, 132(3), (March, 2005), pp. 741–754.

Surmeier, D. J.; Guzman, J. N.; Sanchez-Padilla, J. & Goldberg, J. A. (2010). What causes the death of dopaminergic neurons in Parkinson's disease? *Progress in Brain Research*, 183(1), (January, 2010), pp. 59-77.

Verzi, D. W.; Rheuben, M. B. & Baer, S. M. (2004). Impact of time-dependent changes in spine density and spine shape on the input-output properties of a dendritic branch: A computational study. *Journal of Neurophysiology*, 93(12), (December, 2004), pp. 2073-2089.

Verzi, D. W. & Baer, S. M. (2005). Calcium-mediated spine stem restructuring. *Journal of Mathematical and Computer Modelling*, 42(1), (February, 2004), pp. 151-165.

4

Parkinson's Disease and Parkin: Insights from *Park2* Knockout Mice

Sarah E.M. Stephenson[1,2], Juliet M. Taylor[2] and Paul J. Lockhart[1,2]
[1]Murdoch Childrens Research Institute
[2]University of Melbourne
Australia

1 Introduction

Parkinson's disease (PD) is a neurodegenerative movement disorder distinguished by resting tremor, bradykinesia, rigidity, postural instability and gait disturbances. Non-motor symptoms including dysfunction of the autonomic nervous system, neuropsychiatric changes, sensory and sleep disturbances are also common. PD may be diagnosed at any age but is most common in aged populations - affecting approximately 1% of individuals over 60 years of age and rising to approximately 4% in age groups above 85 years of age (de Lau and Breteler, 2006; Van Den Eeden et al., 2003). It has become apparent that differential subgroups may be categorised by age of onset, dominant symptoms and progression. Two key subsets include late- and early-onset PD. Late-onset PD is typically identified in individuals over the age of 70 and is characterised by postural imbalance and gait impairment with accompanying rigidity and akinesia. Early-onset PD is typified by a dominant tremor and slow progression in motor decline, and is primarily identified in individuals less than 50 years of age (Lewis et al., 2005; Selikhova et al., 2009).

The lead pathological identifier of PD is moderate to severe dopaminergic neuronal loss within the substantia nigra pars compacta with accompanying Lewy pathology in surviving neurons (Daniel and Lees, 1993; Dickson et al., 2009; Gelb et al., 1999). It is thought that the combination of Lewy pathology and dopaminergic cell loss in PD leads to striatal dopamine depletion, and this accounts for the motor symptoms (Obeso et al., 2008). Earlier diagnosis of PD is important as motor symptoms do not become apparent until approximately 60% of dopaminergic neurons are lost (Fearnley and Lees, 1991; Pakkenberg et al., 1991).

Current treatments are available to manage the symptoms of PD. Medications such as the dopamine precursor L-3,4-dihydroxyphenylalanine (L-DOPA) and inhibitors of dopamine metabolism are used to supplement the reduced dopamine level. Deep brain stimulation is an alternative treatment. The patient undergoes surgery to implant an electrical stimulation device into the affected region of the basal ganglia. The electrical impulses generated by the device interfere with the abnormal signals that are causing the tremor, thereby alleviating some of the symptoms of the disease (reviewed in (Hurelbrink and Lewis, 2010)). To identify treatments that address or arrest the progressive nature of PD, an understanding of the molecular mechanisms responsible for the loss of nigrostriatal dopaminergic neurons and associated Lewy pathology must be delineated.

The aetiology of the majority of PD cases remain unknown, however, gene mutations in familial forms of PD account for up to 10% of cases. Over 15 PD loci have been reported and greater than 10 genes have been identified (reviewed in (Shulman et al., 2010)). Mutations in *alpha-synuclein* and *LRRK2* are the predominant cause of autosomal dominant PD, while mutations in *parkin* and *PINK1* cause autosomal recessive PD. Several genome wide association studies using large idiopathic PD cohorts have demonstrated an unequivocal role for common genetic variation in familial PD genes in the aetiology of idiopathic PD, and identified new genetic players including *microtubule associated protein tau* in sporadic disease aetiology (Satake et al., 2009; Simon-Sanchez et al., 2009).

Mutations in *PARK2* (*parkin*) account for 50% of all familial early-onset PD cases, at least 20% of young-onset sporadic PD and also contribute to late onset sporadic disease (Foroud et al., 2003; Lucking et al., 2000; Mata et al., 2004). *Parkin* encodes a 465 amino acid multi-domain protein with homology to a class of enzymes termed E3 ubiquitin-protein ligases that function in the ubiquitin proteasome system (UPS) (Shimura et al., 2000). The UPS is the predominant cellular pathway for the turnover of misfolded and short-lived intracellular proteins (Ciechanover et al., 2000). Parkin mediates the formation of a lysine-48 polyubiquitin chain linked to the target protein, which functions as a signal for degradation by the proteasome. Parkin is also capable of alternative modes of ubiquitination including monoubiquitination and lysine-63 polyubiquitination, which appear to function in signalling and autophagy, respectively (Chew et al., 2011; Olzmann and Chin, 2008).

The pathological hallmark of many neurodegenerative diseases is the accumulation of proteins in aggregates/inclusions. There is very little information about the neuropathology observed in the brains of individuals with *parkin*-proven PD as only a seven cases have gone to autopsy. These cases displayed variable degree of cell loss in the substantia nigra pars compacta, and in some cases the locus coeruleus. Several cases displayed evidence of gliosis and astrocytosis. With the exception of two cases, Lewy pathology was not identified. Evidence of other types of protein aggregation including neurofibrillary tangles, alpha-synuclein-positive dendritic inclusions and tau accumulation were evident to varying degrees (reviewed in (Cookson et al., 2008)). As Lewy pathology is often cited as a significant pathological difference between idiopathic and *parkin*-proven PD some have hypothesised that parkin may play an integral role in Lewy formation (von Coelln et al., 2006). However, due to the small number of autopsies and the limitations of studying end stage disease tissues, animal and cell models provide a more detailed mechanistic understanding of *parkin*-mediated PD and the contribution of parkin to idiopathic PD.

A number of animal and cellular models of parkin dysfunction have been described. Parkin knockout flies demonstrated a reduced lifespan, muscle degeneration mitochondrial abnormalities, sensitivity to oxidative stress and male infertility (Greene et al., 2003; Pesah et al., 2004). While the first reports suggested *parkin* deficient drosophila did not have significant loss of dopaminergic neurons, a subsequent study utilising more sensitive analytical techniques indicated a reduction in the number of a subtype of dopaminergic neurons (Whitworth et al., 2005). *Park2* knockout mice did not appear to display extensive behavioural or dopaminergic abnormalities. As such the utility of such models to evaluate new pharmaceutical agents is unclear. A number of independent *parkin* deficient mouse models have now been generated. This review will outline the insights provided and look ahead to how *Park2* knockout mice may help to better understand *parkin*-mediated PD and by extension idiopathic PD.

2. *Parkin* mouse models

To date, eleven models of parkin dysfunction have been reported, seven of which are independently generated *Park2* knockout models. Studies on these mice will provide the basis of the discussion within. Models noted that are outside the scope of this paper include the quaking viable mouse which is a knockout of *parkin* and *PArkin Co-Regulated Gene* with dysregulation of *quaking* gene (Lockhart et al., 2004; Lorenzetti et al., 2004;), a recently identified spontaneous CH3-*Park2^{E398Q}* mutant (Ramsey and Giasson, 2010), a model of transgenic overexpression of a parkin truncated mutant (Lu et al., 2009) and a model of overexpression of wildtype parkin (Yoshida et al., 2010).

The majority of *parkin*-proven PD cases are the result of large genomic alterations (deletion, duplication or inversion) that affect one or more exons. *PARK2* spans an exaggerated genomic interval of approximately 1.4 Mb due to super-expanded introns and is located in a region of genomic instability (Denison et al., 2003; Palumbo et al., 2010). Several mouse models were generated to replicate known deletions that affect a single exon. Exons targeted in the *Park2* knockout models were exon 2, exon 3 or exon 7, which are predicted to result in a peptide/protein of 4aa, 57aa or 243aa truncated, respectively (Table 1). This suggests that parkin function would be abrogated in all of these models in the event translation occurs. Consistent with loss of function, immunoreactivity corresponding to full length parkin could not be detected in any of the knockout mice lines (Table 1 for references).

2.1 Behavioural characteristics

PD is a progressive adult onset neurodegenerative disorder, therefore, it would be anticipated that disease associated mutations within animal models would replicate this feature. For this reason it is important to consider mouse to human age equivalents. It is generally considered that between the ages of 3-6 months mice have finished development, the rapid maturational growth of most biological processes and structures, but are not affected by senescence. These mice are considered to represent 'mature adults' equivalent to a 20-30 year old human. Changes in senescence can be detected in some but not all mice between the ages of 10-15 months, which is considered 'middle age' and corresponds to 38-47 years in humans. Senescence markers can be detected in almost all 'old' mice between 18-24 months of age and these represent approximately 56-69 years in humans. Although for each inbred strain it varies, the average life span (50% survivorship) of a laboratory mouse is 28 months and the upper limit near 36 months, considered the equivalent of approximately 78 and 94 human years, respectively (Harrison, 2011).

Park2 knockout mice appear to develop normally, have normal general motor function and do not show any obvious clinical phenotype or behavioural abnormality. In one study, Kaplan-Meier survival analysis using the *Park2^{tm1Roo}* knockout model suggested an increase in mortality, which is consistent with data from PD patients' pre-L-DOPA therapy (Rodriguez-Navarro et al., 2007). However, in another study using the *Park2^{tm1Roo}* knockout model on a different background a difference in survival was not found (Guerrero et al., 2008). A reduction in body weight was identified in three lines but was not replicated in three other lines (Table 2) (Itier et al., 2003; Oyama et al., 2010; Palacino et al., 2004; Perez and Palmiter, 2005; Von Coelln et al., 2004; Zhu et al., 2007). In addition, a reduced body temperature was detected in *Park2^{tm1Roo}* knockout mice but was not replicated in the *Park2^{tm1Rpa}* knockout line. The findings for adhesive-removal tests and acoustic-startle were also conflicting (Goldberg et al., 2003; Itier et al., 2003; Perez and Palmiter, 2005; Von Coelln et al., 2004).

B6;129S2-*Park2*[tm1Roo] (Itier et al., 2003)[1]

Partial replacement of exon 3 with PGK-Neo[R] cassette resulting in a truncated protein. If exon 3 is skipped, the predicted result is a frame shift after parkin amino acid 57 with the addition of 49 novel amino acids.

B6;129S4-*Park2*[tm1Shn] (Goldberg et al., 2003)

Partial replacement of exon 3 with in frame insertion of EGFP followed by PGK-Neo[R] cassette resulting in a truncated protein consisting of the first 95 amino acids of parkin followed by EGFP (expression of EGFP protein was not detected). If exon 3 skipping occurs, the predicted result is a frameshift after parkin amino acid 57 with the addition of 49 novel amino acids.

B6;129S7/S4-*Park2*[tm1Tmd] (Von Coelln et al., 2004)[2]

Cre-mediated deletion of exon 7 resulting in a frameshift after parkin amino acid 243 with the addition of 8 novel amino acids.

B6;129S4-*Park2*[tm1Rpa] (Perez and Palmiter, 2005)[1]

Complete replacement of exon 2 with Polr2a-Neo[R] cassette. If exon 2 is skipped, the predicted result would be a change in the reading frame producing a 4-aa peptide.

B6;CBA-*Park2*[tm1Hn] (Sato et al., 2006)[3]

Partial replacement of exon 2 with in frame insertion of tauGFP fusion protein followed by MC1-Neo[R] cassette to produce tauGFP driven by the parkin promoter (expression of tauGFP protein was not detected). If exon 2 skipping occurs, the predicted result would be a change in the reading frame producing a 4-aa peptide.

B6;129P2-*Park2*[tm1Oga](Kitao et al., 2007)

Complete replacement of exon 3 with PGK-Neo[R] cassette. If exon 3 is skipped, the predicted result is a frame shift after parkin amino acid 57 with the addition of 49 novel amino acids.

B6;129S1/X1-*Park2*[tm1Ccs] (Stichel et al., 2007)

Complete replacement of exon 3 with a Neo[R] cassette. If exon 3 is skipped, the predicted result is a frame shift after parkin amino acid 57 with the addition of 49 novel amino acids.

Table 1. *Park2* knockout mouse models
Nomenclature guidelines for naming genetically modified mouse strains were followed. Information regarding the genetic background of the mouse strain was extracted from the embryonic stem cell line strain and strain used in initial chimeric breeding. Only the first reported mouse strain is indicated, mutant alleles may have subsequently been bred to other strains or isogenicity for subsequent publications. [1]Also reported the allele on 129 isogenic background but unless indicated experiments were performed on a mixed background. [2]Strain information was obtained from Perez and Palmiter (2005) Supplementary Table 3. [3]A laboratory code for Nobutaka Hattori, the corresponding author of the publication by Sato et al., (2006) could not be identified with the Institute for Laboratory Animal Research (ILAR) therefore his initials (Hn) were used. This is only for the purposes of differentiating these strains in this chapter and does not represent the true allele designation.

It was anticipated that *parkin*-deficient mouse models would display motor defects, which would validate their suitability for PD research. Initial experiments indicated that only *Park2*[tm1Roo] knockout line showed a basal reduction in locomotion (Table 3) (Itier et al., 2003). However, when investigated in the same line at 24 months, only a non-significant tendency for reduced locomotion was reported (Rodriguez-Navarro et al., 2007). The *Park2* knockout lines did not show significant deficits on the rotarod, which is used to measure balance,

	Body weight		Body temperature		Adhesive-removal		Acoustic-startle	
Park2tm1Roo	↓	1-16	↓	4				
Park2tm1Shn	↓	1-12			↓[3]	2-7		
Park2tm1Tmd	−	NA					↓	9
Park2tm1Rpa	−[1]	3-24	−	3, 22	−	19	−[2]	12-15
Park2tm1Hn								
Park2tm1Oga	↓	NA						
Park2tm1Ccs	−	6, 18						

Table 2. General behavioural attributes of Park2 knockout mice
Attributes investigated in two or more Park2 knockout models. Park2 knockout showed no difference (-) or a significant difference compared to wildtype (decreased = ↓, increased = ↑). The age(s) of mice (in months) is indicated, if unreported it is shown as not available (NA). Gray cells indicate that attribute has not been reported. [1]Decrease in weight was identified at 6 months of age in the B6:129S4 background but was not reproduced in the 129S4 background. [2]An increased sensitivity was detected in the B6:129S4 background but was not reproduced in the 129S4 background. [3]A significant decrease was not identified at 18 months. The table should be used as a guide only as methodology and analysis varies for each model.

	Locomotion		Amphetamine response		Rotarod		Balance-beam		Pole Test	
Park2tm1Roo	↓	6	↓	6						
Park2tm1Shn	−	6-18			−	6-18	↓	2-18		
Park2tm1Tmd	−	18			−	3-24				
Park2tm1Rpa	−[1]	3-22	−	3	−[3]	3-18	−	19	↓	6, 18
Park2tm1Hn	−	12	−	12	−	12				
Park2tm1Oga					−	3-12			−	3-12
Park2tm1Ccs	−	6-21	↓[2]	3	−	6-24				

Table 3. Motor function of Park2 knockout mice.
Attributes investigated in two or more Park2 knockout models. Park2 knockout showed no difference (-) or a significant difference compared to wildtype (decreased = ↓, increased = ↑). The age(s) of mice (in months) is indicated. Gray cells indicate that attribute has not been reported. [1]Park2tm1Rpa knockout mice exhibited greater locomotor activity specifically during the second dark cycle at 12 months only. [2]Reported as a lack of amphetamine to induce thigmotaxic behaviour. [3]Park2tm1Rpa knockout mice were more likely to grip the rotarod at 6 months. The table should be used as a guide only as methodology and analysis varies for each model.

coordination, physical condition, and motor-planning (Goldberg et al., 2003; Oyama et al., 2010; Perez and Palmiter, 2005; Sato et al., 2006; Von Coelln et al., 2004; Zhu et al., 2007). Two of the *Park2* knockout models appeared to have a reduced response to amphetamine, which increases the amount of dopamine in the synaptic cleft and enhances the response of post-synaptic neurons, whereas another two did not (Itier et al., 2003; Perez and Palmiter, 2005; Sato et al., 2006; Zhu et al., 2007). Furthermore, alternative results were reported for motor co-ordination determined by the balance beam test and the pole test (Goldberg et al., 2003; Oyama et al., 2010; Perez and Palmiter, 2005).

Cognitive function has been investigated in three of the *Park2* knockout lines (Table 4). Two of the models displayed a reduction in exploratory behaviour which was suggestive of an increased anxiety (Itier et al., 2003; Zhu et al., 2007). However, in other tests of cognition, including light/dark exploration and T-maze alteration the finding varied depending on the *Park2* knockout model analysed (Itier et al., 2003; Perez and Palmiter, 2005; Zhu et al., 2007).

For the most part, based on the aforementioned investigations of the behavioural attributes of the *Park2* knockout mouse lines it would appear that *parkin* deficiency does not cause a PD-like phenotype in mice. The discrepancies reported for the *Park2* knockout lines may be attributable to the genetic background of the mouse strain harbouring the mutant allele (discussed in (Perez and Palmiter, 2005)). The relative inability to identify a significant difference from wildtype for a number of the attributes investigated may be because the effect of parkin deficiency is very subtle and the experimental approach lacks the required sensitivity. As PD is a progressive disorder, an alternative explanation may be the age of *Park2* knockout model when the attribute was investigated. For example, 18 month old *Park2*^{tm1Roo} knockout mice showed a significant decrease in the length of their hind limb stride, and at 24 months a number of motor and non-motor irregularities were apparent in the *Park2*^{tm1Roo} knockout line that were suggested to parallel symptoms observed in PD sufferers (Rodriguez-Navarro et al., 2007). Further investigation when *parkin* deficiency is combined with old age in the *Park2* knockout models is required to address this issue.

	Refuse to perform tests		T-maze alternation		Exploratory behaviour		Light/dark exploration		Morris water maze	
Park2^{tm1Roo}	↓	15	↓	4	↓	6				
Park2^{tm1Shn}										
Park2^{tm1Tmd}										
Park2^{tm1Rpa}	−	3-22	−	12-20			−	12,18	−	18
Park2^{tm1Hn}										
Park2^{tm1Oga}										
Park2^{tm1Ccs}					↓	3	↓	3	↑	NA

Table 4. Cognitive-related behaviour in *Park2* knockout mice.
Attributes investigated in two or more *Park2* knockout models. *Park2* knockout showed no difference (-) or a significant difference compared to wildtype (decreased = ↓, increased = ↑). The age(s) of mice (in months) is indicated, if age was unreported it is shown as not available (NA). Gray cells indicate that attribute has not been reported. The table should be used as a guide only as methodology and analysis varies for each model.

2.2 Pathology

The pathological hallmark of PD is the loss of dopaminergic neurons within the substantia nigra and Lewy pathology. Other regions may also display loss of neurons and/or Lewy pathology, including the locus ceruleus, the hypothalamus and some regions of the cortex (Halliday and McCann, 2010). The cell body of dopaminergic neurons are predominantly localised to three regions of the brain: the substantia nigra pars compacta, the ventral tegmental area and the hypothalamus. These neurons project into the putamen to form the nigrostriatal dopaminergic system, the ventral striatum or the cortex to form the mesolimbic or the mesocortical dopaminergic pathways, and the pituitary gland to form the tuberoinfundibular pathway, respectively. In contrast, the largest population of noradrenergic neurons is found in the locus ceruleus, and these project to most central nervous system areas (Grimm et al., 2004).

The number and morphology of tyrosine hydroxylase staining neurons in the substantia nigra of *Park2* knockout mice was not found to be remarkably different from wildtype mice (Table 5). However, in the *Park2tm1Roo* knockout line age was an important factor influencing loss of dopaminergic neurons. When examined at 2 or 15 months there was no difference in the

	Morphology of tyrosine hydroxylase staining neurons		Number of tyrosine hydroxylase staining neurons			
Park2tm1Roo	–	2, 15 C, BS, H, SN, ST	–	2, 15 SN	↓1	18, 24
Park2tm1Shn	–	NA LC, SN, ST	–			12-24 SN
Park2tm1Tmd	–	18 SN, ST	–	12-18 SN	↓2	2,12-18 LC
Park2tm1Rpa	–	NA SN	–			NA SN
Park2tm1Hn	–	3 SN	–			3 LC, SN
Park2tm1Oga			–			26 SN
Park2tm1Ccs	–	6-18 LC, SN, ST	–			6-18 LC, SN

Table 5. Catecholaminergic neuron pathology in *Park2* knockout mice.
The morphology and number of catecholaminergic neurons in *Park2* knockout mice were identified by staining with anti-tyrosine hydroxylase antibody. *Park2* knockout showed no difference (-) or a significant difference compared to wildtype (decreased = ↓, increased = ↑) The age(s) of mice (in months) is indicated, if unreported it is shown as not available (NA). Gray cells indicate that attribute has not been reported. Brain stem (BS), cerebellum (C), locus ceruleus *(LC)*, hippocampus (H), substantia nigra (SN), striatum (ST). [1]Significant reduction in the number of tyrosine hydroxylase staining neurons at 18 month was only identified in female *Park2tm1Roo* knockout mice. [2]Phenotype shows reduced penetrance, ~30% of *Park2tm1Tmd* knockout do not show a significant reduction in the number of tyrosine hydroxylase staining neurons in the LC. The table should be used as a guide only as methodology and analysis varies for each model.

number of dopaminergic neurons in the substantia nigra, but when investigated at 24 months a loss of ~35% of neurons was detected (Itier et al., 2003; Rodriguez-Navarro et al., 2007). In addition, a significant loss of tyrosine hydroxylase reactivity was demonstrable at 18 months in females but not males mice (Rodriguez-Navarro et al., 2008). Notably, in two other models examined at or above 24 months no significant loss of dopamineric neurons in the substantia nigra was reported (Goldberg et al., 2003; Kitao et al., 2007). Alternatively, in ~70% of *Park2tm1Tmd* knockout mice there was significant reduction in the number of catecholaminergic neurons in the locus coeruleus. Such pathology was present at 2 months of age, suggesting dysfunctional development of catecholaminergic neurons in the locus ceruleus (Von Coelln et al., 2004). As ~30% *Park2tm1Tmd* knockout mice showed no significant decrease, it is indicative of reduced penetrance and suggests other factors must also influence the trait.

It is generally considered that *parkin* deletion alone in humans is sufficient to cause PD with the onset of symptoms typically earlier than observed for idiopathic PD. The analyses summarised in Tables 2 to 5 suggests mouse models of *parkin* deficiency do not replicate this phenotype. However, some of the *Park2* knockout models display subtle behavioural and pathological phenotypes that parallel PD. Therefore, *parkin* deficiency in the mouse may alter pathways common to human pathogenesis but for as yet unknown reasons do not cause a pronounced PD-like phenotype. Observations reported suggest that the mechanistic pathways in which parkin functions are conserved between the human and mouse, and *Park2* knockout mice may be a useful model to further refine the function of parkin and its role in disease pathogenesis.

2.3 Neurochemistry

It is hypothesised that dysfunction in dopamine metabolism may precede loss of dopaminergic neurons and represent a presymptomatic disease state. This is supported by studies of dopamine metabolism using positron emission tomography in both *parkin*-proven and idiopathic Parkinson's disease, and unaffected individuals with heterozygous mutations in *Parkin* and *PINK1* (Guo et al., 2010; Sioka et al., 2010; Tang et al., 2010). The biosynthetic pathway for dopamine production in catecholaminergic neurons is the sequential conversion of phenylalanine to tyrosine, dihydroxyphenylalanine (L-DOPA) and dopamine. In dopaminergic neurons the synthesis of dopamine is the final product of the process whereas in noradrenergic neurons dopamine may be further modified to norepinephrine (Daubner et al., 2011). Within dopaminergic neurons, newly synthesised cytoplasmic dopamine is translocated by vesicular monoamine transporter 2 (VMAT2) into vesicles for storage until synaptic release. Synaptic dopamine interacts with D1 and D2 receptors on postsynaptic neurons in the striatum, which mediate the direct and indirect dopaminergic pathways, respectively. Within the substantia nigra and the basal ganglia synaptic dopamine is inactivated primarily via reuptake by the dopamine transporter (DAT) on presynaptic neurons. Intracellular dopamine is then sequestered in vesicles via VMAT for re-use or converted by monoamine oxidase (MAO) to 3,4-dihydroxyphenylacetic acid (DOPAC) for degradation. DOPAC then diffuses out of the nerve terminal and into the extracellular space, where it can be transformed into the more stable metabolite homovanillic acid (HVA) via catechol-*O*-methyltransferase (COMT). To a lesser extent, extracellular dopamine can be metabolised without reuptake into presynaptic neurons. In this process, extracellular dopamine is converted to 3-methoxytyramine (3-MT) by COMT then to HVA by MAO (reviewed in (Standaert and Galanter, 2007)).

Investigation of the levels of dopamine and its metabolites DOPAC and HVA in the striatum of the *Park2* knockout lines did not reveal significant alterations (Table 6) (Itier et al., 2003; Oyama et al., 2010; Palacino et al., 2004; Perez and Palmiter, 2005; Von Coelln et al., 2004). The notable exception was the increase in HVA in the *Park2tm1Ccs* model (Zhu et al., 2007). In addition, in a later study, a significant increase in DOPAC and HVA in the striatum at 3 months old *Park2tm1Roo* knockout mice was reported (omitted from table) (Menendez et al., 2006). This may be reflective of an increase dopamine metabolism. Likewise, an increase in the ratio of DOPAC to dopamine or 3-MT was identified in the striatum of the *Park2tm1Roo* knockout line, perhaps indicative of increased intracellular dopamine metabolism via MAO as opposed to extracellular metabolism via COMT (Itier et al., 2003). Although no significant difference of total dopamine levels were identified in the striatum of the *Park2tm1Shn* knockout model, the amount of extracellular dopamine in this region was significantly increased. In addition, dopamine reuptake was unaltered, which suggests that the increased extracellular dopamine was due to increased release of dopamine from presynaptic dopaminergic neurons (Goldberg et al., 2003). In contrast, in the striatum of the *Park2tm1Hn* knockout model a reduction in dopamine synthesis and an increase in D1 and D2 receptor

	Dopamine		DOPAC		HVA		Noradrenaline	
Park2tm1Roo	− 11 BS, D, ST	↑ 11 L	− 11 BS, D, ST	↑ 11 L	− 11 BS, D, L, ST		− 11 BS, D, L, ST	
Park2tm1Shn	− 6-24 ST		− 6-24 ST					
Park2tm1Tmd	− 18 ST		− 18 ST		− 18 ST		− 18 BS, C, CC, D, H, PC	↓ 18 OB, SC
Park2tm1Rpa	− 22 ST		− 22 MB, ST		− 22 ST		− 18-22 OB, SC, ST	
Park2tm1Hn	↑ 12 MB	− 12 ST	− 12 MB, ST		− 12 MB, ST			
Park2tm1Oga	− 3-12 ST		− 3-12 ST		− 3-12 ST			
Park2tm1Ccs	− NA ST		− NA ST		↑ NA ST			

Table 6. Neurochemical analysis of *Park2* Knockout mice
The level of dopamine, its metabolites 3,4-Dihydroxyphenylacetic acid (DOPAC) and homovanillic acid (HVA) and its derivate noradrenaline were analysed. *Park2* knockout showed no difference (-) or a significant difference compared to wildtype (decreased = ↓, increased = ↑). The age(s) of mice (in months) is indicated, if unreported it is shown as not available (NA). Gray cells indicate that attribute has not been reported. Brain stem (BS), cerebral cortex (CC), cerebellum (C), diencephalon (D), hippocampus (H), limbic region (L), olfactory bulb (OB), midbrain (MB), prefrontal cortex (PC), spinal cord (SC), substantia nigra (SN), striatum (ST). The table should be used as a guide only as methodology and analysis varies for each model.

binding was detected using receptor specific antagonists. This suggests decline in striatal dopamine release may result in decreased synaptic dopamine (Sato et al., 2006). Similar analysis in the $Park2^{tm1Shn}$ knockout line however, did not indicate an alteration in the amount of D1 or D2 receptor binding in the striatum (Goldberg et al., 2003; Kitada et al., 2009a). In the $Park2^{tm1Hn}$ line the binding index of DAT and VMAT was unchanged and suggests that the levels of these proteins are not altered (Sato et al., 2006). Likewise, the level of DAT in the $Park2^{tm1Shn}$ knockout mice, measured using radiolabeled dopamine uptake, suggested that DAT levels were not altered (Kitada et al., 2009a). However, a reduction of the DAT and VMAT protein levels were identified in the $Park2^{tm1Roo}$ line (Itier et al., 2003).

Alterations in dopamine metabolism were also found in other brain regions. An increase in the level of dopamine and DOPAC was identified in the limbic region from $Park2^{tm1Roo}$ knockout mice, and an increase in dopamine but not DOPAC was identified in the midbrain, which includes the limbic region, from the $Park2^{tm1Hn}$ knockout line (Itier et al., 2003; Sato et al., 2006). In addition, in the $Park2^{tm1Tmd}$ knockout model, which showed loss of noradrenergic neurons within the locus coeruleus, a significant reduction in the dopamine derivative norepinephrine was identified in two regions that are innervated by the locus ceruleus, the olfactory bulb and the spinal cord (Von Coelln et al., 2004). Although a number of discrepancies related to dopamine metabolism are evident between the different $Park2$ knockout models, collectively these analyses have suggested parkin may play a role in the presynaptic release of dopamine. The loss of parkin function may alter dopamine release, potentially by affecting vesicular packaging. Furthermore, they suggest that alterations in presynaptic dopamine function are evident prior to the development of PD-associated pathology.

2.4 Synaptic transmission

Deficits in dopamine-related synaptic transmission have been identified in *parkin*-mediated PD (Guo et al., 2010). Studies in a number of the $Park2$ knockout lines suggest the presynaptic dopamine transmission is perturbed. In the $Park2^{tm1Shn}$ knockout line, the evoked dopamine signal of medium spiny-neurons, the major class of striatal neurons whose excitability is influenced by dopamine levels, was reduced and could not be restored with DAT inhibition, suggesting dopamine re-uptake was not affected (Goldberg et al., 2003). Long term depression (LTD), which is activity-dependent reduction in the efficacy of neuronal synapses that lasts for an extended period, was also found to also be dysfunctional in these neurons. LTD could be restored by increasing synaptic dopamine with amphetamine but not by inhibition of dopamine re-uptake by antagonism of DAT. In addition, simultaneous antagonism of both D1 and D2 receptors, but not individual receptor antagonism, was required to restore LTD, and L-DOPA treatment was also effective. Furthermore, using primary dissociated adrenal chromaffin cells, which enable real time analysis of catecholamine release from single vesicles, exocytosis was found to be reduced (Kitada et al., 2009a). These observations suggest neurons from $Park2^{tm1Shn}$ knockout have an intrinsic impairment in synaptic transmission that may result from defective presynaptic dopamine release.

The amplitude and half-life of evoked dopamine overflow was reduced in nigrostriatal fibers of the medial forebrain bundle of $Park2^{tm1Oga}$ knockout mice. These are reflective of competing mechanisms of synaptic release and re-uptake, indicating that these mice also have alterations in dopamine synaptic transmission. Furthermore, a progressive age related reduction in facilitation of these neurons was identified, which may be reflective of presymptomatic age-related changes (Oyama et al., 2010). The synaptic strength of hippocampal neurons from $Park2^{tm1Rpa}$ line was significantly weaker in mice carrying one $Park2^{tm1Rpa}$ mutant allele but not two mutant alleles. Hemizygous mice consistently showed reduced pair-pulse ratio whereas $Park2^{tm1Rpa}$ knockout mice were only affected under small inter-stimulus ranges. Changes in pulse-pair ratio are consistent with presynaptic abnormalities, suggesting that in $Park2^{tm1Rpa}$ mouse line parkin deficiency also affects presynaptic process.

Long term potentiation (LTP) is a long-lasting enhancement in signal transmission between two neurons that results from stimulating them synchronously, and is considered one of the major cellular mechanisms that underlies learning and memory. In the $Park2^{tm1Rpa}$ knockout line, the LTP of 24 month old, but not 2 month old, appeared to be more robust, which may suggest that there is an absence of normal age related decline in the hippocampus of these mice (Hanson et al., 2010). In contrast, LTP was unchanged in the hippocampus of $Park2^{tm1Roo}$ knockout line of a similar age (Itier et al., 2003). Furthermore, LTP was also unaltered in the hippocampus of $Park2^{tm1Shn}$ knockout mice but could not be induced in striatal medium spiny neurons (Kitada et al., 2009a). Studies carried out to date on Park2 knockout mice suggest that these mice have presynaptic abnormalities affecting dopamine function, which may be differentially modulated by the homozygous or heterozygous state of the mutant allele, cellular and regional specificity and/or age.

2.5 Neuroinflammation

Neuroinflammation is the chronic presence of activated microglia and reactive astrocytes, and associated mediators of the immune response in the central nervous system (reviewed in (Lee et al., 2009)). Postmortem analyses have demonstrated activated glia in both the striatum and in the substantia nigra of patients with idiopathic PD and in *parkin*-proven PD (reviewed in (Cookson et al., 2008; Lee et al., 2009)).

In vivo, $Park2^{tm1Ccs}$ and $Park2^{tm1Roo}$ knockout mice did not appear to have increased astrocytic or microglial markers in the substantia nigra, striatum or midbrain (Rodriguez-Navarro et al., 2007; Schmidt et al., 2011). However, a significant increase in the number of astrocytes in the striatum and the number of microglia in the midbrain occurs with age in the $Park2^{tm1Roo}$ mice, independent of parkin deficiency, indicating an age-associated increase in the inflammatory environment may contribute to neuronal degeneration (Rodriguez-Navarro et al., 2007). *In vitro* however, alterations of glial populations are evident. Neuronal enriched cultures derived from $Park2^{tm1Roo}$ knockout embryos appear to be enriched for microglial and glial progenitor cells (Casarejos et al., 2005), and glial cultures appear to have a reduced proportion of astrocytes compared to wildtype derived cultures (Solano et al., 2008). Furthermore, glial conditioned medium from $Park2^{tm1Roo}$ and $Park2^{tm1Ccs}$ knockout mice were found to have reduced neuroprotective capabilities that suggest a reduction in a trophic factor production or excretion by astrocytes (Schmidt et al., 2011; Solano et al., 2008).

$Park2^{tm1Shn}$ knockout mice have been used to investigate if parkin deficiency can affect vulnerability to inflammation-mediated dopaminergic degeneration, using sustained low dose intraperitoneal injection of lipopolysaccaride (LPS). LPS is a bacterial endotoxin that is used as a glial activator for the induction of inflammatory dopaminergic neurodegeneration (Dutta et al., 2008). $Park2^{tm1Shn}$ knockout mice showed increased vulnerability to LPS treatment and developed fine motor deficits and a loss of dopaminergic neurons (Frank-

Cannon et al., 2008). This suggests that *parkin* deficiency selectively increases the vulnerability of dopaminergic neurons to the effects of LPS induced inflammatory dopaminergic neurodegeneration. Collectively, these studies suggest that there may be inherent dysregulation of glial cells in *parkin* deficiency. Alterations in the function of these mediators of neuroinflammation within *parkin*-proven PD, together with endogenous age related changes in the neuroimmune system may play a role in the pathogenesis of PD.

2.6 Oxidative stress

Oxidative stress occurs when there is an imbalance between the production of reactive oxygen species (ROS) and the ability to rapidly detoxify the reactive intermediates or repair the resulting damage to cellular constituents. Markers of oxidative stress are increased in PD patients (reviewed in (Tobon-Velasco et al., 2010)), and dopamine metabolism facilitates production of ROS (Lotharius and Brundin, 2002). Glutathione (GSH) is a free radical scavenger that acts on redox reactive molecules. Both astrocytes and neurons have the capacity to synthesis GSH, but astrocytes are known to play an important role in supply of GSH and other substrates to neurons. One of the earliest biochemical changes observed in PD patients is a decrease in GSH levels. It is thought the decrease in GSH levels may be due to increased oxidative stress and recent research suggests that GSH depletion itself may have a role in the pathogenesis of PD (reviewed in (Martin and Teismann, 2009)). *Park2tm1Roo* knockout mice aged 2 months were found to have significantly increased GSH in the midbrain, striatum and limbic system (Itier et al., 2003; Rodriguez-Navarro et al., 2007). However, when GSH levels were investigated in *Park2tm1Roo* knockout mice aged 24 months, the level of GSH in the midbrain was not significantly different from either the 24 month old wildtype or 2 month old knockout mice. While GSH levels in the striatum of 24 month *Park2tm1Roo* knockout mice were significantly reduced compared to 2 month old knockout mice they were not significantly different to 24 month old wildtype mice. In the limbic system of 24 month old *Park2tm1Roo* knockout mice the level of GSH was significantly increased compared to 24 month old wildtype mice. Therefore, regional and age-related alterations of GSH are present in the *Park2tm1Roo* knockout mouse line. Consistent with these observations, *in vitro* age-related studies of alterations in GSH levels have been identified in glial cells derived from *Park2tm1Roo* knockout mice. When knockout glia are cultured for an extended period (6-9 months) the intracellular levels of GSH were significantly reduced compared to wildtype control glia, whereas knockout glia cultured for a shorter time (1-3 months) were shown to have a significant increase in the level of intracellular GSH compared to wildtype (Solano et al., 2008). However, conditioned media generated from glial cultures derived from *Park2tm1Roo* knockout mice that had been cultured for a shorter period had lower levels of GSH and higher levels of hydrogen peroxide, and appeared to be less neuroprotective to wildtype neurons than conditioned media from wildtype glial cultures (Solano et al., 2008). These observations suggest that although intracellular GSH levels are increased in 2 month old *Park2tm1Roo* knockout, there may be defective exocytosis of GSH out of the glia and into the extracellular space.

Mitochondria are a major source of ROS within cells and mitochondrial dysfunction has been robustly implicated with PD. The capacity for electron transport in mitochondria was found to be impaired in the *Park2tm1Shn* and *Park2tm1Ccs* knockout mice (Palacino et al., 2004; Stichel et al., 2007). Dopaminergic neurons in the *Park2tm1Rpa* and *Park2tm1Tmd* knockout lines do not appear to be more sensitive to the mitochondrial toxin MPTP (Perez et al., 2005;

Thomas et al., 2007). However, glial cultures derived from $Park2^{tm1Roo}$ knockout mice appeared more sensitive to MPTP (Solano et al., 2008). Furthermore, neuronal cultures derived from $Park2^{tm1Roo}$ knockout mice were more sensitive to the mitochondrial toxin rotenone. Co-culture of glia from $Park2^{tm1Roo}$ knockout mice with neurons derived from wildtype mice increased the sensitivity of wildtype neurons to rotenone (Casarejos et al., 2006). Furthermore, wildtype neurons exhibited significantly shorter processes and smaller neuronal areas when they were co-cultured with $Park2^{tm1Ccs}$ knockout derived astrocytes as opposed to wildtype astrocytes (Schmidt et al., 2011). Collectively, this suggests that lack of parkin leads to a functional disturbance of neuron-glia interactions, and that environmentally induced mitochondrial dysfunction when combined with parkin deficiency may be detrimental to dopaminergic neurons and stimulatory of neuroinflammatory processes.

The ultrastructure of mitochondria from $Park2^{tm1Ccs}$ knockout mouse has been investigated in both neuronal and glial populations *in vivo*. Compared to 3 month old mice, neurons in the substantia nigra of 12 month old $Park2^{tm1Ccs}$ knockout mice displayed an increased proportion of abnormal mitochondria. This age related change was not identified in wildtype mice (Stichel et al., 2007). Mitochondria within glial populations of $Park2^{tm1Ccs}$ knockout mice were found to exhibit an elevated number of structural deficits that included abnormal disintegration, a reduction of mitochondrial cristae and mitochondrial enlargement. The proportion of abnormal mitochondria identified in $Park2^{tm1Ccs}$ knockout glia depended on both age and glial cell type. Nonetheless, the amount of mitochondrial damage was significant at just 16 days of age in all glial cell types, and the mitochondrial burden was much greater in glial than neuronal cells (Schmidt et al., 2011). Oxidative stress is thought to be a major contributor to the development of PD. Several pathways associated with oxidative stress, notably GSH and the mitochondria, may be dysfunctional within $Park2$ knockout mice. Furthermore, it appears that a number of factors including age and cell type may mediate the extent of dysfunction associated with lack of parkin.

2.7 Ubiquitin Proteasome System (UPS)

Parkin was originally identified as an E3 ubiquitin ligase that functions in the UPS, and a number of putative interacting proteins and substrates have subsequently been identified (reviewed in (Dawson and Dawson, 2010)). Knockout mice allow the *in vivo* analysis of interacting proteins, substrates and pathway deficits that have been identified *in vitro*. A simple working hypothesis is that if a protein is a substrate of parkin mediated ubiquitination and subsequent degradation via the UPS, that protein would be expected to accumulate in a $Park2$ knockout mouse model. A number of groups have investigated some of the putative parkin substrates in $Park2$ knockout mice, but in general very few studies have replicated the *in vitro* results and shown increased levels of putative substrates *in vivo*. Two comprehensive analyses of parkin substrates have been reported using the $Park2^{tm1Tmd}$ knockout mice. The steady state level of aminoacyl-tRNA synthetase cofactor (AIMP2) was increased in the ventral midbrain/hindbrain of $Park2^{tm1Tmd}$ knockout mice but no alteration in the amount of seven other putative parkin substrates, including β-tubulin and α-synuclein, was identified. An accumulation of AIMP2 in brain tissue from individuals with *parkin*-proven PD was also shown, and AIMP2 was shown to interact with parkin *in vitro*, suggesting that AIMP2 is an authentic substrate of parkin (Ko et al., 2005). AIMP2 is a known interacting protein of far upstream element (FUSE)-binding protein 1 (FBP1), promoting its ubiquitination and degradation. Subsequent studies demonstrated that the level of FBP1 was increased in the brain stem and cortex of Park2^{tm1Tmd} knockout mice and also patients with *parkin*-proven PD (Ko et al., 2006). In contrast to the results in the ventral midbrain/hindbrain of Park2^{tm1Tmd} knockout mice, the level of AIMP2 in the cortex, cerebellum, brain stem, and striatum, and the level of FBP1 in the ventral midbrain, cerebellum or striatum was not altered (Ko et al., 2006; Ko et al., 2005). This may imply functional redundancy for turnover of these proteins in some regions of the brain. However, an alternative explanation may be that the rate of new protein synthesis is greater than the rate of protein degradation in these regions and so the effect of parkin absence is masked. A similar phenomenon was observed with estrogen related receptor (ERR) isoforms and α-tubulin. The consequence of loss of parkin on accumulation of ERRs and α-tubulin was only demonstrated after new protein synthesis was inhibited by treatment with puromycin (Ren et al., 2010).

In general, *in vitro* studies suggesting a role for parkin in the turnover of putative substrates have not been replicated in the different *in vivo* models. However the extent to which investigation has been reported is limited. Such apparent discrepancy between *in vitro* and *in vivo* models may due in part to experimental methodology. For example, the *in vitro* data suggesting a role for parkin in ubiquitin-proteasome mediated degradation may be an artefact of exogenous expression of parkin and putative substrates, or due to specificity of the cell type utilised. In addition, there is compelling evidence to suggest that parkin is able to function as a multifaceted ubiquitin ligase, capable of modulating alternative forms of ubiquitination not associated with ubiquitin-proteasome mediated degradation of proteins.

2.8 Autophagy

For a substrate to be recognised by the proteasome it needs to labelled with at least four ubiquitin molecules attached via lysine-48 linkage. Most recently, parkin-mediated lysine-63 polyubiquitylation was shown to be an important mediator of the aggregation and turnover of damaged mitochondria via autophagy (Geisler et al., 2010; Narendra et al., 2008; Narendra et al., 2010; Suen et al., 2010). Autophagy is the major pathway involved in the degradation of long-lived proteins and organelles and has been shown to play an integral role in protection against neurodegeneration (Hara et al., 2006; Komatsu et al., 2006). It is comprised of three distinct pathways, macroautophagy, microautophagy and chaperone-mediated autophagy. Macroautophagy (hereafter referred to as autophagy) involves the sequestration of organelles and proteins in a double-membrane vesicle, called an autophagosome or autophagic vacuole, which subsequently fuses with a lysosome and the contents are degraded by lysosomal hydrolases (reviewed in (Klionsky and Emr, 2000)). Emerging data suggests that the UPS and autophagy are functionally coupled and inhibition of the UPS can result in aggresome formation and elevated autophagy (Pandey et al., 2007). Several markers of the autophagic pathway have been shown to be elevated in the substantia nigra of PD cases and it has been proposed that Lewy bodies may be the *in vivo* representation of aggresome. It is not yet clear if the elevated numbers of autophagosomes identified in PD brains represent increased autophagy induction or impaired completion of autophagic degradation (reviewed in (Chu, 2011)). However, the ability of the autophagic vacuole to engulf organelles and large protein aggregates suggests upregulation of autophagy may represent a therapeutic target for PD (reviewed in ((Arduino et al., 2010; Banerjee et al., 2010)). Recent studies have defined a pathway linking parkin and PINK1 to mitophagy, a form of autophagy selective for mitochondria. Depolarisation of mitochondria results in the accumulation of parkin at the mitochondrion in a PINK1-dependent manner with subsequent degradation via mitophagy (Kawajiri et al., 2010; Narendra et al., 2008; Narendra et al., 2010; Vives-Bauza et al., 2010).

The effect of parkin deficiency on autophagy in *Park2* knockout mice has not been extensively reported. However, one study has investigated autophagy in neuronal cultures derived from *Park2tm1Roo* knockout mice. Midbrain neuronal cultures derived from *Park2tm1Roo* knockout mice were treated with epoxomicin to partially inhibit the proteasome. *Park2tm1Roo* knockout cultures appeared to be less susceptible to the toxic effects of proteasomal inhibition. The autophagic substrate p62 was increased in wildtype neuronal cultures but not in *Park2tm1Roo* knockout neuronal cultures, suggestive of increased autophagic activity. A second indicator of autophagic activity is the relative ratio of LC3I and LC3II. LC3 II is generated by site specific proteolysis and lipidation of LC3I and serves as a specific marker of autophagic activation. In basal conditions, the LC3II/I ratio was unchanged in neuronal cultures derived from wildtype mice, but it was significantly increased in cultures from derived *Park2tm1Roo* knockout mice, and this was further potentiated by epoxomicin treatment. These observations suggest that neuronal cultures derived from *Park2tm1Roo* knockout mice have increased autophagy and that partial proteasomal inhibition further potentiates autophagy in this model (Casarejos et al., 2009). The majority of cell culture models have suggested that Parkin regulates mitochondrial degradation through autophagy, and an early step in this process is the requirement for PINK1 to recruit Parkin to the mitochondria (Vives-Bauza et al., 2010). Therefore, it seems counter intuitive that neuronal cultures derived from *Park2tm1Roo* knockout mice would display increased autophagy following proteasomal inhibition. However, a study of neurons taken from rat substantia nigra suggested that mitophagy was parkin independent in these cells. It was suggested that the difference in neurons may be due to the high dependence of neurons on mitochondrial respiration (Van Laar et al., 2011). Much of what is currently understood about the potential role of parkin in autophagy is derived from studies in cell culture models. However, this is an expanding field in PD research and future studies utilising *Park2* knockout mice will provide considerable insight into the significance of this role *in vivo*.

2.9 Trafficking/signalling

Parkin-mediated ubiquitination has also been suggested to play a role in signal transduction and trafficking. Monoubiquitination is associated with the regulation of endocytosis of membrane proteins and signalling (Mukhopadhyay and Riezman, 2007). The interaction between parkin and PICK1 is an example of this function. PICK1 regulates the trafficking and stability of a number of synaptic proteins, including neurotransmitter receptors, transporters and ion channels (Madsen et al., 2005). *In vitro* analysis suggested that parkin monoubiquitinated rather than polyubiquitinated PICK1. In neurons derived from *Park2tm1Roo* knockout mice steady-state PICK1 levels were not altered, suggesting turnover of the protein is independent of parkin. PICK1 has been shown to interact with the proton-gated ion channel ASIC2a, and potentiation of ASIC2a currents is suggested to be PICK1 dependent. Hippocampal neurons from *Park2tm1Roo* knockout mice show deficits of ASIC2a current potentiation, which suggest that monoubiquitination of PICK1 by parkin is required for ASIC2a channel function (Joch et al., 2007).

The interaction of parkin and the endocytic protein Endophilin A1 provides additional evidence that the ubiquitination activity of parkin is not limited to proteasome turnover. Endophilin A1 is a protein that is abundant in neural synapses and is involved in formation of presynaptic endocytic vesicles. Limited ubiquitination of Endophilin A1 by parkin was shown *in vitro* and Endophilin A1 did not appear to accumulate in synapses from *Park2tm1Roo* knockout mice. *In vivo* the interaction of the two proteins appears to promote co-localisation from the cytosol to the plasma membrane and synaptic vesicle enriched fractions. In synaptosome preparations from wildtype mice relocalisation leads to increased ubiquitination of synaptic proteins, however, this effect is abrogated in *Park2tm1Roo* knockout mice (Trempe et al., 2009). Further understanding of the functional deficits associated with this loss of relocalisation and ubiquitination activity in *Park2* knockout mice may shed light on the defects in synaptic transmission observed in both *Park2* knockout mice and *parkin*-mediated PD.

2.10 Genetic modification of *Park2* knockout mice

Mutations in the genes *parkin*, *PINK1* and *DJ-1* have been associated with familial recessive early-onset PD. A number of lines of evidence suggest that these genes may function in a common pathway(s) important for mitochondrial function (Geisler et al., 2010; Narendra et al., 2010; Thomas et al., 2011). The effect of knockout of all three genes in a single mouse model revealed that *Park2tm1Shn/Pink1/Dj-1* knockout mice at 24 months of age do not show significant dopaminergic degeneration (Kitada et al., 2009b). This may suggest a functional redundancy between these genes. An alternative interpretation may be that these genes are not essential for neuronal survival, but rather may play a protective role against cellular insults.

A major component of Lewy bodies in PD is alpha-synuclein, which is also genetically linked with autosomal dominant PD and sporadic PD (reviewed in (Obeso et al., 2010). The effect of parkin deficiency combined with dysregulation of α-synuclein has been reported for three *Park2* knockout mouse lines. The *Park2tm1Tmd* knockout mouse was crossed with a transgenic mouse overexpressing familial mutant A53T α-synuclein under the control of the mouse prion promoter [Tg(PRP-SNCA^A53T)]. In this model, parkin deficiency did not appear to exacerbate attributes previously recognised in Tg(PRP-SNCA^A53T) mice. Likewise, Tg(PRP-SNCA^A53T) did not potentiate the locus coeruleus degeneration of the *Park2tm1Tmd* knockout line (von Coelln et al., 2006). The *Park2tm1Roo* knockout mouse was crossed with a transgenic mouse overexpressing familial mutant A30P α-synuclein under the control of the thymus cell antigen 1 promoter [Tg(THY1-SNCA^A30P)]. In contrast to the previous model, parkin deficiency appeared to delay the progressive neurodegenerative motor phenotype of Tg(THY1-SNCA^A30P) mice, and decreased neuritic pathology that is associated with these symptoms. Furthermore, co-staining of ubiquitin with phosphorylated α-synuclein positive structures was reduced in this model (Fournier et al., 2009). The *Park2tm1Ccs* knockout mouse was crossed with two different mutant α-synuclein lines. Both lines expressed human α-synuclein carrying two familial mutations, A30P and A53T, under the control of either the chicken beta-actin (BA) promoter [Tg(BA-SNCA^A30/PA53T)] or the mouse tyrosine hydroxylase (TH) promoter [Tg(TH-SNCA^A30/PA53T)]. The most prominent feature identified in neurons from these mutant mice was an age-related increase in the proportion of abnormal mitochondria and a reduction in mitochondrial complex I activity in the substantia nigra (Stichel et al., 2007). Collectively, these studies suggest that the effect of parkin deficiency on α-synuclein mediated phenotypes may be independent (von Coelln et al., 2006), delayed (Fournier et al., 2009) or enhanced (Stichel et al., 2007). Whether this is related to differential attributes of the *Park2* knockout mice or the differential regional effects of α-synuclein overexpression remains to be investigated.

The normal age related increase of tau pathology is potentiated in the *Park2*tm1Roo knockout mouse (Rodriguez-Navarro et al., 2007). Tauopathies are neurodegenerative diseases principally identified by dementia and Parkinsonism. Idiopathic forms are thought to be due to post-translational alteration of tau whereas familiar tauopathies are the result of mutations in the gene encoding tau, *microtubule associated protein tau (MAPT)* (Avila et al., 2004; Hutton et al., 1998). *MAPT* has also recently been genetically implicated in sporadic PD aetiology (Satake et al., 2009; Simon-Sanchez et al., 2009) and aggregation of tau has been shown to be a feature of some cases of *parkin*-proven PD (reviewed in (Cookson et al., 2008).

The consequence of combining the over-expression of a human 4-repeat tau isoform with known familial alterations G2727V, P301L, R406W under the control of human thymus cell antigen 1 promoter [Tg(THY1-TauVLW)] with the *Park2*tm1Roo knockout mouse was investigated. Like *Park2*tm1Roo knockout mice, Tg(THY1-TauVLW) mice have slight behavioural and molecular changes that do not manifest in a clinical phenotype. However, when combined a number of age-progressive behavioural attributes including reduced hind limb length, uncontrolled movements, loss of balance and postural abnormalities as well as increased self-injury of the face that is a reflection of compulsive long-term grooming, were identified. This was coupled with a significant loss of motor neurons, and dopaminergic neurons in the substantia nigra. In addition, tau pathology was identified, as was abnormal expression glia in the substantia nigra and the hippocampus (Menendez et al., 2006; Rodriguez-Navarro et al., 2008a). Furthermore, phosphorylated tau plaques and tangles, as well as endogenous β-amyloid plaques were found in the hippocampus. Notably, dietary supplementation with the disaccharide trehalose, which is thought to enhance autophagy, was found to ameliorate the severity of the symptoms and pathology in this model. (Rodriguez-Navarro et al., 2010). By combining parkin deficiency with abnormal tau expression, a number of attributes that were modestly perturbed in the single monogenetic mutants were significantly dysregulated. This suggests that parkin and tau may be functionally coupled *in vivo*, and their perturbation is capable of eliciting a progressive neurodegenerative phenotype with characteristics of both PD and Alzheimer's disease.

Alzheimer disease is a degenerative dementia characterised by loss of neurons in the cerebral cortex. Pathological features include extracellular amyloid plaques, which are composed predominately of β-amyloid, and intracellular neurofibrillary tangles that mainly consist of hyperphosphorylated tau. The identification of β-amyloid plaques in the *Park2*tm1Roo/Tg(THY1-TauVLW) mouse led to the investigation of the effect of parkin deficiency on β-amyloid expression. The APP_{swe} is a transgenic mouse line that overexpresses the β-amyloid precursor protein containing two mutations, K670N and M671L, under the control of the prion protein promoter. Parkin deficiency appears to reduce the severity of behavioural deficits of APP_{swe} mice including reduced weight gain, exploratory activity and working memory. Furthermore, parkin deficiency appears to reduce β-amyloid plaque pathology within the cerebral cortex and hippocampus, and in the hippocampus the amount of astrogliosis and phosphorylated tau was also reduced. This was coupled with alterations in a number of autophagic markers consistent with induction of autophagy (Perucho et al., 2010).

Therefore, in contrast to the $Park2^{tm1Roo}$/Tg(THY1-Tau^{VLW}) mouse, where combining the two mutant alleles appeared to enhanced the disease process, parkin deficiency combined with APP$_{swe}$ over-expression can ameliorate a number of pathological characteristics of these mice. Consequently, it appears parkin has the potential to be both neuroprotective and a neurotoxic to the neurodegenerative process, depending on context. Furthermore, the effect of active autophagy when either APP$_{swe}$ or Tg(THY1-Tau^{VLW}) were combined with $Park2^{tm1Roo}$ knockout appears to be protective. This suggests further investigation into factors that enhance autophagy may identify potential treatments for individuals with PD and other neurodegenerative disorders.

3. Discussion

PD is differentiated from other neurodegenerative disorders by defined motor disturbances resulting from the pathological loss of dopaminergic neurons. Seven *Park2* knockout models have been generated and characterised. In the current context, loss of function of parkin in these mouse models does not appear to reproduce a PD-like phenotype that is reflective of *parkin*-proven PD. However, two models showed a significant loss of catecholaminergic neurons, one in the substantia nigra and the other in the locus coeruleus. Notably, the extent of neuronal loss within the substantia nigra was not equivalent to that associated with the onset of symptomatic PD in humans. However, both neurochemical and electrophysiological studies have identified disturbances in dopamine pathways in *Park2* knockout mice that are consistent with altered presynaptic release of dopamine. Glial and redox dysfunction was also identified, indicating that the capacity to protect neurons against cellular insult may be diminished in *Park2* knockout mice. Furthermore, mitochondrial abnormalities highlight the importance of parkin function in maintaining mitochondrial integrity. Accumulation of specific proteins within *Park2* knockout mice has confirmed *in vivo* that parkin functions as an E3 ubiquitin ligase in the UPS. The additional role of parkin in autophagy and trafficking/signalling pathways are indicative of a broad role in normal cellular function. With regard to the involvement of parkin with neurodegeneration the most important findings were identified by genetic modification of *Park2* knockout mice. *Park2* knockout mice, when combined with other mutant transgenic models, appeared to have the capacity to both exacerbate and ameliorate disease associated characteristics in a context dependent manner. Therefore, dysfunction of parkin has the potential to be both neuroprotective and neurotoxic.

The inability of *Park2* knockout mice to adequately recapitulate the clinical and pathological manifestation of PD is not an isolated observation. Knockout of other PD associated genes such as *Pink1*, *a-synuclein* and *Lrrk2* also fail to produce robust PD-like phenotypes, and the results of transgenic overexpression of disease associated genes and mutants vary considerably depending on the promoter used to drive expression (reviewed in (Dawson et al., 2010)). In addition, a knockin model of a common pathogenic variant of LRRK2 does not show evidence of dopaminergic degeneration. However, like *Park2* knockout mice these *Lrrk2* knockin mice appear to have dysregulation of the dopamine system (Tong et al., 2009). In addition, a number of other features identified in *Park2* knockout mice, including alterations of the neuroimmune system, mitochondrial dysfunction and oxidative stress are shared between the models. These observations suggest a commonality to the perturbations that occur prior to manifestation of pathogenic phenotypic features.

An explanation as to why *Park2* knockout mice fail, for the most part, to recapitulate the loss of dopaminergic neurons that is a feature of human disease may be the short lifespan of the species. Aging research carried out in mice indicate that a number of molecular markers of aging follow a similar course to that observed in humans, although over a shorter duration. (reviewed ((Yuan et al., 2011)). This suggests that at the cellular and systemic level aging follows a parallel path in mice and humans. The symptoms of *parkin*-mediated PD typically present before 45 years of age. However, there is considerable disparity in age of onset, presentation, progression and response to drug treatment, even for patients within the same sibship, with the same mutations (reviewed in (Mata et al., 2004)). Therefore, loss of function of parkin alone may not be responsible for dopaminergic neuronal loss in individuals with *parkin*-mediated PD. Three lines of evidence from studies carried out in *Park2* knockout mice support this notion. 1) A significant loss (35%), of dopaminergic neurons occurs in the substantia nigra of the *Park2*[tm1Roo] knockout in an age-related progressive manner over the duration of the life-span of the mouse, although not to the extent that is observed (~60%) at symptom onset in humans. This indicates that parkin deficiency can cause dopaminergic neuronal loss in a mouse model. 2) The loss of catecholaminergic neurons in the locus coeruleus in the *Park2*[tm1Tmd] knockout line shows reduced penetrance. This suggests that additional factors mediate this trait. 3) The increased vulnerability of *Park2*[tm1Shn] knockout mice to loss of dopaminergic neurons in the substantia nigra induced by repeated low-dose systemic LPS treatment. This indicates that in this model, although parkin deficiency alone was not sufficient to cause dopaminergic neuronal loss, dopaminergic integrity was compromised in a neuroinflammatory environment.

A number of the phenotypic discrepancies between the *Park2* knockout mice may be attributable to differences between the genetic background of the mouse strains used (discussed in (Perez and Palmiter, 2005)). The majority of studies used mice of variable mixed backgrounds. Isogenic strains are preferred when investigating the effect of gene knockout as genetic similarity tends to result in phenotypic uniformity, increasing the power to identify significant effects. It would be an advantage when comparing traits between different knockout mice for them to be on the same isogenic background, particularly if the genetic effect is modest, as appears to be the case of *parkin*. Therefore, until these carefully controlled studies are undertaken, it remains difficult to determine which of the identified phenotypic features are likely to be attributable to parkin.

Isogenic strains may also be a hindrance if pathogenicity has undefined multigenic influences, as potentially could be the case for parkin. During the process of generating an inbred strain, mice undergo a process called inbreeding depression. In this process the reproductive fitness reduces as homozygosity increases because repressive alleles are unmasked. Therefore, founders of an inbred strain and their offspring must be considered selective survivors of the inbreeding process, and as such have a level of fitness that does not reflect the species as a whole (McClearn and McCarter, 2011). In a multifaceted disease such as PD, other genetic factors may contribute to disease progression. Therefore, the isogenic inbred strains could limit the affect of *Park2* knockout. However, the negative effects associated with inbreeding depression can be overcome by generating F1 hybrids of two different inbred strains. In the context of the *Park2* knockout models, it may be noteworthy that the only strain that demonstrates significant loss of dopaminergic neurons in the substantia nigra, the *Park2^{tm1Roo}* knockout mouse, was reported in a mixed 129S2/C57BL6 (50/50) genetic background.

Another factor that could be significant in the development of a disease phenotype is the environmental differences between laboratory mice and humans. It is clear that environmental factors influence PD development, and in some cases may cause PD. Laboratory mice are housed in controlled environments, often pathogen free, with none or limited exposure to environmental toxins or stresses. Therefore these mice may not be exposed to the appropriate triggers that are necessary for dopaminergic protective mechanisms to fail. Loss of parkin may result in a pre-degenerative state where neurons are under stress but not sufficiently compromised as to cause significant loss. Other cues, such as pro-inflammatory factors, could provide the additional stimulus required for degeneration to occur. This model may better explain an inherited autosomal recessive trait that takes multiple decades to manifest symptoms.

The *Park2* knockout mice are useful to understand the mechanistic consequence of loss of parkin function in a mammalian species. An improved understanding of the effect of *parkin* deletion on neuron and glial populations will provide considerable insight into the pathogenesis of PD, and the contribution that dopamine dysregulation plays in the pathogenic process. Cellular models have provided a great deal of information about the role of parkin in the turnover of protein and cellular constituents, in particular mitochondria, via the UPS and autophagy. The *Park2* knockout models provide a sophisticated platform to refine and advance these studies, for example using neuronal and glial cultures derived from *Park2* knockout mice.

There are a number of avenues that can be explored to potentially develop a *Park2* knockout model with a pathological phenotype of clinical relevance. Crossing the *Park2* knockout mice with α-synuclein, tau and β-amyloid models has provided enormous insight into the role of parkin in the neurodegenerative process *in vivo*. Further research following on from these studies, including breeding to the conditional α-synuclein knockin model currently in development (NIH project No. 1R21NS057795-01A1), has the potential to develop these mice into a more clinically relevant model. Likewise, the role of neuroinflammation in the neurodegenerative process could be further explored using *Park2* knockout mice. This could be achieved by breeding to genetic models with perturbations in the inflammatory response or treatment with agents such as LPS. In addition, a second rodent model, knockout of parkin in the rat, has recently been developed (SAGE Labs). The phenotypic outcome will be of great interest to compare and contrast with the results already obtained in mouse models.

4. Conclusion

A quote by Michael FW Festing, an expert in the field of laboratory animal genetics, eloquently encapsulates the use of mouse models in disease research. *"Models are subject to improvement through further research. A lot of animal research is aimed at understanding the animal as a potential model for particular human conditions, without being too precise as to what those conditions might be. Models are not just found. They need to be developed, and this requires an understanding of the biology of the species and the effects of various interventions such as inactivating specific genes or manipulating the environment. As our understanding increases, so the chance of choosing the most appropriate models for a specific disease increases"* (Festing, 2011). To date, seven *Park2* knockout mice have been generated but *Park2* knockout models still need to be developed in order to understand the clinical manifestation of *parkin*-mediated PD and the contribution of parkin to idiopathic PD.

5. References

Chew, K.C., N. Matsuda, K. Saisho, G.G. Lim, C. Chai, H.M. Tan, K. Tanaka, and K.L. Lim. 2011. Parkin mediates apparent e2-independent monoubiquitination in vitro and contains an intrinsic activity that catalyzes polyubiquitination. *PLoS One.* 6:e19720.

Chu, C.T. 2011. Diversity in the regulation of autophagy and mitophagy: lessons from Parkinson's disease. *Parkinsons Dis.* 2011:789431.

Ciechanover, A., A. Orian, and A.L. Schwartz. 2000. Ubiquitin-mediated proteolysis: biological regulation via destruction. *Bioessays.* 22:442-51.

Cookson, M.R., J. Hardy, and P.A. Lewis. 2008. Genetic neuropathology of Parkinson's disease. *Int J Clin Exp Pathol.* 1:217-31.

Daniel, S.E., and A.J. Lees. 1993. Parkinson's Disease Society Brain Bank, London: overview and research. *J Neural Transm Suppl.* 39:165-72.

Daubner, S.C., T. Le, and S. Wang. 2011. Tyrosine hydroxylase and regulation of dopamine synthesis. *Arch Biochem Biophys.* 508:1-12.

Dawson, T.M., and V.L. Dawson. 2010. The role of parkin in familial and sporadic Parkinson's disease. *Mov Disord.* 25 Suppl 1:S32-9.

Dawson, T.M., H.S. Ko, and V.L. Dawson. 2010. Genetic animal models of Parkinson's disease. *Neuron.* 66:646-61.

de Lau, L.M., and M.M. Breteler. 2006. Epidemiology of Parkinson's disease. *Lancet Neurol.* 5:525-35.

Denison, S.R., G. Callahan, N.A. Becker, L.A. Phillips, and D.I. Smith. 2003. Characterization of FRA6E and its potential role in autosomal recessive juvenile parkinsonism and ovarian cancer. *Genes Chromosomes Cancer.* 38:40-52.

Dickson, D.W., H. Braak, J.E. Duda, C. Duyckaerts, T. Gasser, G.M. Halliday, J. Hardy, J.B. Leverenz, K. Del Tredici, Z.K. Wszolek, and I. Litvan. 2009. Neuropathological assessment of Parkinson's disease: refining the diagnostic criteria. *Lancet Neurol.* 8:1150-7.

Dutta, G., P. Zhang, and B. Liu. 2008. The lipopolysaccharide Parkinson's disease animal model: mechanistic studies and drug discovery. *Fundam Clin Pharmacol.* 22:453-64.

Fearnley, J.M., and A.J. Lees. 1991. Ageing and Parkinson's disease: substantia nigra regional selectivity. *Brain.* 114 (Pt 5):2283-301.

Festing, M.F.W. (2011) Animal models in research, In: *Isogenic.info.* May 2011, available from: http://isogenic.info/index.html

Foroud, T., S.K. Uniacke, L. Liu, N. Pankratz, A. Rudolph, C. Halter, C. Shults, K. Marder, P.M. Conneally, and W.C. Nichols. 2003. Heterozygosity for a mutation in the parkin gene leads to later onset Parkinson disease. *Neurology.* 60:796-801.

Gelb, D.J., E. Oliver, and S. Gilman. 1999. Diagnostic criteria for Parkinson disease. *Arch Neurol.* 56:33-9.

Goldberg, M.S., S.M. Fleming, J.J. Palacino, C. Cepeda, H.A. Lam, A. Bhatnagar, E.G. Meloni, N. Wu, L.C. Ackerson, G.J. Klapstein, M. Gajendiran, B.L. Roth, M.F. Chesselet, N.T. Maidment, M.S. Levine, and J. Shen. 2003. Parkin-deficient mice exhibit nigrostriatal deficits but not loss of dopaminergic neurons. *J Biol Chem.* 278:43628-35.

Greene, J.C., A.J. Whitworth, I. Kuo, L.A. Andrews, M.B. Feany, and L.J. Pallanck. 2003. Mitochondrial pathology and apoptotic muscle degeneration in Drosophila parkin mutants. *Proc Natl Acad Sci U S A.* 100:4078-83.

Grimm, J., A. Mueller, F. Hefti, and A. Rosenthal. 2004. Molecular basis for catecholaminergic neuron diversity. *Proc Natl Acad Sci U S A.* 101:13891-6.

Guerrero, R., P. Navarro, E. Gallego, J. Avila, J.G. de Yebenes, and M.P. Sanchez. 2008. Park2-null/tau transgenic mice reveal a functional relationship between parkin and tau. *J Alzheimers Dis.* 13:161-72.

Guo, J.F., L. Wang, D. He, Q.H. Yang, Z.X. Duan, X.W. Zhang, L.L. Nie, X.X. Yan, and B.S. Tang. 2010. Clinical features and [11C]-CFT PET analysis of PARK2, PARK6, PARK7-linked autosomal recessive early onset Parkinsonism. *Neurol Sci.* 32:35-40.

Halliday, G.M., and H. McCann. 2010. The progression of pathology in Parkinson's disease. *Ann N Y Acad Sci.* 1184:188-95.

Hanson, J.E., A.L. Orr, and D.V. Madison. 2010. Altered hippocampal synaptic physiology in aged parkin-deficient mice. *Neuromolecular Med.* 12:270-6.

Harrison, D.E. (2011) Maximum Lifespan As a Biomarker of Aging, In: *The Jackson Laboratory, May 2011,* available from: http://www.jax.org/

Hurelbrink, C.B., and S.J. Lewis. 2010. Pathological considerations in the treatment of Parkinson's disease: more than just a wiring diagram. *Clin Neurol Neurosurg.* 113:1-6.

Itier, J.M., P. Ibanez, M.A. Mena, N. Abbas, C. Cohen-Salmon, G.A. Bohme, M. Laville, J. Pratt, O. Corti, L. Pradier, G. Ret, C. Joubert, M. Periquet, F. Araujo, J. Negroni, M.J. Casarejos, S. Canals, R. Solano, A. Serrano, E. Gallego, M. Sanchez, P. Denefle, J. Benavides, G. Tremp, T.A. Rooney, A. Brice, and J. Garcia de Yebenes. 2003. Parkin gene inactivation alters behaviour and dopamine neurotransmission in the mouse. *Hum Mol Genet.* 12:2277-91.

Kitada, T., A. Pisani, M. Karouani, M. Haburcak, G. Martella, A. Tscherter, P. Platania, B. Wu, E.N. Pothos, and J. Shen. 2009a. Impaired dopamine release and synaptic plasticity in the striatum of parkin-/- mice. *J Neurochem.* 110:613-21.

Kitada, T., Y. Tong, C.A. Gautier, and J. Shen. 2009b. Absence of nigral degeneration in aged parkin/DJ-1/PINK1 triple knockout mice. *J Neurochem.* 111:696-702.

Kitao, Y., Y. Imai, K. Ozawa, A. Kataoka, T. Ikeda, M. Soda, K. Nakimawa, H. Kiyama, D.M. Stern, O. Hori, K. Wakamatsu, S. Ito, S. Itohara, R. Takahashi, and S. Ogawa. 2007. Pael receptor induces death of dopaminergic neurons in the substantia nigra via endoplasmic reticulum stress and dopamine toxicity, which is enhanced under condition of parkin inactivation. *Hum Mol Genet.* 16:50-60.

Klionsky, D.J., and S.D. Emr. 2000. Autophagy as a regulated pathway of cellular degradation. *Science*. 290:1717-21.

Ko, H.S., S.W. Kim, S.R. Sriram, V.L. Dawson, and T.M. Dawson. 2006. Identification of far upstream element-binding protein-1 as an authentic Parkin substrate. *J Biol Chem*. 281:16193-6.

Lee, J.K., T. Tran, and M.G. Tansey. 2009. Neuroinflammation in Parkinson's disease. *J Neuroimmune Pharmacol*. 4:419-29.

Lewis, S.J., T. Foltynie, A.D. Blackwell, T.W. Robbins, A.M. Owen, and R.A. Barker. 2005. Heterogeneity of Parkinson's disease in the early clinical stages using a data driven approach. *J Neurol Neurosurg Psychiatry*. 76:343-8.

Lotharius, J., and P. Brundin. 2002. Pathogenesis of Parkinson's disease: dopamine, vesicles and alpha-synuclein. *Nat Rev Neurosci*. 3:932-42.

Lu, X.H., S.M. Fleming, B. Meurers, L.C. Ackerson, F. Mortazavi, V. Lo, D. Hernandez, D. Sulzer, G.R. Jackson, N.T. Maidment, M.F. Chesselet, and X.W. Yang. 2009. Bacterial artificial chromosome transgenic mice expressing a truncated mutant parkin exhibit age-dependent hypokinetic motor deficits, dopaminergic neuron degeneration, and accumulation of proteinase K-resistant alpha-synuclein. *J Neurosci*. 29:1962-76.

Lucking, C.B., A. Durr, V. Bonifati, J. Vaughan, G. De Michele, T. Gasser, B.S. Harhangi, G. Meco, P. Denefle, N.W. Wood, Y. Agid, and A. Brice. 2000. Association between early-onset Parkinson's disease and mutations in the parkin gene. *N Engl J Med*. 342:1560-7.

Martin, H.L., and P. Teismann. 2009. Glutathione--a review on its role and significance in Parkinson's disease. *FASEB J*. 23:3263-72.

Mata, I.F., P.J. Lockhart, and M.J. Farrer. 2004. Parkin genetics: one model for Parkinson's disease. *Hum Mol Genet*. 13 Spec No 1:R127-33.

McClearn, G.E., and R.J. McCarter. 2011. Heterogeneous stocks and selective breeding in aging research. *ILAR J*. 52:16-23.

Menendez, J., J.A. Rodriguez-Navarro, R.M. Solano, M.J. Casarejos, I. Rodal, R. Guerrero, M.P. Sanchez, J. Avila, M.A. Mena, and J.G. de Yebenes. 2006. Suppression of Parkin enhances nigrostriatal and motor neuron lesion in mice over-expressing human-mutated tau protein. *Hum Mol Genet*. 15:2045-58.

Mukhopadhyay, D., and H. Riezman. 2007. Proteasome-independent functions of ubiquitin in endocytosis and signaling. *Science*. 315:201-5.

Obeso, J.A., M.C. Rodriguez-Oroz, B. Benitez-Temino, F.J. Blesa, J. Guridi, C. Marin, and M. Rodriguez. 2008. Functional organization of the basal ganglia: therapeutic implications for Parkinson's disease. *Mov Disord*. 23 Suppl 3:S548-59.

Obeso, J.A., M.C. Rodriguez-Oroz, C.G. Goetz, C. Marin, J.H. Kordower, M. Rodriguez, E.C. Hirsch, M. Farrer, A.H. Schapira, and G. Halliday. 2010. Missing pieces in the Parkinson's disease puzzle. *Nat Med*. 16:653-61.

Olzmann, J.A., and L.S. Chin. 2008. Parkin-mediated K63-linked polyubiquitination: a signal for targeting misfolded proteins to the aggresome-autophagy pathway. *Autophagy*. 4:85-7.

Oyama, G., K. Yoshimi, S. Natori, Y. Chikaoka, Y.R. Ren, M. Funayama, Y. Shimo, R. Takahashi, T. Nakazato, S. Kitazawa, and N. Hattori. 2010. Impaired in vivo dopamine release in parkin knockout mice. *Brain Res.* 1352:214-22.

Pakkenberg, B., A. Moller, H.J. Gundersen, A. Mouritzen Dam, and H. Pakkenberg. 1991. The absolute number of nerve cells in substantia nigra in normal subjects and in patients with Parkinson's disease estimated with an unbiased stereological method. *J Neurol Neurosurg Psychiatry.* 54:30-3.

Palacino, J.J., D. Sagi, M.S. Goldberg, S. Krauss, C. Motz, M. Wacker, J. Klose, and J. Shen. 2004. Mitochondrial dysfunction and oxidative damage in parkin-deficient mice. *J Biol Chem.* 279:18614-22.

Palumbo, E., L. Matricardi, E. Tosoni, A. Bensimon, and A. Russo. 2010. Replication dynamics at common fragile site FRA6E. *Chromosoma.* 119:575-87.

Perez, F.A., and R.D. Palmiter. 2005. Parkin-deficient mice are not a robust model of parkinsonism. *Proc Natl Acad Sci U S A.* 102:2174-9.

Perucho, J., M.J. Casarejos, I. Rubio, J.A. Rodriguez-Navarro, A. Gomez, I. Ampuero, I. Rodal, R.M. Solano, E. Carro, J. Garcia de Yebenes, and M.A. Mena. 2010. The effects of parkin suppression on the behaviour, amyloid processing, and cell survival in APP mutant transgenic mice. *Exp Neurol.* 221:54-67.

Pesah, Y., T. Pham, H. Burgess, B. Middlebrooks, P. Verstreken, Y. Zhou, M. Harding, H. Bellen, and G. Mardon. 2004. Drosophila parkin mutants have decreased mass and cell size and increased sensitivity to oxygen radical stress. *Development.* 131:2183-94.

Ren, Y., H. Jiang, D. Ma, K. Nakaso, and J. Feng. 2010. Parkin degrades estrogen-related receptors to limit the expression of monoamine oxidases. *Hum Mol Genet.* 20:1074-83.

Rodriguez-Navarro, J.A., M.J. Casarejos, J. Menendez, R.M. Solano, I. Rodal, A. Gomez, J.G. Yebenes, and M.A. Mena. 2007. Mortality, oxidative stress and tau accumulation during ageing in parkin null mice. *J Neurochem.* 103:98-114.

Rodriguez-Navarro, J.A., R.M. Solano, M.J. Casarejos, A. Gomez, J. Perucho, J.G. de Yebenes, and M.A. Mena. 2008. Gender differences and estrogen effects in parkin null mice. *J Neurochem.* 106:2143-57.

Satake, W., Y. Nakabayashi, I. Mizuta, Y. Hirota, C. Ito, M. Kubo, T. Kawaguchi, T. Tsunoda, M. Watanabe, A. Takeda, H. Tomiyama, K. Nakashima, K. Hasegawa, F. Obata, T. Yoshikawa, H. Kawakami, S. Sakoda, M. Yamamoto, N. Hattori, M. Murata, Y. Nakamura, and T. Toda. 2009. Genome-wide association study identifies common variants at four loci as genetic risk factors for Parkinson's disease. *Nat Genet.* 41:1303-7.

Sato, S., T. Chiba, S. Nishiyama, T. Kakiuchi, H. Tsukada, T. Hatano, T. Fukuda, Y. Yasoshima, N. Kai, K. Kobayashi, Y. Mizuno, K. Tanaka, and N. Hattori. 2006. Decline of striatal dopamine release in parkin-deficient mice shown by ex vivo autoradiography. *J Neurosci Res.* 84:1350-7.

Schmidt, S., B. Linnartz, S. Mendritzki, T. Sczepan, M. Lubbert, C.C. Stichel, and H. Lubbert. 2011. Genetic mouse models for Parkinson's disease display severe pathology in glial cell mitochondria. *Hum Mol Genet.* 20:1197-211.

Selikhova, M., D.R. Williams, P.A. Kempster, J.L. Holton, T. Revesz, and A.J. Lees. 2009. A clinico-pathological study of subtypes in Parkinson's disease. *Brain.* 132:2947-57.

Shimura, H., N. Hattori, S. Kubo, Y. Mizuno, S. Asakawa, S. Minoshima, N. Shimizu, K. Iwai, T. Chiba, K. Tanaka, and T. Suzuki. 2000. Familial Parkinson disease gene product, parkin, is a ubiquitin-protein ligase. *Nat Genet.* 25:302-5.

Shulman, J.M., P.L. De Jager, and M.B. Feany. 2010. Parkinson's Disease: Genetics and Pathogenesis. *Annu Rev Pathol.* 6:193-222.

Simon-Sanchez, J., C. Schulte, J.M. Bras, M. Sharma, J.R. Gibbs, D. Berg, C. Paisan-Ruiz, P. Lichtner, S.W. Scholz, D.G. Hernandez, R. Kruger, M. Federoff, C. Klein, A. Goate, J. Perlmutter, M. Bonin, M.A. Nalls, T. Illig, C. Gieger, H. Houlden, M. Steffens, M.S. Okun, B.A. Racette, M.R. Cookson, K.D. Foote, H.H. Fernandez, B.J. Traynor, S. Schreiber, S. Arepalli, R. Zonozi, K. Gwinn, M. van der Brug, G. Lopez, S.J. Chanock, A. Schatzkin, Y. Park, A. Hollenbeck, J. Gao, X. Huang, N.W. Wood, D. Lorenz, G. Deuschl, H. Chen, O. Riess, J.A. Hardy, A.B. Singleton, and T. Gasser. 2009. Genome-wide association study reveals genetic risk underlying Parkinson's disease. *Nat Genet.* 41:1308-12.

Solano, R.M., M.J. Casarejos, J. Menendez-Cuervo, J.A. Rodriguez-Navarro, J. Garcia de Yebenes, and M.A. Mena. 2008. Glial dysfunction in parkin null mice: effects of aging. *J Neurosci.* 28:598-611.

Standaert, D.G., and J.M. Galanter. (2007) Pharmacology of dopaminergic neurotransmission. In: *Principles of pharmacology: the pathophysiologic basis of drug therapy.* Golan, D.E., editor. pp. 185-200, Lippincott Williams & Wilkins, 0781783550, United Kingdom.

Stichel, C.C., X.R. Zhu, V. Bader, B. Linnartz, S. Schmidt, and H. Lubbert. 2007. Mono- and double-mutant mouse models of Parkinson's disease display severe mitochondrial damage. *Hum Mol Genet.* 16:2377-93.

Tong, Y., A. Pisani, G. Martella, M. Karouani, H. Yamaguchi, E.N. Pothos, and J. Shen. 2009. R1441C mutation in LRRK2 impairs dopaminergic neurotransmission in mice. *Proc Natl Acad Sci U S A.* 106:14622-7.

Van Den Eeden, S.K., C.M. Tanner, A.L. Bernstein, R.D. Fross, A. Leimpeter, D.A. Bloch, and L.M. Nelson. 2003. Incidence of Parkinson's disease: variation by age, gender, and race/ethnicity. *Am J Epidemiol.* 157:1015-22.

von Coelln, R., B. Thomas, S.A. Andrabi, K.L. Lim, J.M. Savitt, R. Saffary, W. Stirling, K. Bruno, E.J. Hess, M.K. Lee, V.L. Dawson, and T.M. Dawson. 2006. Inclusion body formation and neurodegeneration are parkin independent in a mouse model of alpha-synucleinopathy. *J Neurosci.* 26:3685-96.

Von Coelln, R., B. Thomas, J.M. Savitt, K.L. Lim, M. Sasaki, E.J. Hess, V.L. Dawson, and T.M. Dawson. 2004. Loss of locus coeruleus neurons and reduced startle in parkin null mice. *Proc Natl Acad Sci U S A.* 101:10744-9.

Whitworth, A.J., D.A. Theodore, J.C. Greene, H. Benes, P.D. Wes, and L.J. Pallanck. 2005. Increased glutathione S-transferase activity rescues dopaminergic neuron loss in a Drosophila model of Parkinson's disease. *Proc Natl Acad Sci U S A.* 102:8024-9.

Yoshida, T., T. Mizuta, and S. Shimizu. 2010. Neurodegeneration in mnd2 mutant mice is not prevented by parkin transgene. *Biochem Biophys Res Commun.* 402:676-9.

Yuan, R., L.L. Peters, and B. Paigen. 2011. Mice as a mammalian model for research on the genetics of aging. *ILAR J.* 52:4-15.

Zhu, X.R., L. Maskri, C. Herold, V. Bader, C.C. Stichel, O. Gunturkun, and H. Lubbert. 2007. Non-motor behavioural impairments in parkin-deficient mice. *Eur J Neurosci.* 26:1902-11.

5

Bilateral Distribution of Oxytocinase Activity in the Medial Prefrontal Cortex of Spontaneously Hypertensive Rats with Experimental Hemiparkinsonism

Manuel Ramírez[1] et al. *
[1]Unit of Physiology, Department of Health Sciences, University of Jaén, Jaén, Spain

1. Introduction

Oxytocin and vasopressin are important modulators of diverse social and anxiety-related behaviors (Insel, 2010). The enzyme that regulates the function of both peptides, called oxytocinase (OX) or vasopressinase, is also involved in cognitive functions (Stragier et al., 2008; Banegas et al., 2010). Normotensive male Wistar rats exhibited a marked left predominance of OX in the medial prefrontal cortex (mPFC), an area implicated in cognitive functions and reward-related mechanisms in the rat brain and characterized by its asymmetrical organization. Brain dopamine (DA) content as well as the functions in which this neurotransmitter is involved, are asymmetrically organized in physiologic conditions (reviewed by Ramírez et al., 2004). Therefore, Parkinson's disease (PD) represents a disruption of this bilateral pattern of brain DA. Indeed, the disease normally begins unilaterally in the early stages. Animals with hemi-parkinsonism, induced by unilateral nigrostratal lesions using 6-hydroxydopamine (6-OHDA), showed several behavioral abnormalities, not only linked to a disruption of the normal bilateral distribution of brain DA, but probably also by the alteration of other factors such as the disruption of the striking basal left predominance of OX observed in both the left and right sham controls. The bilateral distribution in lesioned animals was altered differently depending on the injured hemisphere. These results may reflect changes in the levels of oxytocin and vasopressin in the mPFC and consequently in the functions in which they are involved and might account, in part, for the cognitive abnormalities observed in hemi-parkinsonism (Henderson et al., 2003). The spontaneously hypertensive rat (SHR), is a recognised model for studies of hypertension. This strain of rat also display major symptoms of the attention-deficit/hyperactivity disorder (ADHD) such as deficits in attention, impulsivity and hyperactivity when compared to Wistar-Kyoto rats (Russell, 2007). Indeed, SHR have been shown to have also disturbances in the dopaminergic system (Russell, 2007). The aim of this

*Inmaculada Banegas[1], Ana Belén Segarra[1], Rosemary Wangesteen[1], Marc de Gasparo[2], Raquel Durán[3], Francisco Vives[3], Antonio Martínez[1], Francisco Alba[3] and Isabel Prieto[1]
[2]Rue es Planches 5, 2842 Rossemaison, Switzerland.
[3]Instituto de Neurociencias 'Federico Oloriz', University of Granada, Granada, Spain.

study was to analyze OX in the left and right mPFC of SHR with left or right hemi-parkinsonism, induced by intrastriatal injections of 6-OHDA, and compared with sham controls. The results dramatically differed from those obtained in Wistar normotensive rats. SHR demonstrated a slighter basal left predominance of OX, only significant in left sham controls. The bilateral distribution in lesioned animals was differently altered depending on the injured hemisphere but in a way dissimilar to the one observed in Wistar. Thus, the hemi-parkinsonism induced in animals with cognitive and behavioral abnormalities such as ADHD induces a different brain bilateral response in OX than the one observed in Wistar. These results suggest that the cognitive consequences of hemi-parkinsonism differed between both Wistar and SHR rats. It is proposed that increased OX in mPFC is related to decreased cognitive process.

1.1 Brain asymmetry and cognitive functions

The brain asymmetry, understood as an anatomical, functional or neurochemical difference between the two hemispheres, is a dynamic phenomenon, modulated by both exogenous and endogenous factors. Increasing evidences suggest that under the anatomical and functional asymmetries underlie neurochemical brain lateralizations. However, the link between these three aspects of the brain asymmetry concept as well its own physiological meaning is not yet well understood (Ramírez et al., 2004). In addition, the impairment of cognitive functions, such as occurs during aging, is linked to vascular dementia (Vallesi et al., 2010; Xu et al., 2008). This is also related to some brain disorders, such as PD or ADHD, both characterized by disruptions in the specific physiological bilateral organization of the brain (Ramírez et al., 2004; Banegas et al., 2010; Shaw et al., 2009). Analyzing how brain bilaterality changes in specific conditions may help us to understand its meaning and its importance in physiology and pathology.

1.2 Brain asymmetry and dopamine function

Numerous studies of the DA content in the striatum in relationship with the rotation (circling behaviour) that the rats exhibited spontaneously and after drug induction (Zimmerberg et al., 1974; Glick et al., 1974; Shapiro et al., 1986) were performed to attempt to relate a neurochemical asymmetry with a lateralized function in physiologic conditions. Zimmerberg et al. (1974) demonstrated that DA levels in the striatum were significantly higher in the contralateral side to which the rats choose in a T-maze test. The concentration of DA between the two hemispheres differed by 15%. However, when high doses of amphetamine were administrated to the animals, this bilateral difference was increased up to 25% (Glick et al., 1974). For these and later studies, the model of rotational behaviour in rodents was used and revised by Shapiro et al. in 1986. The animals with 6-OHDA-induced unilateral lesions of the substantia nigra exhibited a circling behavior in response to several drugs. It was postulated that animals rotated mainly contralaterally to the side containing a higher content of DA or a higher number of activate postsynaptic DA receptors. Xu et al., (2005) compared, by quantitative autoradiography, the changes in DA receptor binding in the left and right striatum in rats after unilateral DA depletion. In comparison with control levels, DA D_1-like receptor binding in the dorsal striatum was reduced 2 weeks after unilateral lesions of the substantia nigra (SN) with 6-OHDA. Remarkably, D_1-like receptor binding was decreased in the ipsilateral striatum following unilateral lesions of either the left or right SN. Also, the left and right striatum responded similarly to unilateral SN lesions, as there were no significant differences in the percent decrease in D_1-like binding in the two striata. In contrast, D_2-like receptor binding was significantly increased in the dorsal striatum following an ipsilateral SN lesion. Furthermore, the up-regulation of D_2-like receptors in the right striatum was significantly greater than that in the left striatum after an ipsilateral lesion. The authors speculated that the asymmetrical up-regulation of striatal D_2 receptors after DA depletion may contribute to the lateralization of the nigrostriatal system observed in some pathological conditions.

1.3 Parkinson's disease, brain asymmetry and cognitive functions

Parkinson's disease is the second most common neurodegenerative disorder (Dorsey et al., 2007). Despite the intensive efforts, progresses in the fight against this disease are slow and new strategies for early diagnosis and treatment to prevent its progression are required (George et al., 2009). A deep knowledge of its pathophysiology is essential to achieve this goal. Although symmetric at the later stages, the damage observed in PD begins asymmetrically (Djaldetti et al., 2006). Therefore, there exist in PD a disruption of the physiologic bilateral distribution of DA content as well as a bilateral disturbance of other neurochemical factors (Banegas et al., 2010). Animal models of PD, such as the experimental hemiparkinsonism after unilateral intrastriatal injections of 6-OHDA, could simulate the initial phase of PD. In the early stages, PD patients exhibit cognitive and behavioral impairments unrelated to the motor symptoms, and involving frontal lobe dysfunction (Brück et al., 2004; Farina et al., 1994; Zgaljardic et al., 2006). They are the result of damage of a specific hemisphere (Cubo et al., 2010). In addition, hemiparkinsonism has been associated with asymmetrical cognitive changes (Huber et al., 1992; Piacentini et al., 2010). Studies in animals with induced hemi-parkinsonism have reported several behavioral abnormalities (Henderson et al., 2003). The mPFC, a part of the mesocorticolimbic system, is involved in cognitive functions and reward-related mechanisms in the rat brain (Tzschentke, 2000). Interestingly, the mesocortical dopamine system, particularly the mPFC, is characterized by its asymmetric organization (Sullivan, 2004).

1.4 Vascular damage, cognitive impairment and brain asymmetry

Cerebral capillary damage occurs not only in neurodegenerative disorders such as in Alzheimer's disease and PD but also in hypertension. Thus, it was hypothesized that ultrastructural abnormalities of cerebral capillaries were related to decreased cerebral blood flow that favors neurodegenerative mechanisms leading to the development of dementia (Farkas et al., 2000). Clearly, hypertension is involved in the development of vascular cognitive impairment and vascular dementia (Amenta et al., 2003). Indeed, an impairment of cognitive functions was described in elderly hypertensive individuals (Vinyoles et al., 2008) as well as in childhood (Adams et al., 2010). The SHR is a recognized animal model of cognitive decline associated with hypertension (Diana, 2002). These animals present abnormal dopaminergic transmission and altered neuronal dendrite morphology of the mPFC (Sánchez et al., 2011). Therefore, there exists a connection between hypertension, vascular dementia, cognitive impairment and a modification of the basal brain asymmetry (Xu et al., 2008; Vallesi et al., 2010; Bergerbest et al., 2009).

In the ADHD, characterized by impaired sustained attention, impulsivity and hyperactivity, a disruption of the physiological cortical asymmetry has been implicated in its pathogenesis (Shaw et al., 2009). The SHR, largely used as a model for hypertension, also display major symptoms of the ADHD (Russel, 2007) when compared with normotensive rats. Indeed,

SHR have also disturbances in the dopaminergic system. Therefore, it could be hypothesized that their brain bilateral functioning for cognitive processes may differ from the brain bilateral behaviour of normotensive rats.

1.5 Oxytocin, oxytocinase, cognitive functions and brain asymmetry

It was proposed that systems other than the dopaminergic pathway may also be involved in the behavioral abnormalities observed in PD (Lang & Obeso, 2004; Banegas et al., 2010). Oxytocin and vasopressin as well as the enzyme that regulates their functions, called oxytocinase (OX) or vasopressinase are involved in cognitive functions. Normotensive male Wistar rats exhibit a marked left predominance of OX in the mPFC, an area implicated in cognitive functions and reward-related mechanisms in the rat brain and characterized by its asymmetrical organization as already mentioned (Sullivan, 2004). Changes in this basal pattern of bilateral organization may cause disorders in brain function (Ramírez et al., 2004). Normotensive animals with hemi-parkinsonism induced by unilateral nigrostratal lesions using 6-OHDA showed several behavioral abnormalities and a disruption of the striking basal left predominance of OX as observed in both the left and right sham controls. The bilateral distribution in lesioned animals was altered differently depending on the injured hemisphere. These results may reflect changes in the levels of oxytocin and vasopressin in the mPFC and consequently, in their functions. This could account, in part, for the cognitive abnormalities observed in hemi-parkinsonism (Banegas et al., 2010).

Therefore, considering that background, it was indicated to analyze OX in the left and right mPFC of SHR with left or right hemi-parkinsonism, induced by intrastriatal injections of 6-OHDA, and compare its activity in sham SHR controls. These results will be discussed with those obtained previously in normotensive rats using the same protocol (Banegas et al., 2010). This approach should give precious indications on the behavior of brain bilaterality in two strains of rat that clearly differ in their cognitive status.

2. Materials and methods

2.1 Animals

Three-month-old male SHR (systolic blood pressure: 164.1 ± 4.2 mmHg; n=40) weighing 250 g at the beginning of the study were used for both sham and lesioned groups. During the experimental period, food and water were available *ad libitum*. The animals were housed under standard conditions of light (12 h of light from 7.00 h to 19.00 h and 12 h of dark from 19.00 h to 7.00 h) and temperature (22° C).

2.2 Surgical procedure

Degeneration of the left or right nigrostriatal dopaminergic pathway was accomplished via neurochemical lesions induced with the catecholaminergic toxin 6-OHDA (Jolicoeur and Rivest, 1992). All animals were anesthetized with 2 ml/kg body weight equithensin (42.5 g/L chloralhydrate dissolved in 19.76 mL ethanol, 9.72 g/L Nembutal®, 0.396 L/L propylenglycol and 21.3 g/L magnesium sulfate in distilled water) and placed in a stereotaxic instrument (David Kopf Instruments, Palo Alto, CA, USA). A 2 mm burr hole was drilled through the skull at horizontal coordinates approximating the position of the striatum (AP 0 mm, L or R 3 mm and H –5 mm) according to the atlas by Paxinos and Watson (1998). Infusion of 4 µL of 6-OHDA (8 mg dissolved in 1 mL of cold saline with 0.02% ascorbic acid to inhibit oxidation) was administered into the left or right striatum

(Jolicoeur & Rivest, 1992). The control rats were operated the same manner but they received 4 μl of saline with 0.02% ascorbic acid.

2.3 Motor behaviour in experimental hemiparkinsonism

Normal rats exhibit a spontaneous turning behaviour, the levels of DA being higher in the contralateral striatum than the side of the turning preference (Glick, 1983). Therefore, animals with experimental hemiparkinsonism turn ipsilaterally to the side of lesion. This turning behavior was amplified after amphetamine administration that increases dopamine in the synaptic cleft. Assessment of the ipsilateral rotational behavior allowed us to verify the efficacy of the 6-OHDA-induced lesions. Four weeks post-surgery and three days before sacrifice, animals were given D-amphetamine sulfate (5 mg/kg s.c.) to enhance the turning behaviour (Robinson et al., 1994) while placed in a 30 cm diameter bowl. Number of turns was determined in 6 periods of 10 min. during 1 h. Sufficiently rotating animals were included in lesion group. Sham-lesioned rats underwent the same surgery and rotational testing but did not demonstrate sufficient rotational behaviour to qualify as parkinsonian models. Most animals exceeded the 100 % of turns from mean of control and were considered with hemiparkinson. Lesioned animals that did not presented turning behaviour but exhibited rigidity after D-amphetamine injection also were considered with hemiparkinson. Compared with sham controls, a marked ipsilateral rotational behavior was observed in left- and right-lesioned animals (Banegas et al., 2009) (figure 1).

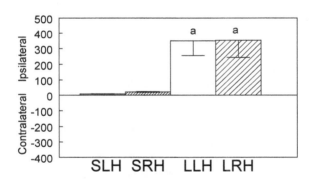

Fig. 1. Turning behaviour in the groups studied.

Turning behaviour in lesioned left (LL) or lesioned right (LR) and sham left (SL) or sham right (SR) spontaneously hypertensive rats (H). Number of turns were determined individually in 6 periods of 10 min during 1 h. Values represent mean ± SEM (n=10) of the cumulative turns recorded in the 6 periods (modified from Banegas et al., 2009 with permission). a Differences between the same side of lesioned vs sham animals. a p<0.001

2.4 Collection and treatment of tissue samples

The surgical procedure, sacrifice and sample collection were performed under anesthesia between 9.00 h and 11.00 h. Four weeks after receiving the injections, the animals were sacrificed and mPFC samples were obtained from each group as previously described (Banegas et al, 2005a). Briefly, the animals were perfused with saline transcardially under equithensin anaesthesia (2 ml/kg body weight). The brain was quickly removed (less than

60 s) and cooled in dry ice. Left and right brain samples were dissected according to the stereotaxic atlas of Paxinos & Watson (1998). The selected area of mPFC was between 12,70 mm and 11,70 mm anterior to the interaural line. All samples were collected the same day and frozen for assays. Tissue samples were homogenized in 400 µl of 10 mM HCl-Tris buffer (pH 7,4) and ultracentrifugated at 100,000 x g for 30 min. at 4 °C. The pellets were re-homogenized in HCl-Tris buffer (pH 7,4) plus 1% Triton-X-100 to solubilize membrane proteins. After centrifugation (100,000 x g, 30 min., 4 °C the supernatants were shaked in an orbital rotor during 2 h. at 4 °C with the polymeric adsorbent Bio-Beads SM-2 (100 mg/ml) in order to remove the detergent from the sample (Alba et al., 1995). The bio-beads were removed and the supernatants were used to measure in triplicate membrane-bound aminopeptidase activities and protein content. Left or right 6-OHDA-lesioned animals were compared with their corresponding left or right sham-operated animals in which the DA pathways were intact. Because bilateral injuries usually lead to the death of rats due to the occurrence of marked aphagia and adipsia (Ungerstedt, 1971), such control animals were not available.

2.5 Procedures for enzymatic assays
Membrane-bound oxytocinase activity was measured fluorometrically using L-Cys-β-naphthylamide as previously described (Banegas et al., 2005a). Proteins were quantified in triplicate by the method of Bradford (1976) using BSA as a standard. Specific OX was expressed as nanomoles of L-Cys-β-naphthylamide hydrolyzed per minute per milligram of protein. Fluorogenic assays were linear with respect to the time of hydrolysis and protein content.

2.6 Experimental groups
Oxytocinase activity levels were measured in mPFC of the following groups ($n = 10$ for all groups):
a.   Simulated lesion of the left hemisphere with saline (sham left, SL)
b.   Simulated lesion of the right hemisphere with saline (sham right, SR)
c.   Lesion of left hemisphere with 6-OHDA (lesion left, LL)
d.   Lesion of right hemisphere with 6-OHDA (lesion right, LR)
All experimental procedures involving animals, including their use and care, were in accordance with the European Communities Council Directive 86/609/EEC.

2.7 Statistical analysis
We used a one-way analysis of variance (ANOVA) to analyze differences between groups. Post-hoc comparisons were made using the paired Student's t test; p-values below 0.05 were considered significant.

3. Results

Results of the present research are represented in figures 2 and 3. There was an asymmetry of OX in the mPFC of left controls (SL) showing a significant left predominance (41% higher; p<0.01). The right controls (SR) showed a tendency for left predominance (15% higher) without reaching statistical significance. After left lesion (LL), there was an increased left

Bilateral Distribution of Oxytocinase Activity in the Medial Prefrontal Cortex of Spontaneously Hypertensive Rats with Experimental Hemiparkinsonism

95

predominance (75% higher; p<0.001), whereas the OX predominance shifted slightly to the right hemisphere in right lesioned animals (LR) (19% higher; p<0.05) (fig. 2).

Compared with the same side of sham animals, the LL produced a significant increase in OX in the left mPFC (48% higher; p<0.01) and no modification in the right side. The LR decreased OX in the left mPFC (32% lower; p<0.01) but did not modify OX activity in the right side compared to the control.

The percentage differences ([(high/low)-1] x 100) between the left and right values of OX in mPFC for each animal in the four groups are shown in figure 3. In SL and SR, although with low level of percentage, most animals were left predominant. The differences ranged from 11% to 113% higher OX activity in the left mPFC of eight SL animals (p<0.01) and from 4% to 56% in seven SR animals (without significant differences between mean values). In LL animals, the level of percentage for left OX predominance increased slightly, ranging from 18% to 185% (higher) in eight animals (p<0.001). The SHR from the LR group shifted slightly to the right predominance (p<0.05) with seven animals right predominance ranging from 3% to 77%.

The present results are indicative of an influence of DA depletion on the bilateral levels of OX in the mPFC of hypertensive rats, and dramatically differ from the data observed in normotensive Wistar rats (Banegas et al, 2010). These effects are conditioned by the side in which 6-OHDA or saline was administered.

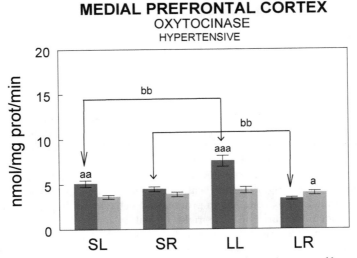

Fig. 2. Oxytocinase activity in the left and right medial prefrontal cortex of hypertensive rats.

Oxytocinase activity in the left (blue bars) and right (rose bars) medial prefrontal cortex of left (SL) or right (SR) sham-operated and left (LL) or right (LR) 6-OHDA lesioned hypertensive rats. (n=10 in each group). Values represent mean ± SEM of specific oxytocinase activity expressed as nanomoles of Cys-β-naphthylamide hydrolyzed per minute per milligram of protein. (a) Differences between left and right sides. (b) Differences in the same side between sham and lesioned animals. Single letter: p<0.05; double letter: p<0.01; triple letter: p<0.001.

Medial Prefrontal Cortex

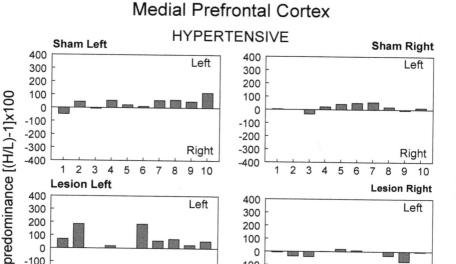

Fig. 3. Percentage differences between the left and right prefrontal cortex of hypertensive rats

Bars represent the percentage differences between the levels of oxytocinase activity of the left and right sides of the prefrontal cortex for each of the hypertensive rats studied in all four groups. H, higher value; L, lower value.

4. Discussion

It has been demonstrated that the PFC plays a critical role in the development of ADHD and that the mesocortical DA system is involved in that process. In addition, previous studies demonstrated that the laterality of the prefrontal function in the rat is also involved in ADHD, particularly the dysregulation of the right PFC having a deficit of its dopaminergic system (Sullivan & Brake, 2003). Indeed, the mPFC DA system exhibits many functional hemispheric asymmetries involving the right mesocortical DA system. Thus, 6-OHDA lesions of the right but not the left frontal cortex conducts to pronounced behavioural hyperactivity and altered subcortical catecholamine function. The right frontal systems play a key role in motor inhibition and the mesocortical DA seems to be an important part of this regulation. It is therefore expected that its impairment may led to hyperactivity behaviour. ADHD children have mainly impaired ability to keep their attention focus due to dysfunctions in the right hemisphere attention systems (Reviewed by Sullivan & Brake, 2003).

Therefore, it is interesting to compare the bilateral behavior of the mPFC after the specific lesion of the right or the left nigrostriatal dopaminergic system in normotensive rats and in an animal model of ADHD: the SHR strain. This could provide valuable information on the bilateral behaviour of the frontostriatal dopaminergic system whose operation is critical for understanding the pathogenesis of disorders such as PD or ADHD.

Bilateral Distribution of Oxytocinase Activity in the Medial Prefrontal Cortex of Spontaneously Hypertensive Rats with
Experimental Hemiparkinsonism

97

The present results obtained in SHR differed substantially from those previously obtained in normotensive rats (Banegas et al, 2010). Most importantly, there is a remarkable lower level of left predominance in sham hypertensive controls (figures 2 and 3), compared with the high one observed in sham normotensive controls (figures 4 and 5). This is in agreement with the reduction of the asymmetry observed in prefrontal cortex and hippocampus in ADHD (Shaw et al., 2009) and during aging and vascular dementia compared to healthy subjects (Xu et al., 2008; Vallesi et al., 2010; Bergerbest et al., 2009). Indeed, disruption of physiological asymmetry has been involved in the pathogenesis of cognitive disorders such as ADHD. An increase in the thickness of the right frontal cortex together with a left-hemispheric increase in the occipital cortical regions characterize the normal bilateral development of children. However, in ADHD, while the posterior component of this bilateral development was intact, the prefrontal one was lost (Shaw et al., 2009). The morphological asymmetry of hippocampus in healthy subjects, assessed by magnetic resonance imaging, is greater than that in Alzheimer's disease and in patients with vascular dementia (Xu et al., 2008). Studying the effects of age on the asymmetry of the motor system, Vallesi et al. (2010) reported that older adults showed a more symmetric pattern than younger subjects. Moreover, an age-associated reduction of asymmetry in prefrontal function has been related to several forms of cognitive impairment (Bergerbest et al., 2009).

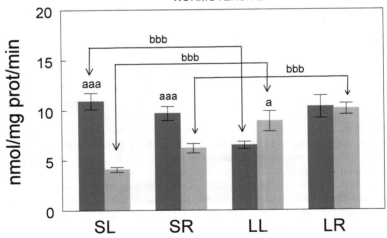

Fig. 4. Oxytocinase activity in the left and right medial prefrontal cortex of normotensive rats

Oxytocinase activity in the left (gray bars) and right (open bars) medial prefrontal cortex of left (SL) or right (SR) sham-operated and left (LL) or right (LR) 6-OHDA lesioned normotensive rats. (n=10 in each group). Values represent mean±SEM of specific oxytocinase activity expressed as nanomoles of Cys-β-naphthylamide hydrolyzed per minute per milligram of protein. (a) Differences between left and right sides. (b) Differences in the same side between sham and lesioned animals. Single letter: p<0.05; triple letter: p<0.001 (from Banegas et al, 2010 with permission).

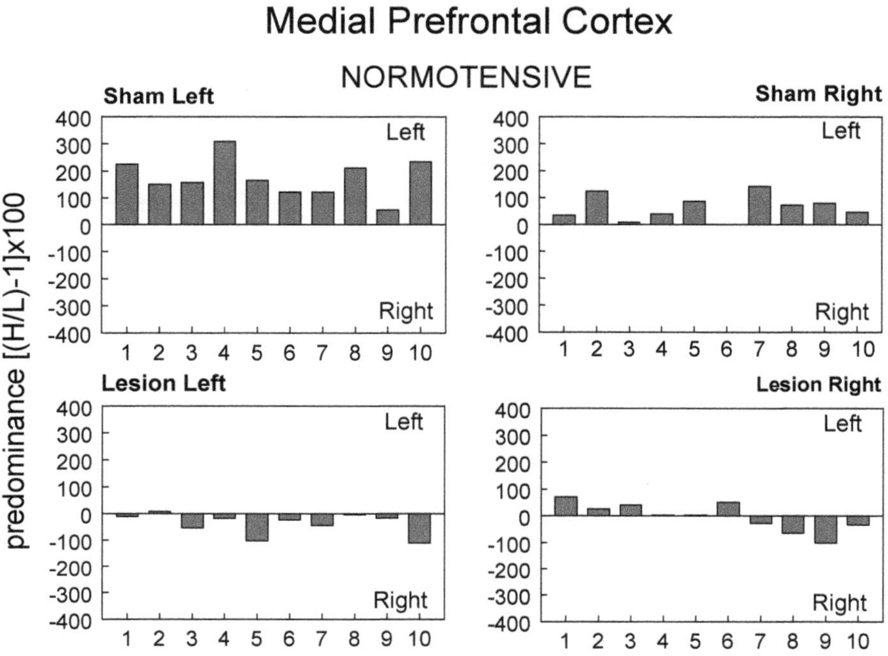

Medial Prefrontal Cortex

Fig. 5. Percentage differences between the left and right prefrontal cortex of normotensive rats.

Bars represent the percentage differences between the levels of oxytocinase activity of the left and right sides of the prefrontal cortex for each of the normotensive rats studied in all four groups. H, higher value; L, lower value.

Especially informative is the comparison of figures 3 and 5 in which we can notice the great difference in the bilateral response of normotensive and SHR. While in SL and SR normotensive rats virtually all the animals were left predominant with a high percentage of difference (figure 5), in SL and SR hypertensive the left predominance is substantially lower (figure 3). Whereas in LL normotensive animals, OX predominance was shifted to the right in nine animals (figure 5), in LL hypertensive rats the left predominance was increased (figure 3). The bilateral response of animals from the LR group of normotensive and hypertensive was quite similar.

The slight difference observed in the bilateral distribution of OX between SL and SR of hypertensive rats could be due to a differential response of the local inflammatory processes following the introduction of the cannula into the left or right hemisphere, as previously suggested by Banegas et al. (2009) in normotensive rats.

The direct effect of lesions in hypertensive animals on OX also differed from the previous observation in normotensive rats. OX decreased in the left side and increased in the right hemisphere of normotensive LL (figure 4). In contrast, in hypertensive LL rats, the enzyme activity increased in the left hemisphere and was not modified in the right one (figure 2).

Clearly, the response to left or right lesions in normotensive rats involved both left and right hemispheres. On the contrary, in hypertensive rats, it only implies changes in the left hemisphere. It is particularly noticeable that the right mPFC was not modified either when left or right lesions were performed, in marked contrast with the important changes that

Bilateral Distribution of Oxytocinase Activity in the Medial Prefrontal Cortex of Spontaneously Hypertensive Rats with Experimental Hemiparkinsonism

99

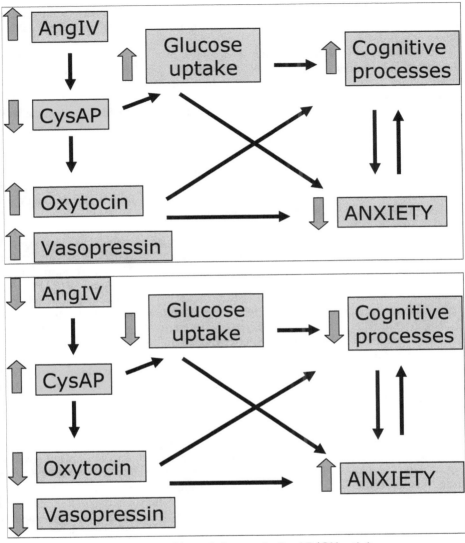

Fig. 6. Hypothetic consequences of frontal changes in CysAP/OX activity

Hypothetic consequences of a reduction (top) or increase (bottom) in the frontal levels of CysAP/OX. Decreased CysAP would imply higher availability of Ang IV as well as lower metabolism/higher availability of its substrates oxytocin and vasopressin. Higher levels of Ang IV could indicate an improvement of cognitive processes (Gard, 2008). The reduction of CysAP may also suggest increased glucose uptake which would also improve cognitive processes (Wenk, 1989). In addition, increased availability of oxytocin or vasopressin would agree with the facilitation of cognitive processes (Gulpinar and Yegen, 2004) as well as a higher anxyolitic effect (Neumann, 2009). Finally, this would support an inverse relationship between cognitive processes and anxiety level (Ouimet et al., 2009). We could suggest contrary effects for an increased frontal level of CysAP.

occurred in normotensive rats (Banegas et al., 2010). This observation may be linked to the reduced volume of right PFC and reduced metabolism in the mPFC in humans with ADHD (Viggiano et al., 2004).

While ADHD have a reduction of left/right asymmetry, as observed in SL and SR, LL return the asymmetrical difference to a degree similar to that observed in normotensive rats. Accordingly, we could hypothesize that LL but not LR balanced the asymmetrical misbalance of SHR/ADHD.

Angiotensin IV (Ang IV) binds specifically to the AT_4 receptor, which is identical to the insulin-regulated aminopeptidase (IRAP) (Albiston et al., 2001). Cystein aminopeptidase (CysAP), also called oxytocinase (OX) or vasopressinase (EC 3.4.11.3), is considered the human variant of IRAP (Stragier et al., 2008). In addition, CysAP was also reported to be identical to the placental leucine aminopeptidase (Tsujimoto et al., 1992). These enzymes can therefore be considered identical and they are located in virtually all regions of the brain, including the cortex (Fernando et al., 2005). In addition, it has been reported that Ang IV increased DA levels in striatum, this effect being mediated by OX/IRAP acting as receptor for Ang IV (Stragier et al., 2007).

Ang IV is thought to play a role in cognitive and behavioral functions. However, the mechanism by which it modulates these functions is not fully understood and several compatible hypothesis have been proposed (Stragier et al., 2008). For example, it was proposed that the binding of Ang IV to its receptor, AT_4 (oxytocinase/CysAP/IRAP), results in the inhibition of the receptor's metabolic activity, reducing the catabolism of its substrates and consequently increasing their availability and extending their action (Stragier et al., 2008). Ang IV could therefore regulate glucose uptake modulating OX activity: OX/IRAP is indeed co-localized with the glucose transporter GLUT4. In the presence of insulin, OX and GLUT4 are expressed in the plasma membrane, where GLUT4 induces glucose uptake. It was suggested that the inhibition of OX, following binding of AngIV, could increase glucose uptake in neurons leading to an improvement of cognitive processes (Gard, 2008; Stragier et al., 2008) (figure 6).

In addition to oxytocin, CysAP/OX hydrolyzes vasopressin, enkephalins and other neuropeptides also involved in cognitive processes (Gard, 2008). Indeed, oxytocin and vasopressin are important modulators of diverse social and anxiety-related behaviors (Veenema & Neumann, 2008). Therefore, a decrease in CysAP/OX activity implies high levels of Ang IV, as well as a lower metabolism and thus a higher availability of its substrates such as oxytocin or vasopressin. Both effects may facilitate cognitive processes (Gard, 2008; Gülpinar & Yegen, 2004) and reduce anxiety levels (Veenema & Neumann, 2008). The contrary is occurring in case of an increase in CysAP/OX. Indeed, the development of cognitive enhancers based on the inhibition of OX has been proposed (Chai et al., 2008) (figure 6).

5. Conclusion

The present results demonstrated that the bilateral behavior of OX in the mPFC differs between normotensive and hypertensive rats and highlights the importance of bilaterality in biology. The functional meaning of bilaterality as well as how its disruption may lead to pathological consequences are unknown. However, we can speculate that brain functions, processed with varying degrees of asymmetry for the two hemispheres, could be under an universal *modus operandi* which would consist in the reciprocal inhibition of homologous centers. The regulationof a large number of brain processes is based on a retro-inhibitor-stimulator *feed-back* system. This could explain the existence of neurochemical imbalances that arise, change their side of prevalence or increase their degree of asymmetry in specific conditions. It could be speculated that imbalances in established brain asymmetries (toward symmetry or toward increasing asymmetry) due to unilateral damage, might lead to neuropathological deviations in brain functions (Ramirez et al., 2004; Banegas-Font et al., 2005b) In any case, these results confirm that studies which are not considering the bilaterality may lead to loss of invaluable informations leading to erroneous conclusions and misinterpretations of the pathophysiological processes.

6. References

Adams, H.R., Szilagyi, P.G., Gebhardt, L. & Lande, M.B. (2010), Learning and attention problems among children with pediatric primary hypertension. *Pediatrics*, Vol. 126, No. 6, (December 2010), pp. 1425-1429. ISSN 0031-4005

Alba, F., Arenas, J.C. & López, M.A. (1995). Properties of rat brain dipeptidyl aminopeptidases in the presence of detergents. *Peptides*, Vol. 16, No. 2, pp. 325-329, ISSN 0196-9781

Albiston, A.L., Mcdowall, S.G., Matsacos, D., Sim, P., Clune, E., Mustafa, T., Lee, J., Mendelsohn, F.A., Simpson, R.J., Connolly, L.M. & Chai, S.Y. (2001), Evidence that the angiotensin IV (AT4) receptor is the enzyme insulin-regulated aminopeptidase. *Journal of Biological Chemistry*, Vol. 276, No. 52, (December 2001), pp. 48623-48626, ISSN 0021-9258

Amenta, F., Di Tullio, M.A. & Tomassoni, D. (2003) Arterial hypertension and brain damage - evidence from animal models. *Clinical and Experimental Hypertension*, Vol. 25, No. 6, (August 2003) pp. 359-380, ISSN 1064-1963

Banegas, I., Prieto, I., Alba, F., Vives, F., Araque, A., Segarra, A.B., Durán, R., de Gasparo, M. & Ramírez, M. (2005a). Angiotensinase activity is asymmetrically distributed in the amygdala, hippocampus and prefrontal cortex of the rat. *Behavioural Brain Research* Vol. 156, No. 2, (January 2005) pp. 321-326, ISSN 0166-4328

Banegas Font I, Prieto Gómez I, Araque Cuenca A, Alba Aragüez F, Vives Montero F, Segarra Robles AB, Durán Ogalla R, Ramírez Sánchez MD & Ramírez Sánchez M. (2005b). [Neurochemical asymmetries in psychiatric alterations] Spanish. *Psiquiatría Biológica*, Vol.12, No.4, (July 2005) pp. 159-165, ISSN 1134-5934

Banegas, I., Prieto, I., Vives, F., Alba, F., de Gasparo, M., Duran, R., Luna, J de D., Segarra, A.B., Hermoso, F. & Ramírez, M. (2009). Asymmetrical response of aminopeptidase A and nitric oxide in plasma of normotensive and hypertensive rats with experimental hemiparkinsonism. *Neuropharmacology*, Vol.56, No3, (Mars 2009), pp. 573-579, ISSN 0028-3908

Banegas, I., Prieto, I., Vives, F., Alba, F., de Gasparo, M., Duran, R., Segarra, A.B. & Ramírez, M. (2010). Lateralized response of oxytocinase activity in the medial prefrontal cortex of a unilateral rat model of Parkinson's disease. *Behavioural Brain Research*, Vol.213, No.2, (December 2010), pp. 328-331, ISSN 0166-4328

Bergerbest, D., Gabrieli, J.D., Whitfield-Gabrieli, S., Kim, H., Stebbins, G.T., Bennett, D.A. & Fleischman D.A. (2009). Age-associated reduction of asymmetry in prefrontal function and preservation of conceptual repetition priming. *Neuroimage*. Vol.45, No.1, (Mars 2009) pp.237-246, ISSN 1053-8119

Bradford, M.M. (1976). A rapid and sensitive method for the quantification of microgram quantities of protein utilizing the principle of protein dye binding. *Analytical Biochemistry* Vol.72, (May 1976) pp.248-254, ISSN 0003-2697

Brück, A., Kurki, T., Kaasinen, V., Vahlberg, T. & Rinne, J.O. (2004). Hippocampal and prefrontal atrophy in patients with early non-demented Parkinson's disease is related to cognitive impairment. *Journal of Neurology, Neurosurgery & Psychiatry*, Vol.75, No.10, (October 2004), pp.1467-1469. ISSN 0022-3050

Chai SY, Yeatman HR, Parker MW, Ascher DB, Thompson PE, Mulvey HT. & Albiston, A.L. (2008), Development of cognitive enhancers based on inhibition of insulin-regulated aminopeptidase. *BMC Neuroscience*, Vol. 9, Suppl. 2, (December 2008), pp. S14, ISSN 1471-2202

Cubo, E., Martin, P.M., Martin-Gonzalez, J.A., Rodriguez-Blazquez, C. & Kulisevsky, J. ELEP Group Members. (2010). Motor laterality asymmetry and nonmotor symptoms in Parkinson's disease. *Movement Disorders*, Vol.25, No.1, (January 2010), pp.70-75. ISSN 0885-3185

Diana, G. (2002). Does hypertension alone lead to cognitive decline in spontaneously hypertensive rats? *Behavioural Brain Research*, Vol.134, No.1-2, (August 2002), pp. 113-121. ISSN 0166-4328

Djaldetti, R., Ziv, I. & Melamed, E. (2006). The mystery of motor asymmetry in Parkinson's disease. *Lancet Neurology*, Vol. 5, No.9, (September 2006), pp.796-802. ISSN 1474-4422

Dorsey, E.R., Constantinescu, R., Thompson, J.P., Biglan, K.M., Holloway, R.G., Kieburtz, K., Marshall, F.J., Ravina, B.M., Schifitto, G., Siderowf, A. & Tanner, C.M. (2007). Projected number of people with Parkinson disease in the most populous nations, 2005 through 2030. *Neurology*, Vol.68, No.5, (January 2007), pp.384-386, ISSN 0028-3878

Farina, E., Cappa, S.F., Polimeni, M., Magni, E., Canesi, M., Zecchinelli, A., Scarlato, G. & Mariani, C. (1994). Frontal dysfunction in early Parkinson's disease, *Acta Neurologica Scandinavica*, Vol.90, No.1, (July 1994) pp. 34-38. ISSN 0365-5598

Farkas, E., De Jong, G.I., Apró, E., De Vos, R.A., Steur, E.N. & Luiten, P.G. (2000). Similar ultrastructural breakdown of cerebrocortical capillaries in Alzheimer's disease, Parkinson's disease, and experimental hypertension. What is the functional link? *Annals of the New York Academy of Sciences*. Vol.903, (April 2000) pp.72-82. ISSN 0077-8923

Fernando, R.N., Lara, J., Albiston, A.L. & Chai, S.Y. (2005). Distribution and cellular localization of insulin-regulated aminopeptidase in the rat central nervous system. *Journal of Comparative Neurology*, Vol.487, No.4, (July 2005), pp. 372–90. ISSN 0021-9967

Gard, P.R. (2008). Cognitive-enhancing effects of angiotensin IV. *BMC Neuroscience*, Vol.9, Suppl.2, (December 2008) pp. S15. ISSN 1471-2202

George, J.L., Mok, S., Moses, D., Wilkins, S., Bush, A.I., Cherny, R.A. & Finkelstein, D.I. (2009). Targeting the progression of Parkinson's disease. *Current Neuropharmacology*, Vol.7, No.1, (Mars 2009) pp.9-36. ISSN 1570-159X

Glick, S.D., Jerussi, T.P., Water, D.H. & Green JP. (1974), Amphetamine-induced changes in striatal dopamine and acetylcholine levels and relationship to rotation (circling behavior) in rats. *Biochemical Pharmacology*. Vol.23, No.22, (November 1974), pp. 3223-3225, ISSN 0006-2952.

Glick, S.D. (1983). Cerebral lateralization in the rat and tentative extrapolations to man. In: *Hemisyndromes: Psychobiology, Neurology, Psychiatry*. M. Myslobodsky (Ed.) pp. 7-26., ISBN 0125124600, Academic Press, London.

Gülpinar, M.A. & Yegen, B.C. (2004). The physiology of learning and memory: role of peptides and stress. *Current Protein and Peptide Science* Vol.5, No.6, (December 2004), pp. 457-473, ISSN 1098-5522

Henderson, J.M., Watson, S., Halliday, G.M., Heinemann, T. & Gerlach, M. (2003). Relationships between various behavioural abnormalities and nigrostriatal

Bilateral Distribution of Oxytocinase Activity in the Medial Prefrontal Cortex of Spontaneously Hypertensive Rats with
Experimental Hemiparkinsonism

103

dopamine depletion in the unilateral 6-OHDA-lesioned rat. *Behavioural Brain Research*, Vol.139, No.1-2, (February 2003) pp. 105-113. ISSN 0166-4328

Huber, S.J., Miller, H., Bohaska, L., Christy, J.A. & Bornstein, R.A. (1992). Asymmetrical cognitive differences associated with hemiparkinsonism. *Archives of Clinical Neuropsychology*, Vol.7, No.6, (November 1992), pp. 471-80. ISSN 0887-6177

Insel, T.R. (2010). The challenge of translation in social neuroscience: a review of oxytocin, vasopressin, and affiliative behavior. *Neuron*, Vol.65 No.6 (Mars 2010), pp.768-779, ISSN 0896-6273.

Jolicoeur, F.B. & Rivest, R. (1992). Rodent model of Parkinson's disease, In: *Neuromethods 21, Animal Models of Neurological Disease I*, A.A. Boulto, G.B. Bakerand a R.F. Butterworth (Eds.). 135-158, Humana Press, ISBN 0-89603-198-5, Totowa, New Jersey

Lang, A.E. & Obeso, J.A. (2004), Challenges in Parkinson's disease: restoration of the nigrostriatal dopamine system is not enough. *Lancet Neurology*, Vol.3, No.5, (May 2004), pp. 309-16, ISSN 1474-4422

Neumann, I.D. (2009). The advantage of social living: brain neuropeptides mediate the beneficial consequences of sex and motherhood. *Frontiers in Neuroendocrinology*, Vol. 30, No.4, (October 2009), pp. 483-496, ISSN 0091-3022

Ouimet, A.J., Gawronski, B. & Dozois, D.J. (2009). Cognitive vulnerability to anxiety: A review and an integrative model. *Clinical Psychology Review*, Vol.29, No.6, (August 2009), pp. 459-470, ISSN 0272-7358

Paxinos, G. & Watson C. (1998). *The rat brain in stereotaxic coordinates*, Academic Press, 4th Ed. ISBN 13: 9780123742438, London, England.

Piacentini, S., Versaci, R., Romito, L., Ferré, F. & Albanese A. (2010) Behavioral and personality features in patients with lateralized Parkinson's disease. *European Journal of Neurology*. (December 2010) [Epub ahead of print], ISSN 1468-1331

Ramírez, M., Prieto, I., Vives, F., de Gasparo, M. & Alba, F. (2004). Neuropeptides, neuropeptidases and brain asymmetry. *Current Protein and Peptide Science*, Vol.5, No.6, (December 2004), pp. 497-506. ISSN 1098-5522

Robinson, T.E., Noordhoorn, M., Chan, E.M., Mocsary, Z., Camp, D.M, & Whishaw, I.Q. (1994). Relationship between asymmetries in striatal dopamine release and the direction of amphetamine-induced rotation during the first week following a unilateral 6-OHDA lesion of the substantia nigra. *Synapse*, (May 1994)Vol. 17, No.1, pp. 16-25, ISSN 0887-4476

Russell, V.A. (2007). Reprint of "Neurobiology of animal models of attention-deficit hyperactivity disorder". *Journal of Neuroscience Methods*, (November 2007), Vol.166, No.2, pp. I-XIV, ISSN 1872-678X

Sánchez, F., Gómez-Villalobos, M. de J., Juarez, I., Quevedo, L. & Flores, G. (2011). Dendritic morphology of neurons in medial prefrontal cortex, hippocampus, and nucleus accumbens in adult SH rats. *Synapse*. (Mars 2011) Vol.65, No.3, (Mars 2011), pp. 198-206. ISSN 0887-4476

Shapiro, R.M., Glick, S.D. & Hough, L.B. (1986). Striatal dopamine uptake asymmetries and rotational behavior in unlesioned rats: revising the model? *Psychopharmacology (Berl)*, Vol.89, No.1, pp.25-30, *ISSN*: 0033-3158.

Shaw, P., Lalonde, F., Lepage, C., Rabin, C., Eckstrand, K., Sharp, W., Greenstein, D., Evans, A., Giedd, J.N. & Rapoport, J. (2009). Development of cortical asymmetry in typically developing children and its disruption in attention-deficit/hyperactivity disorder. *Archives of General Psychiatry*, Vol.66, No.8, (August 2009), pp.888-896, ISSN 0003-990x

Stragier, B., Demaegdt, H., De Burdel, D., Smolders, I., Sarre, S., Vauquelin, G., Ebinger, G., Micote, Y. & Vanderheyden, P. (2007), Involvement of insulin-regulated aminopeptidase and/or aminopeptidase N in the angiotensin IV-induced effect on dopamine release in the striatum of the rat. *Brain Research*, Vol. 1131 No.1 (February 2007) pp. 97-105. ISSN 00068993.

Stragier, B., De Bundel, D., Sarre, S., Smolders, I., Vauquelin, G., Dupont, A., Michotte, Y. & Vanderheyden, P. (2008). Involvement of insulin-regulated aminopeptidase in the effects of the renin-angiotensin fragment angiotensin IV: a review. *Heart Failure Reviews*, Vol.13, No.3, (September 2008), pp. 321-37. ISSN 1382-4147

Sullivan, R.M. & Brake, W.G. (2003). What the rodent prefrontal cortex can teach us about attention-deficit/hyperactivity disorder: the critical role of early developmental events on prefrontal function. *Behavioural Brain Research*, Vol.146, No.1-2, (November 2003) pp. 43-55, ISSN 0166-4328

Sullivan, R.M. (2004). Hemispheric asymmetry in stress processing in rat prefrontal cortex and the role of mesocortical dopamine. *Stress*, Vol.7, No.2, (June 2004), pp. 131-143. ISSN 1025-3890

Tsujimoto, M., Mizutani, S., Adachi, H., Kimura, M., Nakazato, H. & Tomoda, Y. (1992). Identification of human placental leucine aminopeptidase as oxytocinase. *Archives of Biochemistry and Biophysics*, Vol.292, No.2, (February 1992), pp. 388–392. ISSN 0003-9861

Tzschentke, T.M. (2000). The medial prefrontal cortex as a part of the brain reward system. *Amino Acids*, Vol.19, No.1, pp. 211-219, ISSN 0939-4451

Ungerstedt, U. (1971). Adipsia and aphagia after 6-hydroxydopamine induced degeneration of the nigro-striatal dopamine system. *Acta Physiologica Scandinavica* Vol.367, pp. 95–122, ISSN 0001-6772

Vallesi, A., McIntosh, A.R., Kovacevic, N., Chan, S.C. & Stuss, D.T. (2010). Age effects on the asymmetry of the motor system: evidence from cortical oscillatory activity. *Biological Psychology*, (October 2010) Vol.85, No.2, pp.213-218. ISSN 0301-0511

Veenema, A.H. & Neumann, I.D. (2008). Central vasopressin and oxytocin release: regulation of complex social behaviours. *Progress in Brain Research* Vol.170 pp. 261-276. ISSN 0079-6123

Viggiano, D., Ruocco, L.A., Arcieri, S. & Sadile, A.G. (2004). Involvement of norepinephrine in the control of activity and attentive processes in animal models of attention deficit hyperactivity disorder. *Neural Plasticity*. Vol.11, No.1-2, pp.133-149. ISSN 1687-5443

Vinyoles, E., De la Figuera. M. & Gonzalez-Segura, D. (2008). Cognitive function and blood pressure control in hypertensive patients over 60 years of age: COGNIPRES study. *Current Medical Research and Opinion*. Vol.24, No.12, (December 2008), pp.3331-3339, ISSN 0300-7995

Wenk, G.L. (1989) An hypothesis on the role of glucose in the mechanism of action of cognitive enhancers. *Psychopharmacology* Vol.99, No,4, pp. 431-438. ISSN 0033-3158

Xu, Z.C., Ling, G., Sahr, R.N. & Neal-Beliveau BS. (2005). Asymmetrical changes of dopamine receptors in the striatum after unilateral dopamine depletion. *Brain Research*, (Mars 2005), Vol.1038, No.2, pp.163-70, ISSN: 0006-8993

Xu, Y., Valentino, D.J., Scher, A.I., Dinov, I., White, L.R., Thompson, P.M., Launer, L.J. & Toga, A.W. (2008). Age effects on hippocampal structural changes in old men: the HAAS. *Neuroimage*, Vol.40, No.3, (April 2008) pp. 1003-1015. ISSN 1053-8119

Zgaljardic, D.J., Borod, J.C., Foldi, N.S., Mattis, P.J., Gordon, M.F., Feigin, A. & Eidelberg, D. (2006). An examination of executive dysfunction associated with frontostriatal circuitry in Parkinson's disease. *Journal of Clinical and Experimental Neuropsychology* Vol.28, No.7, (October 2006), pp. 1127-1144. ISSN 1380-3395

Zimmerberg, B., Glick, S.D. & Jerussi, T.P. (1974) Neurochemical correlate of a spatial preference in rats. *Science*. Vol.185, No.151, (August 1974), pp. 623-5, ISSN 0036-8075.

6

Dictyostelium discoideum: A Model System to Study LRRK2-Mediated Parkinson Disease

Arjan Kortholt, Bernd Gilsbach, and Peter J.M. van Haastert
Department of Molecular Cell Biology, University of Groningen
The Netherlands

1. Introduction

Parkinson disease (PD) is a neurodegenerative disease that affects more than 5 million people worldwide and one in hundred people over the age of 60. PD is both a chronic and degenerative disorder that is characterized by loss of dopaminergic neurons in the substantia nigra, associated with the formation of fibrillar aggregates composed of α-synuclein and other proteins (Lees et al., 2009). PD is clinically characterized by tremor, bradykinesia, rigidity and postural instability. Initially PD was considered to have no genetic cause, however many patients have one or more family member with the disease and genome-wide association studies identified a number of genetic factors segregating with PD (Satake et al., 2009; Simon-Sanchez et al., 2009). Therefore, it is now general believed that PD is caused by a combination of genetic and environmental factors. Recently, missense mutations in LRRK2 have been linked to autosomal-dominant, late-onset PD (Zimprich et al., 2004;Paisan-Ruiz et al., 2004). LRRK2 is a member of the novel Roco family of complex Ras-like GTPases that have an unique domain architecture (Fig. 1) (Bosgraaf and van Haastert, 2003). Roco proteins are characterized by the presence of a Ras-like Guanine nucleotide binding domain, called Roc (Ras of complex proteins), followed by a conserved stretch of 300-400 amino-acids with no significant homology to other described protein domains called the COR domain (C-terminal of Roc; Fig. 1). The Roc and COR domains always occurs as a pair, and so far no proteins have been identified containing either the Roc or COR domain alone, suggesting that these two domains function as one inseparable unit. Roco proteins were first identified in the social amoeba *Dictyostelium discoideum* and are found in prokaryotes, plants and metazoa, but not in *Plasmodium* and yeast (Bosgraaf et al., 2003). Besides a Roc and COR domain, all Roco proteins contain an N-terminal stretch of leucine-rich repeats (LRR), which are supposed to be involved in protein-protein interaction. A large group of Roco proteins, which is only present in *Dictyostelium* and metazoan, contains an additional C-terminal kinase domain of the MAPKKK subfamily of kinases. Next to this general domain composition, individual Roco proteins are found to be combined with a diversity of additional domains such as Guanine nucleotide exchange factor (GEF) and Regulator of G-protein Signalling (RGS) domains, implicating a link between traditional G-protein signalling pathways and Roco proteins (Bosgraaf et al., 2003). The identification of missense mutations in LRRK2 has redefined the role of genetic variation in PD susceptibility. LRRK2 mutations initiate a penetrant phenotype with complete clinical and neurochemical overlap with idiopathic disease (Khan et al., 2005;Hernandez et al., 2005;Aasly et al., 2005). The various mutations that have been identified in PD are concentrated in the central region of the protein: one amino acid change within the LRR domain, one amino acid change in the Roc domain, one in the COR domain that can have multiple mutations and two amino acids change in the kinase domain (Fig. 1A, (Cookson, 2010). Identified mutations outside of these domains do not segregate in a Mendelian fashion with PD. The mutations are found in 5-6 % of patients with familial PD, and importantly also have been implicated with sporadic PD with unprecedented 1-2 % prevalence (Gilks et al., 2005). Although much progress has been made during the last few years, the exact pathogenic role and associated biochemical pathways responsible for LRRK2-linked disease are slowly emerging. However, recent evidence suggests that these pathways involve other proteins that have been linked to PD, especially α-synuclein and tau (Cookson and Bandmann, 2010;Cookson, 2010). The considerable number of described disease-linked LRRK2 mutations represent an unique opportunity to biochemically explore the pathogenicity of LRRK2 and identify therapeutic targets for related neurodegenerative disorders. Importantly, all known pathogenic mutations in LRRK2 result in decreased GTPase activity and enhanced kinase activity, suggesting a possible PD-related gain of abnormal/toxic function (West et al., 2005;Greggio et al., 2006;Guo et al., 2007;Ito et al., 2007;Luzon-Toro et al., 2007;Lewis et al., 2007;Li et al., 2007;West et al., 2007). Since LRRK2 kinase activity is critically linked to clinical effects, it presents a viable target for therapeutic modulation.

LRRK2

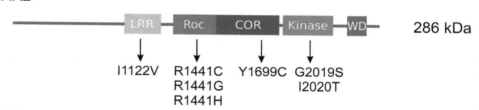

Fig. 1. Domain structure and mutations of LRRK2. The most clearly definined pathogenetic mutations are shown below the diagram.

Attempts to purify mammalian LRRK2 have failed so far in many laboratories. Therefore, the detailed biochemical and structural understanding of LRRK2 is very limited. We have used related proteins, which can serve as models to understand the complex structure and regulatory mechanism of LRRK2. Previously the structure of the Roco protein from the cyanobacterium *Chlorobium tepidum* was elucidated, which revealed that COR is a constitutive dimerization device and that Roco proteins belong to the GAD class of molecular switches (G proteins activated by nucleotide dependent dimerization) (Gotthardt et al., 2008;Gasper et al., 2009). This class also includes proteins such as signal recognition particle, dynamin and septins (Gasper et al., 2009). It is proposed that the juxtaposition of the G domains of two monomers in the complex across the GTP-binding sites activates the GTPase reaction and thereby regulate the biological function of these proteins. The *Chlorobium* Roco structure revealed that the PD-analogous mutations of the Roc and COR domain are in close proximity to each other, and are present in a region of the protein that is strongly conserved between bacteria and man. PD mutations in *Chlorobium*, like that of

LRRK2, decrease the GTPase reaction. Based on the structure and the observed effects of PD-mutations in LRRK2 it is thought that interaction with other proteins modify the dimer interactions resulting in decreased GTPases and enhanced kinase activity (Gotthardt et al., 2008;Gasper et al., 2009). This shows that mechanistic insight can even gained from very distantly related proteins

2. *Dictyostelium discoideum* as model sytem to resolve the function of Roco proteins

This chapter concentrates on *Dictyostelium discoideum* Roco proteins, which are excellent models for LRRK2 and can thus be used to answer key questions for the intramolecular regulation of LRRK2 and give insight in the function of the LRR, the mechanism by which the Roc domain regulates kinase activity, the role that COR plays in this process and how the PD-linked missense mutations alter the interactions between the different domains.

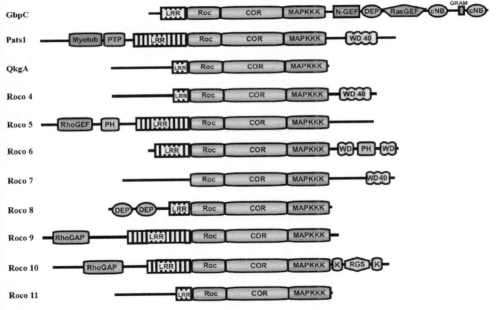

Fig. 2. Domain architecture of the *Dictyostelium* Roco proteins. All proteins contain LRR, the Roc, COR and the kinase domain. Additional a variety of domains are found in specific Roco proteins, such as RasGEFs ,RhoGEFs, RhoGAPs, Regulator of G protein signaling (RGS), and Pleckstrin homology domains (PH).

2.1 Dictyostelium discoideum

Dictyostelium discoideum is a free living soil amoeba. In nature, single *Dictyostelium* cells are feeding on bacteria. They chase bacteria by chemotaxing towards folic acid, which is secreted by the bacteria. Upon starvation cells enter the developmental stage (Kessin, 2000). During development single cells undergo a drastic change in gene expression and start to secrete cAMP. Neighbouring cells respond by migrating toward the chemoattractant cAMP and by secreting cAMP themselves. Thus a cAMP gradient is created around the initiation point. After six hours of starvation, the chemotaxing cells have formed an aggregation centre at the intiation point, which consists of up to 100.000 cells. Differentiation and morphogenesis culminate in the formation of a fruiting body, or stalks of vacuolated dead cells with a spore head on top. These spores can survive long periods without food, high temperatures and drought. Recently the assembly of the *Dictyostelium* genome was completed (Eichinger *et al.*, 2005). The thirty-four Mb genome contains many genes that are homologous to those in higher eukaryotes and are missing in other model system. Due to the availability of the genome sequence, the well established molecular cloning and imaging techniques, *Dictyostelium* provides a well-established model to study the basic aspects of directed cell movement and development (Devreotes and Zigmond, 1988;Van Haastert and Devreotes, 2004). Chemotaxis or directional movement towards a chemical compound is an essential property of many cells and is fundamentally important for processes as diverse as the sourcing of nutrients by prokaryotes, the organisation of the embryo in metazoa, the formation of multicellular structures in protazoa and the migration of lymphocytes during immune response (Baggiolini, 1998;Campbell and Butcher, 2000;Iijima *et al.*, 2002;Crone and Lee, 2002). Chemotaxis is also linked to the development and progression of many diseases including asthma, arthritis, atherosclerosis, and cancers (Trusolino and Comoglio, 2002;Charo and Taubman, 2004;Eccles, 2005). Since the key signalling pathways underlying chemotaxis are essentially similar to those of mammalian cells, *Dictyostelium* has been used to study cell-motility related pathologies, including deficiencies in the immune system and neurological disorders (Carnell and Insall, 2011;Escalante, 2011;Meyer *et al.*, 2011). *Dictyostelium* also has been used as model in pharmacogenomics and to characterize the molecular basis of human diseases associated with the endocytic and secretory pathway (Williams *et al.*, 2006;Van *et al.*, 2007;Francione *et al.*, 2011;Maniak, 2011;Alexander and Alexander, 2011).

2.2 *Dictyostelium discoideum* and the Roco family of proteins

Four Roco proteins are detected in vertebrates, called LRRK1, LRRK2, DAPK1 and MFHAS1. Remarkably, in *Dictyostelium* eleven Roco family members were identified, that all share the characteristic Roc, Cor and kinase domains and most also have LRR (Fig. 2, (Bosgraaf *et al.*, 2003)). *Dictyostelium* Roco proteins are structurally more varied than the Roco proteins found in all the other species together; various domains are additionally fused to the conserved region. Most likely all the *Dictyostelium* Roco genes have evolved quit recently by gene duplication (Marin, 2006). From a functional point of view, the *Dictyostelium* Rocos have provided the most significant data (van Egmond and van Haastert, 2010).

2.2.1 Functions for *Dictyostelium* GbpC in chemotaxis, streaming and osmotic stress

GbpC, also called Roco1, was originally identified in a bioinformatical screen for molecular targets of the second messenger cGMP and is the founding member of the Roco family of proteins (Bosgraaf *et al.*, 2002;Bosgraaf *et al.*, 2003). Besides the conserved Roco region, GbpC has a unique regulatory C-terminal region, consisting of a Ras Exchange Motif (REM), DEP, CDC25, and two cyclic nucleotide binding (cNB) domains with a GRAM domain inserted in between (Fig. 3,(Goldberg *et al.*, 2002)). In the contrary to LRRK2, the cellular function of GbpC has been characterized in detail. GbpC is the only cGMP-signal transducing protein in

Dictyostelium, it binds to cGMP with high affinity to its cNB domains (Bosgraaf *et al.*, 2002). cGMP mediated GbpC activation is essential for the proper regulation of myosin II during chemotaxis, cell streaming and osmotic-stress (Fig.3, (Kuwayama *et al.*, 1996;Bosgraaf *et al.*, 2002;Goldberg *et al.*, 2002;Veltman and van Haastert, 2008;Araki *et al.*, 2010)). Myosin II is an essential regulator of the cytoskeleton at the rear of moving cells. The establishment of a cellular gradient during chemotaxis leads to major changes in the cytoskeleton; actin polymerization occurs at the leading edge of the cell, while acto-myosin filaments are formed at the rear of the cell. The formed myosin-II filaments are preventing the formation of lateral pseudopods and providing the power to retract the uropod (Levi *et al.*, 2002). In *Dictyostelium*, myosin assembly seems to be strictly dependent on the phosphorylation state of the myosin heavy chain (MHC) (Bosgraaf and van Haastert, 2006). Phosphorylation by MHCKs inhibits filament formation (Cote and Bukiejko, 1987;Kolman *et al.*, 1996), whereas dephosphorylation by protein phosphatase 2A is essential for myosin disassembly (Murphy *et al.*, 1996). Phosphorylation of the myosin light chain (MLC) by MLCKs, promotes myosin motor activity, which is important for supplying contractile force to retract the rear of the cell (De la Roche and Cote, 2001;De la Roche *et al.*, 2002). Cells lacking cGMP formation or GbpC have an impaired recruitment of myosin II to the cytoskeleton and impaired chemotaxis. Cells with elevated levels of cGMP have increased activation of myosin-light-chain kinase A (MLCKa) and subsequently an increased myosin motor activity (Bosgraaf *et al.*, 2002). The role of GbpC, becomes even more evident in longer developed cells, which begin to secrete cAMP, neighbouring cells move towards the cAMP and relay the signal. Due to the resulting wave of cAMP through the population, cells become polarized, connect to each other in a head-to-tail fashion, and form streams of cells. Cells lacking cGMP or GbpC have a severe streaming defect; these cells show extensive stream break up due to reduced cell elongation and the inability to maintain stable head-to-tail cell contacts (Veltman *et al.*, 2008). Together these results show that cGMP and GbpC are important for the formation of stably polarized and elongated cells by regulating myosin filament formation in the posterior of the cell, which is important for both chemotaxis and cell streaming.

The cGMP pathway is not only activated in response to cAMP, but also by folic acid and osmotic stress (Hadwiger *et al.*, 1994;Kuwayama *et al.*, 1996;Kuwayama and van Haastert, 1998). *Dictyostelium* can bind folic acid, secreted by bacteria, to the so far unidentified folic acid receptor, resulting in activation of Gα4 and subsequently activation of the cGMP pathway (Hadwiger *et al.*, 1994). In the contrary, cGMP production in response to osmoshock is independent of heterotrimeric proteins (Kuwayama *et al.*, 1998). Also the kinetics of the cGMP responses are completely different, cGMP production occurs in minutes after osmoshock and in seconds after stimulation with cAMP or folic acid (Kuwayama and van Haastert, 1996). The transcription factor StatC and the protein kinase SAPKα show osmotic stressed-induced phosphorylation (Sun *et al.*, 2003;Araki *et al.*, 2003;Araki *et al.*, 2010). Phosphorylated StatC subsequently translocates to the nucleus to bind its transcriptional targets. Activation of both SAPKα and StatC occurs downstream of cGMP and GbpC; SAPKα and StatC are rapidly phosphorylated after treatment with 8-bromo-cGMP and *gbpC*-null cells are lacking the osmotic-stress-induced StatC translocation (Araki *et al.*, 2010). Although the phosphorylation state of Myosin Light Chain Kinase, the protein kinase SAPKα and transcription factor StatC are cGMP-dependent (Sun *et al.*, 2003;Bosgraaf *et al.*, 2006;Araki *et al.*, 2010), no direct binding of GbpC to these proteins could be detected. To completely understand the function of GbpC in *vivo*, it will be important to identify its direct substrates.

2.2.2 Biological role of QKGA and PATS1

Initially two proteins similar to GbpC were found in *Dictyostelium*, Qkga (now also called Roco3) and Pats1 (now also called Roco2). Qkga (Quick growth factor a) only consist of the central Roco region (Fig. 2), and was first described in a study for a new method to create gene disruptions in *Dictyostelium* (Abe et al., 2003). Cells lacking *qkgA* grow faster suggesting a role in cell proliferation. Consistently, Qkga overexpressed in *qkgA* null cells results in slower groth, indicating that higher amounts of QkgA lead to slower cell proliferation, thus confirming a role for QkgA in this process (van Egmond *et al.*, 2010).

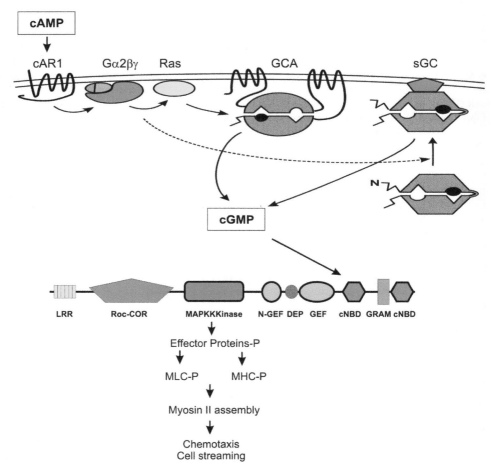

Fig. 3. The cGMP/ GbpC pathway in *Dictyostelium discoideum*. Extracellular cAMP binds to a G-protein coupled receptor cAR1 that stimulates a specific G-protein and Ras. cGMP is synthesised by two guanylyl cyclases, GCA and sGC that are unrelated to mammalian guanylyl cyclases, but are homologs of respectively mammalian membrane and soluble adenylyl cyclase. GbpC, the only target of cGMP, modulates the phosphorylation and assembly of conventional myosin into filaments.

Pats1 was identified in a screen for proteins involved in cytokinesis (Abysalh et al., 2003) and consist, like LRRK2, of LRRs, a ROC, COR, MAPKKK domain and WD40 repeats, and has additionally an N-terminal myotub-related and PTP (Protein Tyrosine Phosphatases) domain (Fig. 2). In a first study, *pats1* was disrupted in DH1 cells, resulting in large multinuclear cells in shaking culture, but these cells divide normally when grown on plate (Abysalh et al., 2003). DH1/*pats1*-null cells show improper localization of MHC to the cleavage furrow and an interaction between the WD40 repeats and the actomyosin was found, suggesting a role for Pats1 in regulating myosin II formation during cytokinesis (Abysalh et al., 2003). In a second study by van Egmond et al., where *pats1* was disrupted in an AX3 background, cells showed large multinuclear cells when grown on plate, but not in shaking culture, which is opposite to *pats1*-null cells that were created in DH1 background (van Egmond *et al.*, 2010). Furthermore, re-expression of the Pats1 kinase domain in *pats1*/DH1 cells, led to rescue of the phenotype and overexpression in DH1 resulted in large multinucleated cells again (Abysalh et al., 2003), whereas no rescue or overexpression effect was observed in the AX3 background (van Egmond *et al.*, 2010). Together these results show that Pats1 has an important role in cytokinesis, but the division-mechanism that it is involved in might vary among different wild-type strains.

2.2.3 Developmental role for Roco4

The complete Roco protein family was identified by Bosgraaf and van Haastert (2003) in a bioinformatic search with the Roc and COR domain of GbpC. Phylogenetic analysis showed that *roco4*, *qkga* and *roco11* are higly similar and are resulting from an ancestor *roco4* gene that was duplicated late in evolution (later than 300 million years ago) (van Egmond *et al.*, 2010). Interestingly, Roco4 has the same domain architecture as LRRK2 (Fig. 1 + 2). The expression of many *Dictyostelium* genes is strictly regulated during the life cycle. RT-PCR experiments showed that *roco4* expression is also developmentally regulated, with a strong elevated expression levels during the slug stage, suggesting a role for Roco4 in late development (van Egmond *et al.*, 2010). To study the function during development, the *roco4* gene was disrupted, and *roco4*-null cells were subjected to starvation on nutrient-free agar plates. During the first hours of development, no difference between *roco4*-null and wild-type could be observed. Cells start to aggregate and form characteristic streams after 6 hours starvation. After 9 hours, aggregation is complete and both cell strains have formed mounds. Developmental defects of *roco4*-null cells become visible after 12 hours of starvation, when wild-type cells are at the onset of forming slugs and form first fingers, while in *roco4*-null this process is first observed after 16 hours of starvation. After 24 hours, wild-type cells culminate in the formation of a fruiting body, while *roco4*-null slugs migrate for many hours before making multiple attempts to culminate, a process that sometimes takes up to 72 hours after the onset of starvation. Eventually, this aberrant culmination results in fruiting bodies consisting of sporeheads that are located on the agar surface, because a proper stalk is not present to lift the sporehead into the air (Fig. 4, (van Egmond *et al.*, 2010)). Re-expression of Roco4 completely rescues the phenotype of *roco4* disruption. Consistent with the developmental defects, Roco4 expression is highly enriched in the prestalk cell and *roco4*-null cells have severely reduced cellulose levels. Cellulose is known in *Dictyostelium* to be the cement of stalking cells, necessary for stability (van Egmond *et al.*, 2010). Together these results show that Roco4 is a prestalk-specific protein involved in the proper production of cellulose.

Wild-type   *roco4*-null   *roco4*-null/Roco4

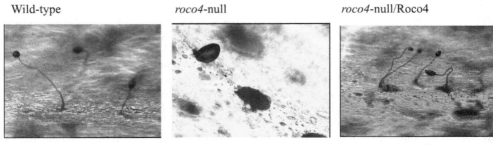

Fig. 4. Phenotype of *roco4*-null cells. Wild-type, *roco4*-null cells, and *roco4*-null cells re-expressing Roco4, were allowed to develop on nutrient-free agar. *roco4*-null cells fail to make a normal fruiting body due to defective synthesis of cellulose.

2.2.4 Function of other *Dictyostelium* Roco proteins

To further investigate the role of Roco proteins during the *Dictyostelium* life cycle, van Egmond et al., (2010) knocked out the 8 remaining *roco* genes and analysed their developmental phenotypes. *Dictyostelium* Roco proteins have distinct expression patterns during development; no major differences in expression were found for Roco5, Roco8 and Roco10 during development. In contrast, Roco6 and Roco11 show, like Pats1, QkgA and Roco4, elevated expression levels during the slug phase. Roco7 and Roco9 are expressed mostly during aggregation, similar to GbpC. Although *roco5*-null cells were previously identified in a large screen for mutants with defects in the developmental cycle (Sawai *et al.*, 2007), they did not show any recognizable developmental phenotype. In the contrary *roco11*-null cells show mild developmental defects: these cells develop significantly larger fruiting bodies; in particular, the multicellular structures have longer stalks compared to wild-type cells, re-expression of Roco11 in *roco11*-null cells rescues this defect. All other *roco*-null mutants did not show any phenotype in development and it will be interesting to see which biological function these proteins have in *Dictyostelium*.

2.3 Activation mechanism of Roco proteins

Pathogenic mutations in LRRK2 result in decreased GTPase activity (West *et al.*, 2005;Greggio *et al.*, 2006;Guo *et al.*, 2007;Ito *et al.*, 2007;Luzon-Toro *et al.*, 2007;Lewis *et al.*, 2007;Li *et al.*, 2007;West *et al.*, 2007). Furthermore, it has been shown that activity of the Roc domain is required to modulate downstream kinase activity, but kinase activity does not have a significant effect on GTP-binding of the Roc domain (Luzon-Toro *et al.*, 2007;West *et al.*, 2007). These results lead to the unifying model that the pathogenetic gain-of-function of LRRK2 relates to increased kinase activity, either directly through mutation of residues in the kinase domain, or indirectly through mutations in the GTPase domain or predicted protein binding domains. However, detailed information about the activation mechanism is missing; it is for example still unclear by which mechanism the Roc domain regulates kinase activity, the role that COR plays in this process and importantly how the PD-linked missense mutations alter the interactions between the different domains. The strong and diverse phenotypes of the *Dictyostelium* Roco disruption mutants provide a strong tool to investigate the activation mechanisms of Roco proteins.

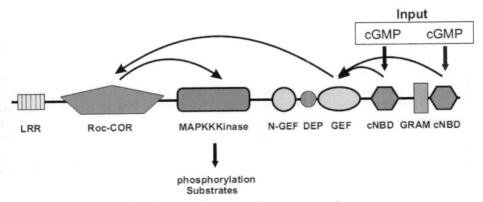

Fig. 5. GbpC: An intramolecular signalling cascade on one protein.

2.3.1 GbpC an intramolecular signaling cascade on one protein

The biochemical properties of GbpC were investigated by rescue analysis of the chemotactic defects of *gbpC*-null cells (van Egmond *et al.*, 2008). Whereas, re-expression of GbpC completely rescued the phenotype, mutants that lack a functional GEF, Roc or kinase domain are inactive. G-proteins function as molecular switches; they cycle between an active GTP- and inactive GDP-bound state. Consistently, in GbpC and LRRK2 the Roc domain is also activated upon GDP/GTP exchange, which subsequently increases kinase activity. The conventional Ras cycle is strictly regulated by guanine nucleotide exchange factors (GEFs) that catalyze the exchange of GDP for GTP, thereby activating the Ras protein. GTPase activating proteins (GAPs) stimulate an otherwise low intrinsic GTPase activity by many orders of magnitude, reverting the conformation back to the inactive GDP-bound form (Bourne *et al.*, 1991). So far it is unclear whether the GDP/GTP cycle of Roco proteins is regulated by GEFs and GAPs, and which structural consequences the GDP and GTP binding has. GbpC differs from the other Roco family members, in the sense that it already contains its own putative GEF domain (Bosgraaf *et al.*, 2003). In vitro nucleotide exchange assays showed that the RasGEF of GbpC specifically activates its own Roc domain. Furthermore, cGMP-binding to GbpC strongly stimulates binding of GbpC to GTP-agarose. Together these results suggest that GbpC contains a complete intramolecular signal transduction pathway; cGMP-binding to the cNB domains causes activation of the GEF domains, the subsequent GDP/GTP exchange of the Roc-COR domain, leading to the activation of the MAPKKK domain and phosphorylating downstream targets (Fig. 5, (van Egmond *et al.*, 2008).

2.3.2 Roc and kinase activities

Dictyostelium Roco4 has the same domain architecture as LRRK2, but in contrast to LRRK2, Roco4 is biochemically and structurally more tractable. The strong developmental phenotype of *roco4*-null cells was used to determine essential structural elements in the protein. Furthermore, high yields of Roco4 and combinations of its domains can be produced in *E. coli*. Similar to LRRK2, a functional Roco4 Roc domain is essential for kinase activity, the COR domain functions as dimerization device and disruption of Roc or the kinase domain by a single point mutation leads to the complete inactivation of the protein, which was also found for all other biochemically studied Roco proteins so far. Also, kinase inactivation does not lead to loss of GTP-binding, thus suggesting that Roc activation occurs upstream of kinase activity. These results indicate that Roco4 has properties very much resembling those described for LRRK2, indicating that Roco4 protein can serve as a valid model to understand the complex structure and regulatory mechanism of LRRK2. As to the relevance for understanding Parkinson we have demonstrated that all Roco4 PD-related mutants show a decreased GTPase and increased kinase activity, except the Roco4 L1180T mutant (LRRK2 I2020T) which shows a large decrease in kinase activity. Strikingly, also for LRRK2 I2020T a reduced kinase activity has been reported, and it has been postulated that the higher neurotoxicity of this mutant might be due to a higher susceptibility of the mutant to intracellular degradation (Jaleel et al., 2007;Ohta et al., 2010).

2.3.3 Different roles for the WD40 repeats in Roco4 and LRRK2
For LRRK2 it was found that deletion of the WD40 repeats leads to lower kinase activity in vitro, which could be restored by introduction of one of the PD-mutations (Iaccarino et al., 2007). Surprisingly, we found that deletion of the Roco4 WD40 repeats does not lead to effects on Roco4 activity *in vivo* (van Egmond et al., 2010). This suggests that in the contrary to LRRK2, the WD40 repeats of Roco4 are apparently not needed for full activation of the kinase domain. A possible explanation for this discrepancy comes from phylogenetic data; Roco4, QkgA and Roco11 have a common ancestor that was duplicated only relatively recently in evolution. QkgA and Roco11 do not have the WD40 repeats that are present in all Roco4 proteins, suggesting that during or after duplication, *qkgA* and *roco11* have lost the WD40 repeats. Apparently, the WD40 repeats were not important enough for the regulation of Roco proteins, that they had to be maintained during evolution (van Egmond *et al.*, 2010).

2.3.4 The LRR are essential for biological activity
The LRR of LRRK2, and Dictyostelium GbpC and Roco4 are not involved in Roc or kinase activation in vitro, but are absolutely essential for activity of the protein in vivo (Iaccarino et al., 2007;van Egmond et al., 2008). Recent data suggest that the LRR are directly involved in determining input/output specificity of the roco proteins, most likely by binding upstream proteins that activate specifically the Roco protein and/or by selectively binding of the substrate (unpublished data).

2.3.5 Subcellular localization of Roco proteins important for activity and function
Recent data suggest that also the subcellular localization of LRRK2 is important for the activity and function. LRRK2 is present both in the cytosol and at the membrane, and the membrane-associated LRRK2 dimer most likely represents the physiologically active form of the protein (Berger *et al.*, 2010). The regulation of membrane association is not well understood, but probably includes dimerization, post-translational modifications and protein-protein interactions (Sen *et al.*, 2009;Berger *et al.*, 2010;Nichols *et al.*, 2010). To better understand the distribution of Roco proteins in the cell, we studied the localization of GbpC (ms in preparation). In resting cells, the protein is present uniformly in the cytosol, but during stream formation and osmotic stress the protein localizes to the membrane. Also

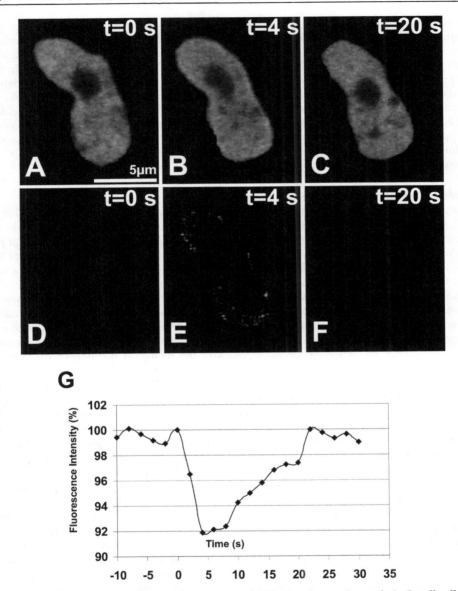

Fig. 6. GbpC translocates to the membrane upon cAMP-stimulation. Starved *gbpC*-null cells expressing GbpC-GFP were stimulated with 10⁻⁶ M cAMP and movies were recorded with time frames of one or two seconds. Shown are confocal images of three frames, at the point of cAMP-stimulation (A; t = 0 s), 4 seconds after stimulation (B), and 20 seconds after stimulation (C). To highlight membrane localization, D-F show equivalents of A-C after subtraction of the average cytosolic fluorescence intensity. Panel (G) shows the decrease of the fluorescence intensity of the cytosol averaged over 8 cells, which was analyzed using ImageJ

stimulation with the chemoattractant cAMP induces a rapid translocation to the cell membrane (Fig 6.). This translocation occurs independent of cGMP and the below described intramolecular signaling cascade in GbpC (van Egmond et al., 2008); GbpC still translocates in mutants that lack cGMP production or a functional GEF, Roc or kinase domain. In the contrary, mutations in the GRAM domain of GbpC lead to disturbed membrane association upon cAMP-stimulation; furthermore, the GRAM domain itself associates with cellular membranes and binds various phospholipids *in vitro*. Furthermore, mutants in the GRAM domain cause inactivation of GbpC *in vivo*. Together, the results show that GbpC receives multiple input signals: cAMP-stimulation induces a cGMP-dependent signaling cascade leading to kinase activity, and independently GRAM-dependent translocation of GbpC to the membrane is needed for proper functional activity.

2.4 Model for the activation of Roco proteins

Together these data show that although there is a high variation of additional regulatory domains among the Roco proteins, the Roco core itself functions in a similar way in all proteins. We have translated our biochemical, genetic and structural data into a model for the regulatory mechanism of LRRK2 (Fig 7). LRRK2 is a constitutive dimer by interaction of the COR domains. In the GDP-bound inactive state the G-domains are flexible, but in the active form the G-domains come in close proximity to each other. This conformational change is transmitted to the kinase domains to allow the activation loops of the two kinase protomers to be autophosphorylated and activated. The GTPase reaction is also dependent on dimerization, because efficient catalytic machinery is formed by complementation of the active site of one protomer with that of the other protomer. In this way the GTPase reaction functions as a timing device for the activation of the kinase and the biological function of the protein. Consistently, PD-related mutations have reduced GTPase activity and enhance kinase activity (unpublished data, (Cookson et al., 2010)). Since the GTPase reaction is regulated by homodimerization and Roco proteins have a low nucleotide affinity (in the μM range), regulation by GEFs and GAPs is not necessary (Gotthardt et al., 2008). However in some transient responses, as shown for GbpC, additional stimulation of the already high intrinsic exchange rate by GEF protein might be required. To completely understand the mechanism it will be important to know how the GDP-GTP cycle changes the RocCOR tandem and how it might influences the output of other parts of the protein. Therefore it will be important to solve structures of wild-type and/or PD-analogous mutants of Roco proteins in the different nucleotide states. The N-terminal segment, including the LRRs, is determining the input/output specificity of the proteins, but the exact mechanism is not clear. We propose two non-exclusive mechanisms: the N-terminal segment may selectively bind its substrates, brings it in close proximity of the Roco kinase domain and is subsequently phosphorylated. Alternatively, the N-terminal segment is binding upstream protein that activates specifically the Roco protein. In the context of LRRK2, 14-3-3 might be one of these upstream regulators: 14-3-3 binds in a phosphorylation dependent way to the N-terminal segment of LRRK2, thereby regulating its subcellular localization (Sen et al., 2009;Nichols et al., 2010).

3. Conclusion

Together, our results show that *Dictyostelium* provides an excellent model to study the function and activation mechanism of LRRK2. Roco proteins are the result of recent gene duplications, and are very homologous to mammalian LRRK2. Disruption of *Dictyostelium*

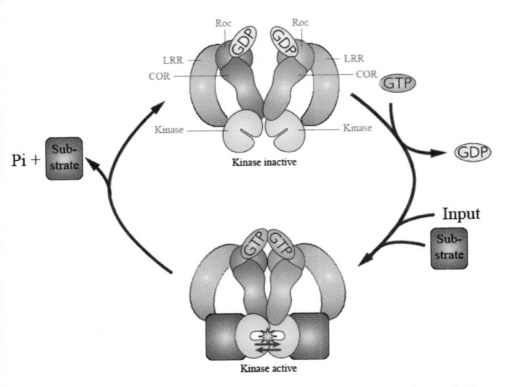

Fig. 7. Proposed model for the function and mechanism of LRRK2. GTP binding to the Roc domain results in dimerization of the Roc domain and subsequently activation of the kinase domain. The GTPase reaction is also dependent on dimerization; the efficient catalytic machinery is formed by complementation of the active site of one protomer with that of the other protomer. The LRR are directly involved in determining input/output specificity of the Roco proteins, most likely by binding upstream proteins that activate specifically the Roco protein and/or by selectively binding of the substrate.

Roco genes leads to very different phenotypes, indicating that they are involved in multiple cellular processes: they participate in cell division, osmotic-stress-response and development (van Egmond et al., 2010). The strong and diverse deletion phenotypes provide a unique opportunity to study PD-related mutations in living cells. These *roco2*- or *roco4*-null cells also provide a tool to express chimera proteins of Roco2, Roco4 and LRRK2 (full length proteins with domains derived from different sources). In contrast to LRRK2, many large parts of Roco4 can be expressed in *E.coli* to high levels in a stable and active form. Sufficient Roco4 protein and combinations of its domains could be purified for biochemical studies and crystallization. All Roco4 constructs both of wild-type and PD-related mutants show properties very much resembling those described for LRRK2. We have translated our results in a model, which can serve as a framework for the basic understanding for the complex regulatory mechanism of LRRK2, and provides a new starting point to answer major questions in the Parkinson field (Cookson, 2010): i) what are the upstream activators of Roco proteins, ii) what is the 3D structure of Roco proteins and how are they activated, iii) what are the output substrates of activated kinase, and iv) can we identify small molecule inhibitors of the activated kinase to revert the activity of the PD-associated mutations. Our studies in *Dictyostelium* might be instrumental in this enterprise and can give important insights in the molecular mechanism of LRRK2 activation, and how mutations of LRRK2 result in neuronal toxicity. In this way we hope to contribute to the understanding of the biochemical pathways responsible for LRRK2-linked PD and help to identify therapeutic targets for PD and related neurodegenerative disorders.

4. Acknowledgment

This work is done in collaboration with Dr. A Wittinghofer (MPI Dortmund) and is supported by the Alexander von Humboldt foundation and the Michael J Fox foundation for Parkinson's disease research. We want to thank Dr. Wouter van Egmond, Dr. Yiu-Fung Ho and Matthieu Bosman for their input in this the project.

5. References

[1] Aasly JO, Toft M, Fernandez-Mata I, Kachergus J, Hulihan M, White LR, and Farrer M (2005) Clinical features of LRRK2-associated Parkinson's disease in central Norway. *Ann Neurol*, 57, 762-765.

[2] Alexander S and Alexander H (2011) Lead genetic studies in Dictyostelium discoideum and translational studies in human cells demonstrate that sphingolipids are key regulators of sensitivity to cisplatin and other anticancer drugs. *Semin Cell Dev Biol*, 22, 97-104.

[3] Araki T, Tsujioka M, Abe T, Fukuzawa M, Meima M, Schaap P, Morio T, Urushihara H, Katoh M, Maeda M, Tanaka Y, Takeuchi I, and Williams JG (2003) A STAT-regulated, stress-induced signalling pathway in Dictyostelium. *J Cell Sci*, 116, 2907-2915.

[4] Araki T, van Egmond WN, van Haastert PJ, and Williams JG (2010) Dual regulation of a Dictyostelium STAT by cGMP and Ca2+ signalling. *J Cell Sci*, 123, 837-841.

[5] Baggiolini M (1998) Chemokines and leukocyte traffic. *Nature*, 392, 565-568.

[6] Berger Z, Smith KA, and Lavoie MJ (2010) Membrane localization of LRRK2 is associated with increased formation of the highly active LRRK2 dimer and changes in its phosphorylation. *Biochemistry*, 49, 5511-5523.

[7] Bosgraaf L, Russcher H, Smith JL, Wessels D, Soll DR, and van Haastert PJ (2002) A novel cGMP signalling pathway mediating myosin phosphorylation and chemotaxis in Dictyostelium. *EMBO J*, 21, 4560-4570.

[8] Bosgraaf L and van Haastert PJ (2003) Roc, a Ras/GTPase domain in complex proteins. *Biochim Biophys Acta*, 1643, 5-10.

[9] Bosgraaf L and van Haastert PJ (2006) The regulation of myosin II in Dictyostelium. *Eur J Cell Biol*, 85, 969-979.

[10] Bourne HR, Sanders DA, and Mccormick F (1991) The Gtpase Superfamily - Conserved Structure and Molecular Mechanism. *Nature*, 349, 117-127.

[11] Campbell JJ and Butcher EC (2000) Chemokines in tissue-specific and microenvironment-specific lymphocyte homing. *Current Opinion in Immunology*, 12, 336-341.

[12] Carnell MJ and Insall RH (2011) Actin on disease--studying the pathobiology of cell motility using Dictyostelium discoideum. *Semin Cell Dev Biol*, 22, 82-88.

[13] Charo IF and Taubman MB (2004) Chemokines in the pathogenesis of vascular disease. *Circ Res*, 95, 858-866.

[14] Cookson MR (2010) The role of leucine-rich repeat kinase 2 (LRRK2) in Parkinson's disease. *Nat Rev Neurosci*, 11, 791-797.

[15] Cookson MR and Bandmann O (2010) Parkinson's disease: insights from pathways. *Hum Mol Genet*, 19, R21-R27.

[16] Cote GP and Bukiejko U (1987) Purification and Characterization of A Myosin Heavy-Chain Kinase from Dictyostelium-Discoideum. *Journal of Biological Chemistry*, 262, 1065-1072.

[17] Crone SA and Lee KF (2002) The bound leading the bound: Target-derived receptors act as guidance cues. *Neuron*, 36, 333-335.

[18] De la Roche MA and Cote GP (2001) Regulation of Dictyostelium myosin I and II. *Biochim Biophys Acta*, 1525, 245-261.

[19] De la Roche MA, Smith JL, Betapudi V, Egelhoff TT, and Cote GP (2002) Signaling pathways regulating Dictyostelium myosin II. *J Muscle Res Cell Motil*, 23, 703-718.

[20] Devreotes PN and Zigmond SH (1988) Chemotaxis in Eukaryotic Cells - A Focus on Leukocytes and Dictyostelium. *Annual Review of Cell Biology*, 4, 649-686.

[21] Eccles SA (2005) Targeting key steps in metastatic tumour progression. *Curr Opin Genet Dev*, 15, 77-86.

[22] Eichinger L, Pachebat JA, Glockner G, Rajandream MA, Sucgang R, Berriman M, Song J, Olsen R, Szafranski K, Xu Q, Tunggal B, Kummerfeld S, Madera M, Konfortov BA, Rivero F, Bankier AT, Lehmann R, Hamlin N, Davies R, Gaudet P, Fey P, Pilcher K, Chen G, Saunders D, Sodergren E, Davis P, Kerhornou A, Nie X, Hall N, Anjard C, Hemphill L, Bason N, Farbrother P, Desany B, Just E, Morio T, Rost R, Churcher C, Cooper J, Haydock S, van Driessche N, Cronin A, Goodhead I, Muzny D, Mourier T, Pain A, Lu M, Harper D, Lindsay R, Hauser H, James K, Quiles M, Babu MM, Saito T, Buchrieser C, Wardroper A, Felder M, Thangavelu M, Johnson D, Knights A, Loulseged H, Mungall K, Oliver K, Price C, Quail MA, Urushihara H, Hernandez J, Rabbinowitsch E, Steffen D, Sanders M, Ma J, Kohara Y, Sharp S, Simmonds M, Spiegler S, Tivey A, Sugano S, White B, Walker D, Woodward J, Winckler T, Tanaka Y, Shaulsky G, Schleicher M, Weinstock G, Rosenthal A, Cox EC, Chisholm RL, Gibbs R, Loomis WF, Platzer M, Kay RR, Williams J, Dear PH, Noegel AA, Barrell B, and Kuspa A (2005) The genome of the social amoeba Dictyostelium discoideum. *Nature*, 435, 43-57.

[23] Escalante R (2011) Dictyostelium as a model for human disease. *Semin Cell Dev Biol*, 22, 69.

[24] Francione LM, Annesley SJ, Carilla-Latorre S, Escalante R, and Fisher PR (2011) The Dictyostelium model for mitochondrial disease. *Semin Cell Dev Biol*, 22, 120-130.

[25] Gasper R, Meyer S, Gotthardt K, Sirajuddin M, and Wittinghofer A (2009) It takes two to tango: regulation of G proteins by dimerization. *Nat Rev Mol Cell Biol*, 10, 423-429.

[26] Gilks WP, bou-Sleiman PM, Gandhi S, Jain S, Singleton A, Lees AJ, Shaw K, Bhatia KP, Bonifati V, Quinn NP, Lynch J, Healy DG, Holton JL, Revesz T, and Wood NW (2005) A common LRRK2 mutation in idiopathic Parkinson's disease. *Lancet*, 365, 415-416.

[27] Goldberg JM, Bosgraaf L, van Haastert PJ, and Smith JL (2002) Identification of four candidate cGMP targets in Dictyostelium. *Proc Natl Acad Sci U S A,* 99, 6749-6754.

[28] Gotthardt K, Weyand M, Kortholt A, van Haastert PJ, and Wittinghofer A (2008) Structure of the Roc-COR domain tandem of C. tepidum, a prokaryotic homologue of the human LRRK2 Parkinson kinase. *EMBO J,* 27, 2239-2249.

[29] Greggio E, Jain S, Kingsbury A, Bandopadhyay R, Lewis P, Kaganovich A, van der Brug MP, Beilina A, Blackinton J, Thomas KJ, Ahmad R, Miller DW, Kesavapany S, Singleton A, Lees A, Harvey RJ, Harvey K, and Cookson MR (2006) Kinase activity is required for the toxic effects of mutant LRRK2/dardarin. *Neurobiol Dis,* 23, 329-341.

[30] Guo L, Gandhi PN, Wang W, Petersen RB, Wilson-Delfosse AL, and Chen SG (2007) The Parkinson's disease-associated protein, leucine-rich repeat kinase 2 (LRRK2), is an authentic GTPase that stimulates kinase activity. *Exp Cell Res,* 313, 3658-3670.

[31] Hadwiger JA, Lee S, and Firtel RA (1994) The G alpha subunit G alpha 4 couples to pterin receptors and identifies a signaling pathway that is essential for multicellular development in Dictyostelium. *Proc Natl Acad Sci U S A,* 91, 10566-10570.

[32] Hernandez DG, Paisan-Ruiz C, Inerney-Leo A, Jain S, Meyer-Lindenberg A, Evans EW, Berman KF, Johnson J, Auburger G, Schaffer AA, Lopez GJ, Nussbaum RL, and Singleton AB (2005) Clinical and positron emission tomography of Parkinson's disease caused by LRRK2. *Ann Neurol,* 57, 453-456.

[33] Iaccarino C, Crosio C, Vitale C, Sanna G, Carri MT, and Barone P (2007) Apoptotic mechanisms in mutant LRRK2-mediated cell death. *Hum Mol Genet,* 16, 1319-1326.

[34] Iijima M, Huang YE, and Devreotes P (2002) Temporal and spatial regulation of chemotaxis. *Developmental Cell,* 3, 469-478.

[35] Ito G, Okai T, Fujino G, Takeda K, Ichijo H, Katada T, and Iwatsubo T (2007) GTP binding is essential to the protein kinase activity of LRRK2, a causative gene product for familial Parkinson's disease. *Biochemistry,* 46, 1380-1388.

[36] Jaleel M, Nichols RJ, Deak M, Campbell DG, Gillardon F, Knebel A, and Alessi DR (2007) LRRK2 phosphorylates moesin at threonine-558: characterization of how Parkinson's disease mutants affect kinase activity. *Biochem J,* 405, 307-317.

[37] Kessin RH (2000) Evolutionary biology. Cooperation can be dangerous. *Nature,* 408, 917, 919.

[38] Khan NL, Jain S, Lynch JM, Pavese N, bou-Sleiman P, Holton JL, Healy DG, Gilks WP, Sweeney MG, Ganguly M, Gibbons V, Gandhi S, Vaughan J, Eunson LH, Katzenschlager R, Gayton J, Lennox G, Revesz T, Nicholl D, Bhatia KP, Quinn N, Brooks D, Lees AJ, Davis MB, Piccini P, Singleton AB, and Wood NW (2005) Mutations in the gene LRRK2 encoding dardarin (PARK8) cause familial Parkinson's disease: clinical, pathological, olfactory and functional imaging and genetic data. *Brain,* 128, 2786-2796.

[39] Kolman MF, Futey LM, and Egelhoff TT (1996) Dictyostelium myosin heavy chain kinase A regulates myosin localization during growth and development. *Journal of Cell Biology,* 132, 101-109.

[40] Kuwayama H, Ecke M, Gerisch G, and van Haastert PJ (1996) Protection against osmotic stress by cGMP-mediated myosin phosphorylation. *Science,* 271, 207-209.

[41] Kuwayama H and van Haastert PJ (1996) Regulation of guanylyl cyclase by a cGMP-binding protein during chemotaxis in Dictyostelium discoideum. *J Biol Chem*, 271, 23718-23724.

[42] Kuwayama H and van Haastert PJ (1998) Chemotactic and osmotic signals share a cGMP transduction pathway in Dictyostelium discoideum. *FEBS Lett*, 424, 248-252.

[43] Lees AJ, Hardy J, and Revesz T (2009) Parkinson's disease. *Lancet*, 373, 2055-2066.

[44] Levi S, Polyakov MV, and Egelhoff TT (2002) Myosin II dynamics in Dictyostelium: Determinants for filament assembly and translocation to the cell cortex during chemoattractant responses. *Cell Motility and the Cytoskeleton*, 53, 177-188.

[45] Lewis PA, Greggio E, Beilina A, Jain S, Baker A, and Cookson MR (2007) The R1441C mutation of LRRK2 disrupts GTP hydrolysis. *Biochem Biophys Res Commun*, 357, 668-671.

[46] Li X, Tan YC, Poulose S, Olanow CW, Huang XY, and Yue Z (2007) Leucine-rich repeat kinase 2 (LRRK2)/PARK8 possesses GTPase activity that is altered in familial Parkinson's disease R1441C/G mutants. *J Neurochem*, 103, 238-247.

[47] Luzon-Toro B, Rubio dIT, Delgado A, Perez-Tur J, and Hilfiker S (2007) Mechanistic insight into the dominant mode of the Parkinson's disease-associated G2019S LRRK2 mutation. *Hum Mol Genet*, 16, 2031-2039.

[48] Maniak M (2011) Dictyostelium as a model for human lysosomal and trafficking diseases. *Semin Cell Dev Biol*, 22, 114-119.

[49] Marin I (2006) The Parkinson disease gene LRRK2: evolutionary and structural insights. *Mol Biol Evol*, 23, 2423-2433.

[50] Meyer I, Kuhnert O, and Graf R (2011) Functional analyses of lissencephaly-related proteins in Dictyostelium. *Semin Cell Dev Biol*, 22, 89-96.

[51] Murphy MB, Cote GP, and Egelhoff TT (1996) Purification and characterization of a myosin heavy chain phosphatase from Dictyostelium. *Molecular Biology of the Cell*, 7, 1153.

[52] Nichols RJ, Dzamko N, Morrice NA, Campbell DG, Deak M, Ordureau A, Macartney T, Tong Y, Shen J, Prescott AR, and Alessi DR (2010) 14-3-3 binding to LRRK2 is disrupted by multiple Parkinson's disease-associated mutations and regulates cytoplasmic localization. *Biochem J*, 430, 393-404.

[53] Ohta E, Kubo M, and Obata F (2010) Prevention of intracellular degradation of I2020T mutant LRRK2 restores its protectivity against apoptosis. *Biochem Biophys Res Commun*, 391, 242-247.

[54] Paisan-Ruiz C, Jain S, Evans EW, Gilks WP, Simon J, van der BM, Lopez de MA, Aparicio S, Gil AM, Khan N, Johnson J, Martinez JR, Nicholl D, Carrera IM, Pena AS, de SR, Lees A, Marti-Masso JF, Perez-Tur J, Wood NW, and Singleton AB (2004) Cloning of the gene containing mutations that cause PARK8-linked Parkinson's disease. *Neuron*, 44, 595-600.

[55] Satake W, Nakabayashi Y, Mizuta I, Hirota Y, Ito C, Kubo M, Kawaguchi T, Tsunoda T, Watanabe M, Takeda A, Tomiyama H, Nakashima K, Hasegawa K, Obata F, Yoshikawa T, Kawakami H, Sakoda S, Yamamoto M, Hattori N, Murata M, Nakamura Y, and Toda T (2009) Genome-wide association study identifies common variants at four loci as genetic risk factors for Parkinson's disease. *Nat Genet*, 41, 1303-1307.

[56] Sawai S, Guan XJ, Kuspa A, and Cox EC (2007) High-throughput analysis of spatio-temporal dynamics in Dictyostelium. *Genome Biol,* 8, R144.

[57] Sen S, Webber PJ, and West AB (2009) Dependence of leucine-rich repeat kinase 2 (LRRK2) kinase activity on dimerization. *J Biol Chem,* 284, 36346-36356.

[58] Simon-Sanchez J, Schulte C, Bras JM, Sharma M, Gibbs JR, Berg D, Paisan-Ruiz C, Lichtner P, Scholz SW, Hernandez DG, Kruger R, Federoff M, Klein C, Goate A, Perlmutter J, Bonin M, Nalls MA, Illig T, Gieger C, Houlden H, Steffens M, Okun MS, Racette BA, Cookson MR, Foote KD, Fernandez HH, Traynor BJ, Schreiber S, Arepalli S, Zonozi R, Gwinn K, van der BM, Lopez G, Chanock SJ, Schatzkin A, Park Y, Hollenbeck A, Gao J, Huang X, Wood NW, Lorenz D, Deuschl G, Chen H, Riess O, Hardy JA, Singleton AB, and Gasser T (2009) Genome-wide association study reveals genetic risk underlying Parkinson's disease. *Nat Genet,* 41, 1308-1312.

[59] Sun B, Ma H, and Firtel RA (2003) Dictyostelium stress-activated protein kinase alpha, a novel stress-activated mitogen-activated protein kinase kinase kinase-like kinase, is important for the proper regulation of the cytoskeleton. *Mol Biol Cell,* 14, 4526-4540.

[60] Trusolino L and Comoglio PM (2002) Scatter-factor and semaphorin receptors: cell signalling for invasive growth. *Nat Rev Cancer,* 2, 289-300.

[61] van Egmond WN, Kortholt A, Plak K, Bosgraaf L, Bosgraaf S, Keizer-Gunnink I, and van Haastert PJ (2008) Intramolecular activation mechanism of the Dictyostelium LRRK2 homolog Roco protein GbpC. *J Biol Chem,* 283, 30412-30420.

[62] van Egmond WN and van Haastert PJ (2010) Characterization of the Roco protein family in Dictyostelium discoideum. *Eukaryot Cell,* 9, 751-761.

[63] Van Haastert PJM and Devreotes PN (2004) Chemotaxis: Signalling the way forward. *Nature Reviews Molecular Cell Biology,* 5, 626-634.

[64] Van DN, Alexander H, Min J, Kuspa A, Alexander S, and Shaulsky G (2007) Global transcriptional responses to cisplatin in Dictyostelium discoideum identify potential drug targets. *Proc Natl Acad Sci U S A,* 104, 15406-15411.

[65] Veltman DM and van Haastert PJ (2008) The role of cGMP and the rear of the cell in Dictyostelium chemotaxis and cell streaming. *J Cell Sci,* 121, 120-127.

[66] West AB, Moore DJ, Biskup S, Bugayenko A, Smith WW, Ross CA, Dawson VL, and Dawson TM (2005) Parkinson's disease-associated mutations in leucine-rich repeat kinase 2 augment kinase activity. *Proc Natl Acad Sci U S A,* 102, 16842-16847.

[67] West AB, Moore DJ, Choi C, Andrabi SA, Li X, Dikeman D, Biskup S, Zhang Z, Lim KL, Dawson VL, and Dawson TM (2007) Parkinson's disease-associated mutations in LRRK2 link enhanced GTP-binding and kinase activities to neuronal toxicity. *Hum Mol Genet,* 16, 223-232.

[68] Williams RS, Boeckeler K, Graf R, Muller-Taubenberger A, Li Z, Isberg RR, Wessels D, Soll DR, Alexander H, and Alexander S (2006) Towards a molecular understanding of human diseases using Dictyostelium discoideum. *Trends Mol Med,* 12, 415-424.

[69] Zimprich A, Biskup S, Leitner P, Lichtner P, Farrer M, Lincoln S, Kachergus J, Hulihan M, Uitti RJ, Calne DB, Stoessl AJ, Pfeiffer RF, Patenge N, Carbajal IC, Vieregge P, Asmus F, Muller-Myhsok B, Dickson DW, Meitinger T, Strom TM, Wszolek ZK, and Gasser T (2004) Mutations in LRRK2 cause autosomal-dominant parkinsonism with pleomorphic pathology. *Neuron,* 44, 601-607.

7

Animal Models of Parkinson's Disease Induced by Toxins and Genetic Manipulation

Shin Hisahara and Shun Shimohama
Department of Neurology, Sapporo Medical University,
Japan

1. Introduction

Parkinson's disease (PD) is one of the most common chronic neurodegenerative disorders. It is characterized by a variety of motor (bradykinesia, rigidity, tremor, and postural instability) and nonmotor (autonomic disturbances and psychosis) symptoms. Although it can be diagnosed accurately, no therapeutic strategies can cure or completely block the progression of PD. Pathologically, PD is characterized by the severe loss of dopaminergic (DAergic) neurons in the pars-compacta nigra and the presence of proteinaceous α-synuclein inclusions, called Lewy bodies (LBs), which are present in neurons of the central nervous system (specific cortical regions, brain stem, and spinal cord), peripheral autonomic nervous system, enteric nervous system (ENS), and cutaneous nerves (Braak et al., 2006; Ikemura et al., 2008; Lebouvier et al., 2009). Similar to other neurodegenerative diseases, such as Alzheimer's disease, age is the major risk factor for PD although 10% of the people with the disease are younger than 45.

Although PD is regarded as a sporadic disorder, remarkably few environmental causes or triggers have been identified (Dick et al., 2007; Tanner, 2003; Taylor et al., 2005). Pesticides and herbicides are the most likely candidates for environmental agents associated with the pathogenesis of PD. On the other hand, PD characteristics are seen in a number of familial motor disorders caused by different genetic factors. Animal models of neurodegenerative diseases, including PD, have in general been quite instructive in understanding their pathogenesis. Ideally, animal models of PD, whether induced by environmental risk factors (neurotoxins) or genetic manipulations, should faithfully reproduce the clinical manifestations (behavioral abnormalities), pathological features, and molecular dysfunctions characterizing the disease. Unfortunately, animal models rarely mimic the etiology, progression, and pathology of PD completely, and in most cases, only partial insight can be gained from these studies. Despite these difficulties, animal models are considered to be very helpful in the development of therapies to treat PD. In this paper, we discuss recently developed neurotoxin-induced and genetic model animals of PD.

Over the years, many chemical compounds and toxin have been identified causative agents of PD. 1-Methyl-4-phenyl-1,2,3,6-tetrahydropyridine (MPTP) is a representative strong neurotoxin that has been recognized from several young drug addicts developed severe parkinsonism. The addicts illegally achieved street preparations of drugs and products were contaminated with MPTP. In addition, epidemiologically, environmental neurotoxins such as agricultural chemicals (pesticides, herbicides, and fungicides) are promising candidates for causative factors of PD. Rotenone and paraquat could promote and accelerate the development of PD. Oxidative stress and mitochondrial dysfunction induced by these toxins could contribute to the progression of PD. While most cases of PD are sporadic, specific mutations in genes that cause familial forms of PD have led to provide new insights into its pathogenesis. Analysis of these gene products may provide vital clues to our understanding of the molecular pathogenesis of dopaminergic neuronal death in PD.

Over 10 causative genes for autosomal-dominant (*α-synuclein, Ubiqitin carboxy-terminal hydrolase L1 (UCHL1)*, and *Leucine-rich repeat kinase 2 (LRRK2)*) or autosomal-recessive (*parkin, phosphatase and tensin homolog deleted on chromosome ten (PTEN)-induced putative kinase 1 (PINK1)*, and *DJ-1* inheritance PD have been identified and classified for PARK loci. Studying animal models are important tools in experimental medical science for understanding the pathogenesis and therapeutic intervention strategies of human diseases, including neurodegenerative diseases such as PD. However, it is quite difficult to completely reproduce symptomatic and pathological features of human disorders. Since many human diseases including PD do not arise spontaneously in animals, in particular, characteristic functional changes have to be mimicked by neurotoxic agents. Nevertheless, recent studies have indicated excellent neurotoxin-induced animal models of PD. In addition, many genetic animal models of familial PD have been generated and recognized valuable tools for investigating and understanding pathophysiology of familial and even sporadic PD. Apart from the obvious preference for vertebrate (rodents and primates) models to investigate PD, an increasing number of studies have also shown a number of advantages and the utility of invertebrate (flies and nematodes) models. The central nervous system of invertebrate animal has a rather small number of neuron and glia as compared to vertebrates, however, essential functional features such as neurotransmitter system of vertebrates and invertebrates are conserved. This chapter focuses on animal models of both toxin-induced and genetically determined PD that have provided significant insight for understanding this disease. We also discuss the validity, benefits, and limitations of representative models.

2. Neurotoxin-induced animal models of PD

PD is currently viewed as a multifactorial disease. Environmental exposures, particularly to pesticides, are thought to be involved in the pathogenesis of sporadic PD. Specifically, the herbicide Paraquat (PQ) and the fungicide Maneb (manganese ethylene-bis-dithiocarbamate) have been associated with the incidence of PD (Ascherio et al., 2006; Ferraz et al., 1988). However, a causal role for pesticides in the etiology of PD has yet to be definitively established. In animal models, PD-like disorders induced by neurotoxins or other chemical compounds have led to a better understanding of the pathophysiology of PD (Table 1).

2.1 1-Methyl-4-Phenyl-1,2,3,6-Tetrahydropyridine (MPTP)

In 1979 and 1983, MPTP was initially identified as a strong neurotoxin when heroin addicts accidentally self-administered MPTP and developed an acute form of parkinsonism that was indistinguishable from idiopathic PD (Davis et al., 1979; Langston et al., 1999). A detailed neuropathological study of MPTP-induced parkinsonism in humans showed severe neuronal degeneration in the substantia nigra and the absence of LBs (Langston, et al., 1999).

Neurotoxin	Behavioral and Pathological Features	Molecular Mechanisms
MPTP	1) Parkinsonism (akinesia, rigidity, and tremor) with acute onset 2) Relatively less potent in rodents 3) Good response to L-DOPA and DA-agonists 4) Loss of TH-neurons (-fibers) and DA-content in nigrostriatal region 5) Loss of TH-neurons (-fibers) in ENS 6) α-Synuclein-positive inclusions 7) No typical LBs	1) Easily crosses the BBB 2) Converted to MPP+ in glial cells 3) Transferred into mitochondria by transporters 4) Inhibits electron transport chain complex I 5) Upregulation of iNOS, NADPH-oxidase, and ROS 6) Microglial activation
6-OHDA	1) Intracerebral administration 2) Quantifiable locomotor abnormalities (rotation, akinsesia) 3) Good response to L-DOPA and DA-agonists 4) Loss of TH-neurons (-fibers) and DA-content in nigrostriatal region 5) No typical LBs	1) Transferred into mitochondria by transporters 2) Inhibits electron transport chain complex I 3) Microglial activation
Rotenone	1) Parkinsonism (bradykinesia, fixed posture, and rigidity) 2) Good response to L-DOPA and DA-agonists 3) Loss of TH-neurons (-fibers) and DA-content in nigrostriatal region 4) α-Synuclein-positive inclusions, resemblance to true LBs 5) Loss of myenteric neurons	1) Easily crosses the BBB 2) Inhibits electron transport chain complex I 3) Upregulation of NADPH-oxidase 4) Microglial activation
Paraquat (+ Maneb)	1) Parkinsonism similar to that of induced by MPTP 2) Loss of DA-content in nigrostriatal region 3) α-Synuclein-positive inclusions with long exposure	1) Crosses the BBB by neutral amino acid transporter 2) Inhibits electron transport chain complex I 3) Reduction of nAchR-mediated DA release 4) Inhibits complex III (Maneb)

Abbreviations: MPTP, 1-Methyl-4-phenyl-1,2,3,6-tetrahydropyridine; 6-OHDA, 6-hydroxy-dopamine; Maneb, manganese ethylene-bis-dithiocarbamate; L-DOPA, L-3,4-dihydroxy-L-phenylalanine; TH, tyrosine hydroxylase; DA, dopamine; ENS, enteric nervous system; LB, Lewy body; BBB, blood-brain barrier; MPP+, 1-methyl-4-phenylpyridinium; iNOS, inducible nitric oxide synthase; ROS, reactive oxygen species; NADPH, nicotinamide adenine dinucleotide phosphate; nAchR, nicotinic acetylcholine receptor

Table 1. Representative neurotoxin-induced mammalian models of PD

The lack of LBs may have reflected the age of the patient and the duration of exposure to MPTP. The tragic results of MPTP poisoning in the heroin addicts led to the development of MPTP-induced rodent and nonhuman primate animal models of PD, which have proved extremely valuable (Chiueh et al., 1984; Kopin & Markey, 1988; Langston et al., 1984; Langston & Irwin, 1986; Markey et al., 1984). The MPTP-exposed primates show good response to therapy with L-3,4-dihydroxy-L-phenylalanine (L-DOPA) and dopamine (DA) receptor agonists (Kopin & Markey, 1988; Langston & Irwin, 1986). However, rats are relatively insensitive to MPTP neurotoxicity compared with primates. Rats given MPTP at doses comparable to those used in mice do not show remarkable neurodegeneration

(Giovanni et al., 1994; Giovanni et al., 1994). Only high doses of MPTP cause DAergic neurodegeneration in rats, indicating that complete blockade of the DA receptors is required for them to display signs of parkinsonism. Mice, like rats, are also less sensitive to MPTP than primates (Przedborski et al., 2001; Schmidt & Ferger, 2001). This model also shows pathological changes in the ENS, as observed in PD. In PD, gastrointestinal (GI) dysfunction was hypothesized to depend on neuronal degeneration in the ENS that is similar to that seen in the CNS. Recent studies show that the administration of MPTP results in decreased tyrosine hydroxylase- (TH-) positive enteric neurons in mice, indicating that the MPTP model mice should be suitable for understanding the extranigral pathophysiology of PD (Anderson et al., 2007; Natale et al., 2010).

2.2 6-Hydroxy-Dopamine (6-OHDA)

Like MPTP, 6-OHDA is a neurotoxin that has been successfully used in induction animal models of PD. 6-OHDA's strong neurotoxic effects were described by Ungerstedt in 1971, in a study presenting the first example of using a chemical agent to produce an animal model of PD (Ungerstedt, 1971). Since 6-OHDA cannot cross the blood-brain barrier (BBB), systemic administration fails to induce parkinsonism. This induction model requires 6-OHDA to be injected into the substantia nigra, medial forebrain bundle, and striatum (Perez & Palmiter, 2005; Przedborski et al., 1995). The effects resemble those in the acute MPTP model, causing neuronal death over a brief time course (12 hours to 2-3 days). Interestingly, the intrastriatal injection of 6-OHDA causes progressive retrograde neuronal degeneration in the substantia nigra and ventral tegmental complex (ST-VTA) (Berger et al., 1991; Przedborski, et al., 1995; Sauer & Oertel, 1994). As in PD, DAergic neurons are killed, and the non-DAergic neurons are preserved. However LBs do not form. Typically, 6-OHDA is used as a hemiparkinson model, in which its unilateral injection into the substantia nigra causes asymmetric motor behavior (turning, rotation) when apomorphine, a DAergic receptor agonist, or amphetamine, a dopamine releasing agent, is given systemically. In this model, the quantifiable motor behavior is a major advantage for screening pharmacological screening agents for their effects on the DAergic system and for testing cell replacement therapies (Beal, 2001; Deumens et al., 2002; Hirsch et al., 2003).

2.3 Rotenone

Rotenone is a naturally occurring complex ketone pesticide derived from the roots of *Lonchocarpus* species. It can rapidly cross cellular membranes without the aid of transporters, including the BBB. Rotenone is a strong inhibitor of complex I, which is located at the innermitochondrial membrane and protrudes into the matrix. In 2000, Betarbet et al. demonstrated in rats that chronic systemic exposure to rotenone causes many features of PD, including nigrostriatal DAergic degeneration (Betarbet et al., 2000). Importantly, pathological features match those seen in typical PD. For example, many of the degenerating neurons have intracellular inclusions that are morphologically similar to LBs. These inclusions also show immunoreactivity for α–synuclein and ubiquitin, like true LBs (Betarbet, et al., 2000; Sherer et al., 2003). The rotenone-administered model animals also reproduce all the behavioral and pathological features seen in the typical form of human PD. However, rotenone-injected rats without nigrostriatal DAergic neuronal loss demonstrate the same abnormal motor behaviors as those with such pathological features (Lapointe et al., 2004; Sherer, et al., 2003). This finding suggested that the abnormal behaviors of PD could depend, at least partly, on the damage to non-DAergic neurons in the nigrostriatal area. Furthermore, rotenone exposure also causes the loss of myenteric neurons in the rat (Drolet et al., 2009).

2.4 Paraquat and maneb

Because of its close structural similarity to 1-methyl-4-phenylpyridinium (MPP+, the active metabolite form of MPTP), an herbicide, 1,1'-dimethyl-4,4'-bipyridinium, named paraquat has been suggested as a risk factor for PD (Di Monte et al., 1986). The systemic administration of paraquat to adult mice results in a significant decrease in substantia nigra DAergic neurons, a decline in striatal dopamine nerve terminal density, and a neurobehavioral syndrome characterized by reduced ambulatory activity (Brooks et al., 1999). These data support the idea that paraquat crosses the BBB to cause destruction of the dopamine neurons in the substantia nigra, like MPP+ (Brooks, et al., 1999). The prolonged exposure to paraquat leads to a remarkable accumulation of α–synuclein-like aggregates in neurons of the substantia nigra pars compacta in mice (Manning-Bog et al., 2002). Chronic exposure to paraquat also reduces the expression of the nicotinic acetylcholine receptor (nAChR) subunit $\alpha 3/\alpha 6\beta 2*$ (the asterisk indicates the possible presence of additional subunits). Normally, the activation of both nAChR subtypes stimulates DA release in the striatum (Khwaja et al., 2007; McCallum et al., 2005; Wonnacott et al., 2000). The injection of paraquat selectively reduces the $\alpha 3/\alpha 6\beta 2*$-mediated DA release from the striatum in primates (O'Leary et al., 2008). Maneb is an organomanganese fungicide that is broadly used in agriculture and is a putative causative agent for PD. Surprisingly, Thiruchelvam et al. found that the neurotoxic effects of maneb or paraquat on the nigrostriatal DA system in mice are synergistically potentiated in combination (Thiruchelvam et al., 2000). Their report argued that this finding has important implications for the human risk of PD, because the marked geographical overlap in the estimated annual agricultural applications of paraquat and maneb means that people living in these areas may be exposed to the synergistic neurotoxicity of these two agents (Thiruchelvam, et al., 2000; Thiruchelvam et al., 2000).

3. Pathophysiological mechanisms of DAergic neurotoxins

All the representative neurotoxin-induced PD models described above show defective mitochondrial function, manifested by the inhibition of mitochondrial complex I or III. MPTP is a highly lipophilic agent. After its systemic administration, MPTP rapidly crosses the BBB. Once in the brain, MPTP is converted to 1-methyl-4-phenyl-2,3- dihydropyridium (MPDP+) in glial cells (astrocytes) and serotonin neurons by monoamine oxidase B (MAO-B) and then spontaneously oxidizes to MPP+ (Nicklas et al., 1985; Przedborski & Vila, 2003). Thereafter, MPP+ is released into the extracellular space. Unlike MPTP, MPP+ is a polar molecule that cannot freely enter DAergic neurons. Thus, a plasma membrane transport system is required. MPP+ has a high affinity for dopamine transporter (DAT) as well as for norepinephrine and serotonin transporters (Bezard et al., 1999; Mayer et al., 1986). Once inside DAergic neurons, MPP+ can accumulate in mitochondria and impair mitochondrial respiration by inhibiting complex I in the electron transport chain (Nicklas, et al., 1985; Ramsay & Singer, 1986), which induces the generation of reactive oxygen species (ROS). MPP+ can also bind to vesicular monoamine transporters (VMATs), which help move selected materials into synaptic vesicles containing DA (Del Zompo et al., 1993). MPP+ can also remain in the cytoplasm and interact with cytosolic enzymes (Klaidman et al., 1993).

Inducible nitric oxide synthase (iNOS) is also involved in the pathogenesis of MPP+-induced parkinsonism in animal models. Increased iNOS has also been found in the substantia nigra of autopsied PD patients, indicating that nitric oxide (NO) overproduction is a feature of the human disease (Huerta et al., 2007; Hunot et al., 1996). Excess NO could contribute to the formation of free radicals, which could damage DAergic neurons, leading to the development of PD symptoms. Mice null for iNOS show a resistance to neuronal damage by MPTP, and iNOS inhibitors protect against the degeneration of DAergic neurons in MPTP-treated mice (Dehmer et al., 2000; Liberatore et al., 1999). Furthermore, microglial cells can be activated by the formation of free radicals and iNOS-mediated damage, and thereby exacerbate the toxicity of MPTP (Barcia et al., 2004; Breidert et al., 2002; Wu et al., 2002). Finally, MPTP can also upregulate nicotinamide adenine dinucleotide phosphate (NADPH)-oxidase in the substantia nigra of mice (Wu, et al., 2002), which is significant because NADPH-oxidase appears to be ubiquitously expressed in all brain regions and metabolizes molecular oxygen, generating superoxide as a product. In fact, MPTP toxicity is diminished in mice lacking functional NADPH-oxidase, indicating a pivotal role for superoxide ions in the neurotoxicity induced by MPTP (Wu, et al., 2002).

The toxicity of 6-OHDA also involves mechanisms of oxidative stress. 6-OHDA can be taken up by DAergic neurons through DAT (Bove et al., 2005; Schober, 2004). Once transported into neurons, 6-OHDA is oxidized like DA. The oxidized molecule generates free radicals inhibits mitochondrial complex I and produces superoxide and hydroxyl radicals (Bove, et al., 2005; Schober, 2004). It is not only toxic to the DAergic neurons but can also induce microglial activation (Bove, et al., 2005).

Like MPTP, the pesticide rotenone is very lipophilic, crosses the BBB, and is distributed evenly throughout the brain (Bove, et al., 2005; Uversky, 2004). It can enter mitochondria, where it inhibits complex I of the electron transport chain with high affinity (Bove, et al., 2005). Interestingly, the inhibition of microglial activation by an antibiotic,minocycline, can attenuate the neurotoxicity of rotenone (Casarejos et al., 2006). Gao et al. also showed that the neurotoxicity of rotenone is reduced in neuron-glia cocultures from NADPH oxidase-null mice (Gao et al., 2003). The DA uptake of the neuron-enriched cultures was not affected by the addition of microglia from NADPH oxidase-null mice, the addition of microglia from wild-type (WT) mice significantly increased the sensitivity of DAergic neurons either from WT or knockout (KO) mice to rotenone neurotoxicity. These data indicate that microglial NADPH oxidase, but not neuronal NADPH oxidase, is responsible for the NADPH oxidase-mediated neurotoxicity of rotenone (Gao, et al., 2003). Paraquat mainly crosses the BBB through the neutral amino acid transporter (McCormack & Di Monte, 2003; Shimizu et al., 2003; Yang & Sun, 1998). Once in the brain, it is selectively taken up by the terminals of DA-containing neurons in the substantia nigra by the DAT, and it inhibits mitochondrial complex I (Shimizu, et al., 2003). Maneb contains a major active fungicidal component, manganese ethylene-bis-dithiocarbamate (Mn–EBDC). In a rat model in which Mn–EBDC is directly delivered to the lateral ventricles, Mn–EBDC causes selective DAergic neurodegeneration (Zhang et al., 2003). Mn–EBDC preferentially inhibits mitochondrial complex III (Zhang, et al., 2003).

4. Genetic animal models of PD

Although the etiopathogenesis (including environmental factors) of PD is not fully understood, the extensive examination of human postmortem material, the genetic analysis of patients, and the study of experimental animal models have shed significant light on the molecular mechanisms involved in its progression. However, since the number of patients with familial PD is extremely low compared to the number with sporadic PD, genetic studies in affected human families are very difficult. Therefore, the development of animal genetic models for PD is especially important, and such models provide an opportunity not only to investigate the genetic etiology of PD but also to identify new factors that could be invaluable in terms of diagnosis, drug design, and/or therapy (Gasser, 2009; Lees et al., 2009). Even invertebrate animals, for example, *Drosophila melanogaster*, are useful models for surveys of human PD. While their numbers of neurons and glia are obviously much smaller than in rodents and primates, *Drosophila* have the same types of neuron-glia systems, and a great number of genes and molecular transduction pathways are conserved between *Drosophila* and humans.

In recent years, several genetic animal models of PD have been reported, including models for autosomal-dominant (AD) inheritance patterns. The genes manipulated in these models include *α-synuclein, LRRK2, UCHL1,* and *high temperature requirement A2 (HTRA2/Omi)* (Table 2). There are also models of autosomal-recessive (AR) inherited PD, which involve KO or knockdown genes for *parkin, DJ-1,* and *PINK1* (Table 3). In addition, we will review a PD mouse model deficient in *nuclear receptor-related 1 (Nurr1)*, also named *nuclear receptor subfamily 4, group A, member 2 (NR4A2)*, which is a susceptibility gene for familial PD (Table 3).

Gene	Animal	Manipulation	DA neuron loss	LB-like inclusions[1]	DA-responsive motor deficits[2]
α-synuclein (*PARK1*)	Nematode	Transgenic	Yes[§]	No	Yes
	Fly	Transgenic	Yes	Yes	Yes
	Mouse	Transgenic	No	Yes[§] (PrP promoter)	Yes[§] (PDGFβ promoter)
	Rat	Transgenic	Yes	No	Yes
	Monkey	Transgenic	Yes	No	ND
UCHL1 (*PARK5*)	Mouse	Transgenic	Yes	No	Yes
LRRK2 (*PARK8*)	Nematode	Transgenic	Yes	ND	ND
	Fly	Transgenic	Yes	No	Yes
	Mouse	Transgenic	No	No	Yes

Abbreviations: UCHL1, ubiquitin carboxy-terminal hydrolase L1; LRRK2, leucine-rich repeat kinase 2; DA, dopamine; LB, Lewy body; ND, not determined; PrP, prion; PDGFβ, platelet-derived growth factor β
1; LB-like inclusions by definition contain filamentous α-synuclein
2; ND could include some degree of behavioral impairment in spontaneous and locomotor activity and in response to sensory stimulation
§; Controversial. The opposite result has also been shown.

Table 2. Autosomal-dominant PD models

Gene	Animal	Manipulation	DA neuron loss	LB-like inclusion[1]	DA-responsive motor deficits[2]
parkin (PARK2)	Nematode	Knockout	No	No	No
	Fly	Knockout	Yes	No	Yes
		Transgenic	Yes	No	Yes
	Mouse	Knockout	No	No	ND
		Transgenic	Yes	Yes	ND
PINK1 (PARK6)	Fly	Knockout	Yes	No	Yes
	Mouse	Knockout	No	No	ND
DJ-1 (PARK7)	Fly	Knockout	Yes	No	Yes
	Mouse	Knockout	No	No	ND
HtrA2/Omi (PARK13)	Fly	Knockout	No	No	No
	Mouse	Knockout	No	No	ND
Nurr1 (NR4A2)	Mouse	Knockout	Yes	No	ND

Abbreviations: PINK1, phosphatase and tensin homolog deleted on chromosome ten (PTEN)-induced putative kinase 1; HtrA2, high temperature requirement A2; Nurr1, nuclear receptor-related 1; NR4A2, nuclear receptor subfamily 4, group A, member 2; DA, dopamine; LB, Lewy body; ND, not determined 1; LB-like inclusions by definition contain filamentous α-synuclein 2; ND could include some degree of behavioral impairment in spontaneous and locomotor activity and in response to sensory stimulation

Table 3. Autosomal-recessive PD models and other causative genes of PD

4.1 α-synuclein

α-synuclein was the first gene linked to an AD-type familial PD, called Park1. The identification of an *α-synuclein* mutation in this family revolutionized PD research, since α-synuclein is the main component of LBs, which are observed in the sporadic PD brain. This striking result strongly indicates that genetic and sporadic PD may share similar etiologies and that investigating α-synuclein-mediated pathogenesis in familial PD could uncover important information about sporadic PD. Three missense mutations of *α-synuclein*, encoding the substitutions A30P, A53T, and E46K, have been identified in familial PD (Gasser, 2009; Kruger et al., 1998; Lees, et al., 2009; Polymeropoulos et al., 1997). Furthermore, the duplication or triplication of *α-synuclein* is sufficient to cause PD, suggesting that the level of α-synuclein expression is a critical determinant of PD progression (Singleton, 2005; Singleton et al., 2003). Even though no direct relationship between sporadic PD and α-synuclein expression has yet been shown, the existence of several polymorphisms in the promoter or 3'-UTR of the *α-synuclein* gene suggests that its expression level might be a risk factor (Holzmann et al., 2003; Pals et al., 2004; Winkler et al., 2007).

Human α-synuclein is an abundant 140-amino acid presynaptic phosphoprotein involved in vesicle handling and neurotransmitter release. Mutations in α-synuclein that increase the propensity for misfolding are probably deleterious, because the misfolded forms are toxic, and they induce cell death *in vitro* (Cookson, 2005; Lee & Trojanowski, 2006). Among the variety of abnormal forms that mutant α-synuclein can adopt, protofibrils and fibrils seem to be the most toxic (Lee & Trojanowski, 2006). These demonstrations of α-synuclein toxicity *in vitro* led to the creation and extensive analysis of many *α-synuclein*-based animal models of PD.

Although flies (*Drosophila*) and nematodes (*C. elegans*) do not have complex nervous systems compared to vertebrates and do not express endogenous α-synuclein, they are useful for identifying genetic and pharmacological modifiers of *α-synuclein* and its product. In *Drosophila*, the overexpression of WT and mutated (A30P, A53T) human α-synuclein causes the age-dependent loss of dorsomedial DAergic neurons, an accumulation of LB-like filamentous inclusions with α-synuclein immunoreactivity, and compromised locomotor activity (climbing ability) (Feany & Bender, 2000). In *C. elegans*, α-synuclein overexpression leads to accelerated DAergic neuronal loss and motor impairment (Kuwahara et al., 2006; Lakso et al., 2003). However, the neurons of these nematodes do not contain notable synuclein-containing inclusions.

Many different mouse lines that overexpress α-synuclein under various promoters have been generated in the last ten years, and most have been described in recent reviews (Chesselet, 2008; Fernagut & Chesselet, 2004; Fleming & Chesselet, 2006). Mice expressing α-synuclein containing two mutations (A30P + A53T) under the TH promoter show progressive declines in locomotor activity and the loss of substantia nigra neurons and striatal DA content (Richfield et al., 2002; Thiruchelvam et al., 2004). Similarly, mice overexpressing WT human (-synuclein under the neuron-specific platelet-derived growth factor β (PDGFβ) promoter show reduced TH immunoreactivity and DA content in the striatum and impaired motor performance (Masliah et al., 2000). Mice overexpressing WT human α-synuclein under another neuron-specific promotor, Thy1, show strong widespread expression in cortical and subcortical neurons, including the substantia nigra pars compacta, but no glial, spinal, or neuromuscular pathology (Kahle et al., 2001; Rockenstein et al., 2002; Song et al., 2004). These mice have an increased sensitivity to mitochondrial damage from low doses of MPTP (Song, et al., 2004). Mice in which the mouse prion promoter (mPrP) is used to drive the expression of α-synuclein A53T show α-synuclein aggregation, fibrils and truncation, α-synuclein phosphorylation, ubiquitination, and progressive age-dependent neurodegeneration, just as in humans (Giasson et al., 2002; Lee et al., 2002).

Several viral vectors, primarily lentiviruses and adenoassociated viruses (AAVs), have been used to drive exogenous α-synuclein. Because viral vector delivery requires stereotactic injections within or near the site of the neuronal cell bodies in the substantia nigra pars compacta, rats are generally used for these studies although the model has been reproduced in other rodents (Kirik et al., 2002; Klein et al., 2002; Lauwers et al., 2003; Lo Bianco et al., 2002). The overexpression of human WT or A53T mutant α-synuclein by AAVs in the SNc neurons of rats causes the progressive age-dependent loss of DA neurons, motor impairment, and α-synuclein-positive cytoplasmic inclusions (Kirik, et al., 2002). Kirik et al. also overexpressed WT or A53T mutant α-synuclein in marmosets (Kirik et al., 2003), in which the α-synuclein protein was expressed in 90%–95% of all substantia nigra DA neurons. The transduced neurons showed evidence of severe pathology, including α-synuclein-positive cytoplasmic inclusions, granular deposits, and loss of the TH-positivity.

It is particularly notable that the phenotypic outcome of α-synuclein overexpression in mice heavily depends on the promoter used to drive transgene expression. Unfortunately, most of these models fail to accurately mimic PD in that there is no progressive loss of DA neurons. The loss of TH-positive cell bodies in the substantia nigra does not necessarily indicate cell death. Despite the lack of overt degenerative pathology in the DA-positive neurons, obvious locomoter abnormalities due to degeneration of the nigrostriatal system and a lack of DA responsiveness are observed in the various mouse α-synuclein models. Thus, most of these lines are excellent models of α-synuclein-induced neurodegenerative disorders, such as PD.

Although mutated α-synuclein causes human familial PD, α-synuclein's physiological roles in PD are not fully understood. In KO mice of α-synuclein, neuronal development and the formation of presynaptic terminals are normal (Abeliovich et al., 2000). Moreover, double KO mice that lack α- and β-synuclein exhibit normal basic brain functions and survive to adulthood (Chandra et al., 2004). Thus, the loss of α-synuclein function is unlikely to play a role in the pathogenesis of α-synuclein-induced neurodegeneration. Meanwhile, α-synuclein KO mice show reduced rearing activity in the open field, decreased DA content in the striatum, and a decrease in the reserve pool of vesicles in the hippocampus (Abeliovich, et al., 2000; Cabin et al., 2002). These results indicate that α-synuclein may play a regulatory role *in vivo*, possibly in the fine tuning of synaptic plasticity and/or vesicle maintenance. Interestingly, several lines of α-synuclein-null mice have a complete or partial resistance to the MPTP (Dauer et al., 2002; Schluter et al., 2003). Dauer et al. showed that this resistance is not due to abnormalities of the DA transporter, which appears to function normally in α-synuclein null mice (Dauer, et al., 2002). These reports indicate that α-synuclein is not obligatorily coupled to MPTP sensitivity, but can influence MPTP toxicity on some genetic background.

4.2 UCHL1

A rare AD-inherited form of PD, PARK5, is caused by a missense mutation in the UCHL1 gene. UCHL1 constitutes 1%-2% of the brain proteins and functions in the ubiquitin-proteasome system. The ubiquitin hydrolase activity of UCHL1 is important for freeing reusable ubiquitin monomers. The missense mutation in PARK5 causes an Ile93Met substitution in the UCHL1 protein (UCHL1Ile93Met), and this mutant was initially shown to have decreased ubiquitin hydrolase activity (Leroy et al., 1998). Interestingly, UCHL1 is detected in LBs in sporadic PD cases (Lowe et al., 1990). These findings initiated a debate on whether the Ile93Met mutation causes a gain of function (toxicity) or loss of function (deficiency).

The gracile axonal dystrophy (*gad*) mouse is an AR-mutant that shows sensory ataxia at an early stage, followed by motor ataxia. Saigoh et al. showed that these mice exhibit spontaneous intragenic deletion of the UCHL1 gene and do not express the UCHL1 protein (Saigoh et al., 1999). These mice do not show obvious pathological changes in the nigrostriatal DA pathway; in particular, there is no loss of DA cell bodies in the substantia nigra. Setsuie et al. generated transgenic mice that overexpressed UCHL1Ile93Met and reported a reduction in the DAergic neurons of the substantia nigra and of the DA content in the striatum (Setsuie et al., 2007). These mice show behavioral and pathological phenotypes of parkinsonism at 20 weeks of age. Moreover, recently, Yasuda et al. performed a viral vector-mediated *α-synuclein* injection into the substantia nigra of the UCHL1Ile93Met transgenic mice (Yasuda et al., 2009). These mice show a significantly enhanced loss of DA-positive cell bodies in the substantia nigra and of DA content in the striatum. The neurotoxicity is enhanced by PARK5-associated UCHL1Ile93Met mutant, but not influenced by the loss of UCH-L1 WT protein *in vivo*, indicating that the UCHL1Ile93Met toxicity results from a gain of function.

4.3 *LRRK2*

The *LRRK2* mutation is another type of ADPD, called *PARK8*. LRRK2 is a large protein containing a serine/threonine kinase and a GTPase domain that is localized to membranous structures (Biskup et al., 2006). The frequency of the common LRRK2 Gly2019Ser mutation was 1% in patients with sporadic PD and, interestingly, 4% of patients with hereditary PD (Healy et al., 2008). The risk of PD when the LRRK2 Gly2019Ser mutation was present was 28% at age 59 years, 51% at 69 years, and 74% at 79 years. The motor symptoms and non-motor symptoms of LRRK2-associated PD are more benign than those of idiopathic PD. In autopsied tissue, the LB pathology was present in a representative LRRK2 G2019S case, indicating that LRRK2 and α-synuclein share some pathogenic mechanisms (Ross et al., 2006). Yet, LRRK2 may play a role in neuronal outgrowth and guidance, and its precise physiological function remains to be clarified (MacLeod et al., 2006).

dLRRK is a *Drosophila* orthologue of LRRK2, and it shows elevated expression in DA neurons of the head (Imai et al., 2008; Lee et al., 2007). Liu et al. overexpressed constructs with mutations similar to those found in patients (G2019S), in *Drosophila* (Liu et al., 2008). The neuronal expression of LRRK2 or LRRK2-G2019S produces an adult-onset selective loss of DAergic neurons, locomotor dysfunction, and early mortality. However, the phenotype caused by the G2019S-LRRK2 mutant is more severe than that cause by the expression of equivalent levels of WT LRRK2. Treatment with L-DOPA improves the mutant LRRK2-induced locomotor impairment but does not prevent the loss of TH-positive neurons. Some fly models that overexpress other LRRK2 mutations, such as I1122V, Y1699C, and I2020T, show similar results, in terms of an age-dependent impairment of locomotor activity that improves with DA stimulation, and the loss of DA neurons (Liu, et al., 2008; Ng et al., 2009; Venderova et al., 2009). Moreover, in transgenic *C. elegans*, DA marker loss is greater in those expressing G2019S LRRK2 than WT LRRK2 (Saha et al., 2009).

Transgenic mice made using bacterial artificial chromosome (BAC) technology and expressing WT LRRK2, or the R1441G or G2091S mutation exhibit mild axonal pathology in the nigrostriatal DA projection (Li et al., 2010; Li et al., 2009). However, the conditional overexpression of neither WT LRRK2 nor its G2019S mutation causes degeneration of the DA-containing neurons (Lin et al., 2009). Interestingly, although the LRRK2 conditional transgenic mice show minimal nigrostriatal pathologies, they exhibit a progressive age-dependent motor impairment that is improved by DA stimulation. LRRK2 involvement in the pathogenesis of PD may be limited, and other genetic and/or environmental factors are probably required to trigger DA neuronal degeneration.

LRRK2 KO mice are viable, have no major abnormalities, and live to adulthood, and there is no significant difference in the susceptibility of LRRK2-deficient and WT mice to MPTP (Andres-Mateos et al., 2009). In *LRRK2-KO Drosophila* models, differing results on the pathology of the DA neurons have been obtained (Imai, et al., 2008; Wang et al., 2008). Lee et al. showed that *LRRK* loss-of-function mutants exhibited severely impaired locomotive activity (Lee, et al., 2007). Moreover, DAergic neurons in *LRRK* mutants showed a severe reduction in tyrosine hydroxylase immunostaining and shrunken morphology. Conversely, Wang et al. demonstrated that mutants lacking *dLRRK* kinase activity are viable with normal development and life span as well as unchanged number and pattern of DAergic neurons (Wang, et al., 2008). Nematode deletion mutants indicate that LRRK2 is dispensable for the development and maintenance of DA neurons (Sakaguchi-Nakashima et al., 2007).

4.4 Parkin

Parkin covers approximately 1.3 Mb of genomic DNA and is the causative gene for representative AR juvenile PD (*PARK2*). Mutations in *parkin* are not only a cause of familial PD but are also seen in 20% of young-onset sporadic PD cases (Lucking et al., 2000). Parkin is an E3 ubiquitin ligase that functions in the ubiquitin-proteasome system. The loss of parkin function is believed to result in abnormal accumulations of parkin's substrates. Springer et al. demonstrated that *pdr-1* (the nematode parkin homolog) mutants are viable and display no obvious morphological defects or alterations in motility, egg-laying behavior, brood size, or life span under standard growth conditions (Springer et al., 2005). Moreover, the authors did not detect any effect of the mutations on the survival of the DA neurons in the worms. However, overexpression of the α-synuclein A53T mutation in *pdr-1* mutants leads to developmental arrest and lethality, indicating this *C. elegans* model recapitulates parkin insolubility and aggregation similar to several AR juvenile PD-linked parkin mutations (Springer, et al., 2005).

Drosophila parkin-null mutants exhibit a reduced lifespan, locomotor defects (flight and climbing abilities), and male sterility (Greene et al., 2003; Whitworth et al., 2005). The locomotor defects derive from the apoptotic cell death of muscle subsets whereas the male sterile phenotype derives from a spermatid individualization defect at a late stage of spermatogenesis. Mitochondrial pathology is the earliest manifestation of muscle degeneration and a prominent characteristic of individualizing spermatids in parkin mutants. These mutants also display a decrement in the TH level and degeneration of a subset of DA neurons in the brain (Whitworth, et al., 2005). Several parkin-null mice have been generated and display motor and cognitive deficits including reduced locomotor activity and decreased spontaneous alteration in the T-maze; however, they show no substantial DAergic behavioral abnormalities (Goldberg et al., 2003; Itier et al., 2003; Perez & Palmiter, 2005; Von Coelln et al., 2004). Pathologically, KO mice exhibit slightly abnormal DA nigrostriatal and locus coeruleus noradrenergic regions (Goldberg, et al., 2003; Von Coelln, et al., 2004).

The overexpression of human mutant *parkin* in *Drosophila* causes an age-dependent, selective degeneration of DA neurons accompanied by progressive motor impairment (Sang et al., 2007; Wang et al., 2007). *Parkin-Q311X* mice also exhibit multiple late-onset and progressive hypokinetic motor deficits (Lu et al., 2009). Stereological analyses revealed that the mutant mice develop age-dependent DA neuron degeneration in the substantia nigra and a significant reduction of the striatal DA level, accompanied by a significant loss of DA neuron terminals in the striatum. These results indicate that *parkin* mutants may play a pivotal role in the dominant-negative etiological mechanisms of PD.

4.5 PINK1

PINK1 is another causative gene for the AR inherited PD called *PARK6*. PARK6 is the second most frequent early-onset AR PD. PINK1 is located in mitochondria and is a putative mitochondrial kinase, because it contains a conserved serine/threonine kinase domain with an N-terminal mitochondrial-targeting motif (Silvestri et al., 2005). Thus, the PD-causative mutations of *PINK1* may cause loss of function. Park et al. and Clark et al. generated and characterized loss-of-function *Drosophila* PINK1 mutants (Clark et al., 2006; Park et al., 2006). These flies exhibit male sterility, apoptotic muscle degeneration, defects in mitochondrial morphology, and increased sensitivity to multiple stresses, including oxidative stress.

Park et al. showed an age-dependent decrease in DA levels and a mild loss of DA neurons in these *Drosophila* mutants (Park, et al., 2006). Notably, the PINK1mutants share marked phenotypic similarities with parkin mutants. Parkin overexpression is able to rescue the mitochondrial defects found in PINK1, although the double mutants do not show an enhanced phenotype. PINK1 overexpression does not rescue parkin phenotypes. Together, the data indicate that parkin and PINK1 function, at least partly, in a common pathway, and PINK1 acts upstream of parkin. Whereas PINK1-deficient mice show age-dependent mitochondrial dysfunction, increased sensitivity to oxidative stress, decreased evoked DA release, and DA receptor agonist-responsive impairment of striatal plasticity, the number of DA neurons, the level of striatal DA, and the level of DA receptors are the same as in WT animals (Gautier et al., 2008; Gispert et al., 2009; Kitada et al., 2007). These phenotypes are similar to those of *parkin*-KO mice.

4.6 *DJ-1*

Deletion or point mutations in *DJ-1* have been identified in early onset AR PD (*PARK7*). DJ-1 plays a role as an antioxidant and chaperone, and it is expressed ubiquitously in the cytosol, mitochondrial matrix, and intermembranous space (Zhang et al., 2005). In vitro, downregulation or KO of the endogenous DJ-1 increases cells' vulnerability to oxidative stress and proteasome inhibition, implicating it in the cellular response to oxidative stress (Martinat et al., 2004; Mitsumoto et al., 2001; Yokota et al., 2003). *Drosophila* possesses two different orthologs of the human DJ-1 gene, named *DJ-1α* and *DJ-1β*. While loss-of-function DJ-1β mutants have normal numbers of DA neurons, classical genetic analyses and RNAi experiments have yielded contradictory results regarding the function of DJ-1α in DA neuron maintenance (Lavara-Culebras & Paricio, 2007; Menzies et al., 2005; Meulener et al., 2005; Park et al., 2005; Yang et al., 2005). However, DA neuron loss cannot be detected inDJ-1α/DJ-1β double-deletion mutants, which are also viable, fertile, and have a normal life span. Some studies have reported a loss of DA neurons upon acute RNA silencing of DJ-1α (Lavara-Culebras & Paricio, 2007; Yang, et al., 2005).

Similar to *α*-synuclein and parkin KO mice, DJ-1 KO mice do not show major DA-agonist-responsive behavioral abnormalities or the loss of nigrostriatal DA neurons (Andres-Mateos et al., 2007; Goldberg et al., 2005; Kim et al., 2005). In particular, although the levels of striatal DA and DA receptors are unchanged, the evoked dopamine release from striatal slices is clearly reduced, most likely as a consequence of increased reuptake. DJ-1 mutant mice also show an increased sensitivity to MPTP (Kim, et al., 2005). This is rescued by restoring the DJ-1 expression in mutant mice, further indicating a role for DJ-1 in the oxidative stress response.

4.7 HtrA2/Omi

HtrA2/Omi has been identified as the causative gene for a rare inherited PD, *PARK13*. HtrA2/Omi has a PDZ (PDZ is based on three proteins that led to its discovery, postsynaptic density protein (PSD-95), *Drosophila* disc large tumor suppressor (DLG1), and zonula occludens-1 protein (ZO-1)) domain in addition to a serine protease domain and is localized to the mitochondrial intermembrane space by its mitochondria-targeting sequence. Whitworth et al. have demonstrated a genetic interaction between *HtrA2/Omi* and *PINK1*, described below, by investigating the eye phenotype of double mutant flies (Whitworth et al., 2008). Their study revealed that *HtrA2/Omi* acts downstream of *PINK1* and is independent of the *parkin* gene. Yet, Yun et al. indicated that *HtrA2/Omi* null fly mutants show neither mitochondrial morphological defects nor DAergic neuronal loss (Yun et al., 2008). They also generated a *Drosophila HtrA2/Omi* mutant analogue to the human mutation G399S, which was identified in *PARK13* patients. HtrA2/Omi G399S retains a significant, if not complete, function of HtrA2/Omi, compared with protease-compromised versions of the protein, indicating that *HtrA2/Omi* is unlikely to play a pivotal role in PD pathogenesis or as an etiological factor. The targeted deletion of *HtrA2/Omi* in mice increases their sensitivity to stress-induced cell death (Jones et al., 2003; Martins et al., 2004). Animals lacking HtrA2/Omi display a progressive movement disorder similar to progressive akinesia, a rigidity syndrome, showing lack of coordination, decreased mobility, bent posture, tremor, and a decreased number of TH-positive striatal neurons (Martins, et al., 2004).

4.8 Nurr1 (NR4A2)
Nurr1 is a member of the nuclear receptor superfamily and is involved in the differentiation and development of nigrostriatal DA neurons. Le et al. identified two mutations in *Nurr1* associated with PD (–291Tdel and –245T→G), which map to the first exon of *NR4A2* and affected one allele in 10 of 107 individuals with familial PD (Le et al., 2003). Mutations in *Nurr1* alter the transcription of *TH* and the DA transporter, suggesting that alterations in Nurr1 may cause chronic DA alterations that could increase susceptibility to PD (Sacchetti et al., 2001). Nurr1 is essential for the development of the ventral mesencephalic DA neurons, because homozygous Nurr1-KO mice do not develop DA neurons in the substantia nigra and die soon after birth (Zetterstrom et al., 1997). Heterozygous Nurr1-KO mice exhibit a significant decrease in rotarod performance and locomotor activities (Jiang et al., 2005). These phenotypes are associated with decreased DA levels in the striatum, decreased numbers of DAergic neurons, and a reduced expression of Nurr1 and DAT in the substantia nigra. Moreover, Le et al. reported that heterozygous Nurr1-KO mice show a significant decrease in the total number of TH-positive neurons in the substantia nigra and reduced DA in the striatum after MPTP administration (Le et al., 1999). Thus, these mice show a progressive DA phenotype that bears some resemblance to that found in α-synuclein-overexpressing and mutant mice. Therefore, *Nurr1*-knockdown mice may provide a good model for investigating the later stages of PD characterized by severe DA neuron loss.

5. Genetic risk factors of PD

The identification and characterization of susceptibility genes for common human disease, including PD, is a difficult challenge. The usual approach of focusing a study on just one or a few candidate genes limits our ability to identify novel genetic effects associated with disease. In addition, many susceptibility genes may exhibit effects that are partially or solely dependent on interactions with other genes and/or the environment. Recently, Genome-wide association studies (GWAS) have been proposed as a solution to these problems. GWAS analyses must embrace abundant clinical and environmental data available to complement the rich genotypic data with the ultimate goal of revealing the genetic and environmental factors important for disease risk.

In 2009, two reports of GWAS demonstrated that several genes and loci could be genetic risk factors for PD in the different population (Satake et al., 2009; Simon-Sanchez et al., 2009). These studies indicated that α-synuclein, LRRK2, and locus on 1q32 (designated as PARK16) showed strong association to PD. Interestingly, BST1 on 4q15 is only identified a new risk locus in the Japanese study (Satake, et al., 2009) and microtubule-associated protein tau (MAPT) is only found association in the European study (Simon-Sanchez, et al., 2009), indicating that population-specific genetic heterogeneity involves in the pathogenesis of PD.

MAPT is primarily expressed in neurons and plays a key role in the organization and integrity of the cytoskeleton and filamentous neuronal tau inclusions define a set of neurodegenerative diseases referred to as the "tauopathies," which include Alzheimer's disease, corticobasal degeneration (CBD), progressive supranuclear palsy (PSP), and frontotemporal dementia with parkinsonism linked to chromosome 17 (FTDP-17). While tau pathology is sometimes found in PD, it is not pathognomic. Thus, the relationship between the MAPT and the pathophysiology of PD still remains to be elucidated, however, brain pathology in Alzheimer's disease cases with amyloid precursor protein mutation exhibits not only β-amyloid deposition, tangle, but also sometimes LB pathology (Hardy, 1994). This finding indicates that there are genetic pathologic connections between α-synuclein and tau. Other GWAS demonstrated that the strongest evidence of association was obtained on chromosome 4p16 in the gene cyclin G associated kinase (GAK), designated as PARK17 (Hamza et al., 2010; Pankratz et al., 2009). This gene might be a promising candidate since the expression of cell cycle regulators altered in the substantia nigra pars compacta with PD (Grunblatt et al., 2004).

More recent GWAS showed a new genetic association with PD in the human leukocyte antigen (HLA)-DRA region (6p21), designated as PARK18 (Hamza, et al., 2010). Interestingly, this result suggests an involvement of immune system in the pathogenesis of PD. Furthermore, genetic variability of HLA region potentially has impact on damage repair and cleaning up risk for disease. The adaptive or innate immune systems had previously been implicated in disease pathology in the late-onset neurodegenerative diseases such as PD and Alzheimer's disease (McGeer et al., 2005).

Gaucher disease (GD) is an autosomal recessive glycolipid storage disorder with multisystemic manifestations caused by loss of function mutations in the glucocerebrosidase (GBA) gene, which encodes the enzyme glucocerebrosidase. A small subset of patients with GD develops parkinsonism with brain stem or diffuses LB-related pathology (Wong et al., 2004). An increased incidence of parkinsonism has also been reported in relatives of patients with PD (Halperin et al., 2006). In 2009, multicenter analysis demonstrated that there is a strong association between GBA mutations (L444P and N370S) and PD (Sidransky et al., 2009). While both gain-of- and loss-of- function hypotheses have been proposed, he mechanism by which GBA mutations increase risk for PD is not fully known (Velayati et al., 2010).

Additional susceptibility loci will likely be uncovered in the near future, as the wealth of recent data from GWASs is further analyzed. Such efforts will include meta-analysis, consideration of gene-gene and gene -environment interaction, and analysis of copy number variation. Although important progress has been made, the mechanisms by which variation in PD-linked genes leads to neurodegeneration remains poorly understood. However, data accumulated thus far has implicated mitochondrial dysfunction, oxidative damage, aberrant protein aggregation, deficits in ubiquitin-mediated protein degradation, and malfunction of immune system as playing key roles in the etiopathogenesis of PD. Actually, animal models of these risk factor gene mutations have been described very few, but once they are available (if pathological features including LB and clinical manifestation are replicated by candidate genes manipulation), they will undoubtedly shed new light on the mechanisms of PD.

6. Concluding remarks

The symptoms of PD become apparent after more than 80% of the DA neurons have died. The rate of substantia nigral cell loss is assumed to be about 2,500 per year in normal people. The loss of DA function can be accelerated by exposure to neurotoxins and by molecular (genetic) abnormalities, leading to a fast and significant decrease in the number of DA neurons. Consequently, these pharmacological and/or genetic insults can cause early onset of PD. This scenario indicates that critical pathological changes could be initiated one or two decades prior to the onset of PD. As described above, whether the causative factor is a toxic compound or a mutated gene, we have no perfect animal models of PD. So far, the neurotoxin-induced vertebrate models of PD are suitable for investigating disease-modifying therapies, since they have already proved predictive. Several genetic animal models of PD are useful for understanding the early processes of degeneration in the nigrostriatal DA system. In particular, transgenic α-synuclein animals are valuable for researching general toxicity effects and the mechanisms of α-synuclein pathology, as well as for confirming potential therapeutic strategies.

Neurotoxic and genetic models of PD have opened new perspectives for modeling and understanding the progression of PD but the advantages and disadvantages of each approach must be carefully considered. As described above, some models of PD induced by toxins and mutations exhibit insoluble α-synuclein inclusions in the pathological feature, however, they fail to exhibit true LBs. It is important to distinguish models that reproduce the progressive degeneration of nigrostriatal DA neurons from those that model disease progression in the whole organism. Genetic modeling of nigrostriatal degeneration complements toxin-induced neuronal loss by reproducing insults that are mechanistically linked to PD in humans. These models can provide useful information on stages of neurodegeneration, in particular on the interplay between protective and detrimental mechanisms, which are likely to contribute to the late onset of the disease and the effect of aging, a main risk factor for PD.

7. References

Abeliovich, A. et al. (2000). Mice lacking alpha-synuclein display functional deficits in the nigrostriatal dopamine system, *Neuron*, Vol. 25, No. 1, pp. 239-252, ISSN 0896-6273

Anderson, G. et al. (2007). Loss of enteric dopaminergic neurons and associated changes in colon motility in an MPTP mouse model of Parkinson's disease, *Experimental Neurology*, Vol. 207, No. 1, pp. 4-12, ISSN 0014-4886

Andres-Mateos, E. et al. (2007). DJ-1 gene deletion reveals that DJ-1 is an atypical peroxiredoxin-like peroxidase, *Proceedings of the National Academy of Sciences of the United States of America*, Vol. 104, No. 37, pp. 14807-14812, ISSN 0027-8424

Andres-Mateos, E. et al. (2009). Unexpected lack of hypersensitivity in LRRK2 knock-out mice to MPTP (1-methyl-4-phenyl-1,2,3,6-tetrahydropyridine), *Journal of Neuroscience*, Vol. 29, No. 50, pp. 15846-15850, ISSN 1529-2401

Ascherio, A. et al. (2006). Pesticide exposure and risk for Parkinson's disease, *Ann Neurol*, Vol. 60, No. 2, pp. 197-203, ISSN 0364-5134

Barcia, C. et al. (2004). Evidence of active microglia in substantia nigra pars compacta of parkinsonian monkeys 1 year after MPTP exposure, *Glia*, Vol. 46, No. 4, pp. 402-409, ISSN 0894-1491

Beal, M. F. (2001). Experimental models of Parkinson's disease, *Nat Rev Neurosci*, Vol. 2, No. 5, pp. 325-334, ISSN 1471-003X

Berger, K. et al. (1991). Retrograde degeneration of nigrostriatal neurons induced by intrastriatal 6-hydroxydopamine injection in rats, *Brain Research Bulletin*, Vol. 26, No. 2, pp. 301-307, ISSN 0361-9230

Betarbet, R. et al. (2000). Chronic systemic pesticide exposure reproduces features of Parkinson's disease, *Nature Neuroscience*, Vol. 3, No. 12, pp. 1301-1306, ISSN 1097-6256

Bezard, E. et al. (1999). Absence of MPTP-induced neuronal death in mice lacking the dopamine transporter, *Experimental Neurology*, Vol. 155, No. 2, pp. 268-273, ISSN 0014-4886

Biskup, S. et al. (2006). Localization of LRRK2 to membranous and vesicular structures in mammalian brain, *Annals of Neurology*, Vol. 60, No. 5, pp. 557-569, ISSN 0364-5134

Bove, J. et al. (2005). Toxin-induced models of Parkinson's disease, *NeuroRx*, Vol. 2, No. 3, pp. 484-494, ISSN 1545-5343

Braak, H. et al. (2006). Gastric alpha-synuclein immunoreactive inclusions in Meissner's and Auerbach's plexuses in cases staged for Parkinson's disease-related brain pathology, *Neuroscience Letters*, Vol. 396, No. 1, pp. 67-72, ISSN 0304-3940

Breidert, T. et al. (2002). Protective action of the peroxisome proliferator-activated receptor-gamma agonist pioglitazone in a mouse model of Parkinson's disease, *Journal of Neurochemistry*, Vol. 82, No. 3, pp. 615-624, ISSN 0022-3042

Brooks, A. I. et al. (1999). Paraquat elicited neurobehavioral syndrome caused by dopaminergic neuron loss, *Brain Research*, Vol. 823, No. 1-2, pp. 1-10, ISSN 0006-8993

Cabin, D. E. et al. (2002). Synaptic vesicle depletion correlates with attenuated synaptic responses to prolonged repetitive stimulation in mice lacking alpha-synuclein, *Journal of Neuroscience*, Vol. 22, No. 20, pp. 8797-8807, ISSN 1529-2401

Casarejos, M. J. et al. (2006). Susceptibility to rotenone is increased in neurons from parkin null mice and is reduced by minocycline, *Journal of Neurochemistry*, Vol. 97, No. 4, pp. 934-946, ISSN 0022-3042

Chandra, S. et al. (2004). Double-knockout mice for alpha- and beta-synucleins: effect on synaptic functions, *Proceedings of the National Academy of Sciences of the United States of America*, Vol. 101, No. 41, pp. 14966-14971, ISSN 0027-8424

Chesselet, M. F. (2008). In vivo alpha-synuclein overexpression in rodents: a useful model of Parkinson's disease?, *Experimental Neurology*, Vol. 209, No. 1, pp. 22-27, ISSN 0014-4886

Chiueh, C. C. et al. (1984). Neurochemical and behavioral effects of 1-methyl-4-phenyl-1,2,3,6- tetrahydropyridine (MPTP) in rat, guinea pig, and monkey, *Psychopharmacology Bulletin*, Vol. 20, No. 3, pp. 548-553, ISSN 0048-5764

Clark, I. E. et al. (2006). Drosophila pink1 is required for mitochondrial function and interacts genetically with parkin, *Nature*, Vol. 441, No. 7097, pp. 1162-1166, ISSN 1476-4687

Cookson, M. R. (2005). The biochemistry of Parkinson's disease, *Annual Review of Biochemistry*, Vol. 74, No. pp. 29-52, ISSN 0066-4154

Dauer, W. et al. (2002). Resistance of alpha -synuclein null mice to the parkinsonian neurotoxin MPTP, *Proceedings of the National Academy of Sciences of the United States of America*, Vol. 99, No. 22, pp. 14524-14529, ISSN 0027-8424

Davis, G. C. et al. (1979). Chronic Parkinsonism secondary to intravenous injection of meperidine analogues, *Psychiatry Res*, Vol. 1, No. 3, pp. 249-254, ISSN 0165-1781

Dehmer, T. et al. (2000). Deficiency of inducible nitric oxide synthase protects against MPTP toxicity in vivo, *Journal of Neurochemistry*, Vol. 74, No. 5, pp. 2213-2216, ISSN 0022-3042

Del Zompo, M. et al. (1993). Selective MPP+ uptake into synaptic dopamine vesicles: possible involvement in MPTP neurotoxicity, *Br J Pharmacol*, Vol. 109, No. 2, pp. 411-414, ISSN 0007-1188

Deumens, R. et al. (2002). Modeling Parkinson's disease in rats: an evaluation of 6-OHDA lesions of the nigrostriatal pathway, *Experimental Neurology*, Vol. 175, No. 2, pp. 303-317, ISSN 0014-4886

Di Monte, D. et al. (1986). Comparative studies on the mechanisms of paraquat and 1-methyl-4-phenylpyridine (MPP+) cytotoxicity, *Biochem Biophys Res Commun*, Vol. 137, No. 1, pp. 303-309, ISSN 0006-291X

Dick, F. D. et al. (2007). Environmental risk factors for Parkinson's disease and parkinsonism: the Geoparkinson study, *Occupational and Environmental Medicine*, Vol. 64, No. 10, pp. 666-672, ISSN 1470-7926

Drolet, R. E. et al. (2009). Chronic rotenone exposure reproduces Parkinson's disease gastrointestinal neuropathology, *Neurobiology of Disease*, Vol. 36, No. 1, pp. 96-102, ISSN 1095-953X

Feany, M. B. & Bender, W. W. (2000). A Drosophila model of Parkinson's disease, *Nature*, Vol. 404, No. 6776, pp. 394-398, ISSN 0028-0836

Fernagut, P. O. & Chesselet, M. F. (2004). Alpha-synuclein and transgenic mouse models, *Neurobiology of Disease*, Vol. 17, No. 2, pp. 123-130, ISSN 0969-9961

Ferraz, H. B. et al. (1988). Chronic exposure to the fungicide maneb may produce symptoms and signs of CNS manganese intoxication, *Neurology*, Vol. 38, No. 4, pp. 550-553, ISSN 0028-3878

Fleming, S. M. & Chesselet, M. F. (2006). Behavioral phenotypes and pharmacology in genetic mouse models of Parkinsonism, *Behavioural Pharmacology*, Vol. 17, No. 5-6, pp. 383-391, ISSN 0955-8810

Gao, H. M. et al. (2003). Critical role for microglial NADPH oxidase in rotenone-induced degeneration of dopaminergic neurons, *Journal of Neuroscience*, Vol. 23, No. 15, pp. 6181-6187, ISSN 1529-2401

Gasser, T. (2009). Molecular pathogenesis of Parkinson disease: insights from genetic studies, *Expert Rev Mol Med*, Vol. 11, No. pp. e22, ISSN 1462-3994

Gautier, C. A. et al. (2008). Loss of PINK1 causes mitochondrial functional defects and increased sensitivity to oxidative stress, *Proceedings of the National Academy of Sciences of the United States of America*, Vol. 105, No. 32, pp. 11364-11369, ISSN 1091-6490

Giasson, B. I. et al. (2002). Neuronal alpha-synucleinopathy with severe movement disorder in mice expressing A53T human alpha-synuclein, *Neuron*, Vol. 34, No. 4, pp. 521-533, ISSN 0896-6273

Giovanni, A. et al. (1994a). Studies on species sensitivity to the dopaminergic neurotoxin 1-methyl-4-phenyl-1,2,3,6-tetrahydropyridine. Part 1: Systemic administration, *Journal of Pharmacology and Experimental Therapeutics*, Vol. 270, No. 3, pp. 1000-1007, ISSN 0022-3565

Giovanni, A. et al. (1994b). Studies on species sensitivity to the dopaminergic neurotoxin 1-methyl-4-phenyl-1,2,3,6-tetrahydropyridine. Part 2: Central administration of 1-methyl-4-phenylpyridinium, *Journal of Pharmacology and Experimental Therapeutics*, Vol. 270, No. 3, pp. 1008-1014, ISSN 0022-3565

Gispert, S. et al. (2009). Parkinson phenotype in aged PINK1-deficient mice is accompanied by progressive mitochondrial dysfunction in absence of neurodegeneration, *PLoS One*, Vol. 4, No. 6, pp. e5777, ISSN 1932-6203

Goldberg, M. S. et al. (2003). Parkin-deficient mice exhibit nigrostriatal deficits but not loss of dopaminergic neurons, *Journal of Biological Chemistry*, Vol. 278, No. 44, pp. 43628-43635, ISSN 0021-9258

Goldberg, M. S. et al. (2005). Nigrostriatal dopaminergic deficits and hypokinesia caused by inactivation of the familial Parkinsonism-linked gene DJ-1, *Neuron*, Vol. 45, No. 4, pp. 489-496, ISSN 0896-6273

Greene, J. C. et al. (2003). Mitochondrial pathology and apoptotic muscle degeneration in Drosophila parkin mutants, *Proceedings of the National Academy of Sciences of the United States of America*, Vol. 100, No. 7, pp. 4078-4083, ISSN 0027-8424

Grunblatt, E. et al. (2004). Gene expression profiling of parkinsonian substantia nigra pars compacta; alterations in ubiquitin-proteasome, heat shock protein, iron and oxidative stress regulated proteins, cell adhesion/cellular matrix and vesicle trafficking genes, *J Neural Transm*, Vol. 111, No. 12, pp. 1543-1573, ISSN 0300-9564

Halperin, A., Elstein, D. & Zimran, A. (2006). Increased incidence of Parkinson disease among relatives of patients with Gaucher disease, *Blood Cells Mol Dis*, Vol. 36, No. 3, pp. 426-428, ISSN, 1079-9796

Hamza, T. H. et al. (2010). Common genetic variation in the HLA region is associated with late-onset sporadic Parkinson's disease, *Nat Genet*, Vol. 42, No. 9, pp. 781-785, ISSN 1546-1718

Hardy, J. (1994). Lewy bodies in Alzheimer's disease in which the primary lesion is a mutation in the amyloid precursor protein, *Neurosci Lett*, Vol. 180, No. 2, pp. 290-291, ISSN 0304-3940

Healy, D. G. et al. (2008). Phenotype, genotype, and worldwide genetic penetrance of LRRK2-associated Parkinson's disease: a case-control study, *Lancet Neurol*, Vol. 7, No. 7, pp. 583-590, ISSN 1474-4422

Hirsch, E. C. et al. (2003). Animal models of Parkinson's disease in rodents induced by toxins: an update, *Journal of Neural Transmission. Supplementum*, Vol. No. 65, pp. 89-100, ISSN 0303-6995

Holzmann, C. et al. (2003). Polymorphisms of the alpha-synuclein promoter: expression analyses and association studies in Parkinson's disease, *Journal of Neural Transmission*, Vol. 110, No. 1, pp. 67-76, ISSN 0300-9564

Huerta, C. et al. (2007). No association between Parkinson's disease and three polymorphisms in the eNOS, nNOS, and iNOS genes, *Neuroscience Letters*, Vol. 413, No. 3, pp. 202-205, ISSN 0304-3940

Hunot, S. et al. (1996). Nitric oxide synthase and neuronal vulnerability in Parkinson's disease, *Neuroscience*, Vol. 72, No. 2, pp. 355-363, ISSN 0306-4522

Ikemura, M. et al. (2008). Lewy body pathology involves cutaneous nerves, *Journal of Neuropathology and Experimental Neurology*, Vol. 67, No. 10, pp. 945-953, ISSN 0022-3069

Imai, Y. et al. (2008). Phosphorylation of 4E-BP by LRRK2 affects the maintenance of dopaminergic neurons in Drosophila, *EMBO Journal*, Vol. 27, No. 18, pp. 2432-2443, ISSN 1460-2075

Itier, J. M. et al. (2003). Parkin gene inactivation alters behaviour and dopamine neurotransmission in the mouse, *Human Molecular Genetics*, Vol. 12, No. 18, pp. 2277-2291, ISSN 0964-6906

Jiang, C. et al. (2005). Age-dependent dopaminergic dysfunction in Nurr1 knockout mice, *Experimental Neurology*, Vol. 191, No. 1, pp. 154-162, ISSN 0014-4886

Jones, J. M. et al. (2003). Loss of Omi mitochondrial protease activity causes the neuromuscular disorder of mnd2 mutant mice, *Nature*, Vol. 425, No. 6959, pp. 721-727, ISSN 1476-4687

Kahle, P. J. et al. (2001). Selective insolubility of alpha-synuclein in human Lewy body diseases is recapitulated in a transgenic mouse model, *American Journal of Pathology*, Vol. 159, No. 6, pp. 2215-2225, ISSN 0002-9440

Khwaja, M. et al. (2007). Nicotine partially protects against paraquat-induced nigrostriatal damage in mice; link to alpha6beta2* nAChRs, *Journal of Neurochemistry*, Vol. 100, No. 1, pp. 180-190, ISSN 0022-3042

Kim, R. H. et al. (2005). Hypersensitivity of DJ-1-deficient mice to 1-methyl-4-phenyl-1,2,3,6-tetrahydropyrindine (MPTP) and oxidative stress, *Proceedings of the National Academy of Sciences of the United States of America*, Vol. 102, No. 14, pp. 5215-5220, ISSN 0027-8424

Kirik, D. et al. (2002). Parkinson-like neurodegeneration induced by targeted overexpression of alpha-synuclein in the nigrostriatal system, *Journal of Neuroscience*, Vol. 22, No. 7, pp. 2780-2791, ISSN 1529-2401

Kirik, D. et al. (2003). Nigrostriatal alpha-synucleinopathy induced by viral vector-mediated overexpression of human alpha-synuclein: a new primate model of Parkinson's disease, *Proceedings of the National Academy of Sciences of the United States of America*, Vol. 100, No. 5, pp. 2884-2889, ISSN 0027-8424

Kitada, T. et al. (2007). Impaired dopamine release and synaptic plasticity in the striatum of PINK1-deficient mice, *Proceedings of the National Academy of Sciences of the United States of America*, Vol. 104, No. 27, pp. 11441-11446, ISSN 0027-8424

Klaidman, L. K. et al. (1993). Redox cycling of MPP+: evidence for a new mechanism involving hydride transfer with xanthine oxidase, aldehyde dehydrogenase, and lipoamide dehydrogenase, *Free Radical Biology and Medicine*, Vol. 15, No. 2, pp. 169-179, ISSN 0891-5849

Klein, R. L. et al. (2002). Dopaminergic cell loss induced by human A30P alpha-synuclein gene transfer to the rat substantia nigra, *Human Gene Therapy*, Vol. 13, No. 5, pp. 605-612, ISSN 1043-0342

Kopin, I. J. & Markey, S. P. (1988). MPTP toxicity: implications for research in Parkinson's disease, *Annual Review of Neuroscience*, Vol. 11, No. pp. 81-96, ISSN 0147-006X

Kruger, R. et al. (1998). Ala30Pro mutation in the gene encoding alpha-synuclein in Parkinson's disease, *Nature Genetics*, Vol. 18, No. 2, pp. 106-108, ISSN 1061-4036

Kuwahara, T. et al. (2006). Familial Parkinson mutant alpha-synuclein causes dopamine neuron dysfunction in transgenic Caenorhabditis elegans, *Journal of Biological Chemistry*, Vol. 281, No. 1, pp. 334-340, ISSN 0021-9258

Lakso, M. et al. (2003). Dopaminergic neuronal loss and motor deficits in Caenorhabditis elegans overexpressing human alpha-synuclein, *Journal of Neurochemistry*, Vol. 86, No. 1, pp. 165-172, ISSN 0022-3042

Langston, J. W. et al. (1984). Selective nigral toxicity after systemic administration of 1-methyl-4-phenyl-1,2,5,6-tetrahydropyrine (MPTP) in the squirrel monkey, *Brain Research*, Vol. 292, No. 2, pp. 390-394, ISSN 0006-8993

Langston, J. W. & Irwin, I. (1986). MPTP: current concepts and controversies, *Clinical Neuropharmacology*, Vol. 9, No. 6, pp. 485-507, ISSN 0362-5664

Langston, J. W. et al. (1999). Evidence of active nerve cell degeneration in the substantia nigra of humans years after 1-methyl-4-phenyl-1,2,3,6-tetrahydropyridine exposure, *Annals of Neurology*, Vol. 46, No. 4, pp. 598-605, ISSN 0364-5134

Lapointe, N. et al. (2004). Rotenone induces non-specific central nervous system and systemic toxicity, *FASEB Journal*, Vol. 18, No. 6, pp. 717-719, ISSN 1530-6860

Lauwers, E. et al. (2003). Neuropathology and neurodegeneration in rodent brain induced by lentiviral vector-mediated overexpression of alpha-synuclein, *Brain Pathology*, Vol. 13, No. 3, pp. 364-372, ISSN 1015-6305

Lavara-Culebras, E. & Paricio, N. (2007). Drosophila DJ-1 mutants are sensitive to oxidative stress and show reduced lifespan and motor deficits, *Gene*, Vol. 400, No. 1-2, pp. 158-165, ISSN 0378-1119

Le, W. et al. (1999). Reduced Nurr1 expression increases the vulnerability of mesencephalic dopamine neurons to MPTP-induced injury, *Journal of Neurochemistry*, Vol. 73, No. 5, pp. 2218-2221, ISSN 0022-3042

Le, W. D. et al. (2003). Mutations in NR4A2 associated with familial Parkinson disease, *Nature Genetics*, Vol. 33, No. 1, pp. 85-89, ISSN 1061-4036

Lebouvier, T. et al. (2009). The second brain and Parkinson's disease, *European Journal of Neuroscience*, Vol. 30, No. 5, pp. 735-741, ISSN 1460-9568

Lee, M. K. et al. (2002). Human alpha-synuclein-harboring familial Parkinson's disease-linked Ala-53 --> Thr mutation causes neurodegenerative disease with alpha-synuclein aggregation in transgenic mice, *Proceedings of the National Academy of Sciences of the United States of America*, Vol. 99, No. 13, pp. 8968-8973, ISSN 0027-8424

Lee, S. B. et al. (2007). Loss of LRRK2/PARK8 induces degeneration of dopaminergic neurons in Drosophila, *Biochemical and Biophysical Research Communications*, Vol. 358, No. 2, pp. 534-539, ISSN 0006-291X

Lee, V. M. & Trojanowski, J. Q. (2006). Mechanisms of Parkinson's disease linked to pathological alpha-synuclein: new targets for drug discovery, *Neuron*, Vol. 52, No. 1, pp. 33-38, ISSN 0896-6273

Lees, A. J. et al. (2009). Parkinson's disease, *Lancet*, Vol. 373, No. 9680, pp. 2055-2066, ISSN 1474-547X

Leroy, E. et al. (1998). The ubiquitin pathway in Parkinson's disease, *Nature*, Vol. 395, No. 6701, pp. 451-452, ISSN 0028-0836

Li, X. et al. (2010). Enhanced striatal dopamine transmission and motor performance with LRRK2 overexpression in mice is eliminated by familial Parkinson's disease mutation G2019S, *Journal of Neuroscience*, Vol. 30, No. 5, pp. 1788-1797, ISSN 1529-2401

Li, Y. et al. (2009). Mutant LRRK2(R1441G) BAC transgenic mice recapitulate cardinal features of Parkinson's disease, *Nature Neuroscience*, Vol. 12, No. 7, pp. 826-828, ISSN 1546-1726

Liberatore, G. T. et al. (1999). Inducible nitric oxide synthase stimulates dopaminergic neurodegeneration in the MPTP model of Parkinson disease, *Nature Medicine*, Vol. 5, No. 12, pp. 1403-1409, ISSN 1078-8956

Lin, X. et al. (2009). Leucine-rich repeat kinase 2 regulates the progression of neuropathology induced by Parkinson's-disease-related mutant alpha-synuclein, *Neuron*, Vol. 64, No. 6, pp. 807-827, ISSN 1097-4199

Liu, Z. et al. (2008). A Drosophila model for LRRK2-linked parkinsonism, *Proceedings of the National Academy of Sciences of the United States of America*, Vol. 105, No. 7, pp. 2693-2698, ISSN 1091-6490

Lo Bianco, C. et al. (2002). alpha -Synucleinopathy and selective dopaminergic neuron loss in a rat lentiviral-based model of Parkinson's disease, *Proc Natl Acad Sci U S A*, Vol. 99, No. 16, pp. 10813-10818, ISSN 0027-8424

Lowe, J. et al. (1990). Ubiquitin carboxyl-terminal hydrolase (PGP 9.5) is selectively present in ubiquitinated inclusion bodies characteristic of human neurodegenerative diseases, *Journal of Pathology*, Vol. 161, No. 2, pp. 153-160, ISSN 0022-3417

Lu, X. H. et al. (2009). Bacterial artificial chromosome transgenic mice expressing a truncated mutant parkin exhibit age-dependent hypokinetic motor deficits, dopaminergic neuron degeneration, and accumulation of proteinase K-resistant alpha-synuclein, *Journal of Neuroscience*, Vol. 29, No. 7, pp. 1962-1976, ISSN 1529-2401

Lucking, C. B. et al. (2000). Association between early-onset Parkinson's disease and mutations in the parkin gene, *New England Journal of Medicine*, Vol. 342, No. 21, pp. 1560-1567, ISSN 0028-4793

MacLeod, D. et al. (2006). The familial Parkinsonism gene LRRK2 regulates neurite process morphology, *Neuron*, Vol. 52, No. 4, pp. 587-593, ISSN 0896-6273

Manning-Bog, A. B. et al. (2002). The herbicide paraquat causes up-regulation and aggregation of alpha-synuclein in mice: paraquat and alpha-synuclein, *Journal of Biological Chemistry*, Vol. 277, No. 3, pp. 1641-1644, ISSN 0021-9258

Markey, S. P. et al. (1984). Intraneuronal generation of a pyridinium metabolite may cause drug-induced parkinsonism, *Nature*, Vol. 311, No. 5985, pp. 464-467, ISSN 0028-0836

Martinat, C. et al. (2004). Sensitivity to oxidative stress in DJ-1-deficient dopamine neurons: an ES- derived cell model of primary Parkinsonism, *PLoS Biol*, Vol. 2, No. 11, pp. e327, ISSN 1545-7885

Martins, L. M. et al. (2004). Neuroprotective role of the Reaper-related serine protease HtrA2/Omi revealed by targeted deletion in mice, *Molecular and Cellular Biology*, Vol. 24, No. 22, pp. 9848-9862, ISSN 0270-7306

Masliah, E. et al. (2000). Dopaminergic loss and inclusion body formation in alpha-synuclein mice: implications for neurodegenerative disorders, *Science*, Vol. 287, No. 5456, pp. 1265-1269, ISSN 0036-8075

Mayer, R. A. et al. (1986). Prevention of the nigrostriatal toxicity of 1-methyl-4-phenyl-1,2,3,6-tetrahydropyridine by inhibitors of 3,4-dihydroxyphenylethylamine transport, *Journal of Neurochemistry*, Vol. 47, No. 4, pp. 1073-1079, ISSN 0022-3042

McCallum, S. E. et al. (2005). Decrease in alpha3*/alpha6* nicotinic receptors but not nicotine-evoked dopamine release in monkey brain after nigrostriatal damage, *Molecular Pharmacology*, Vol. 68, No. 3, pp. 737-746, ISSN 0026-895X

McCormack, A. L. & Di Monte, D. A. (2003). Effects of L-dopa and other amino acids against paraquat-induced nigrostriatal degeneration, *Journal of Neurochemistry*, Vol. 85, No. 1, pp. 82-86, ISSN 0022-3042

McGeer, E. G., Klegeris, A. & McGeer, P. L. (2005). Inflammation, the complement system and the diseases of aging, *Neurobiol Aging*, Vol. 26 Suppl 1, No. pp. 94-97, ISSN 0197-4580

Menzies, F. M. et al. (2005). Roles of Drosophila DJ-1 in survival of dopaminergic neurons and oxidative stress, *Current Biology*, Vol. 15, No. 17, pp. 1578-1582, ISSN 0960-9822

Meulener, M. et al. (2005). Drosophila DJ-1 mutants are selectively sensitive to environmental toxins associated with Parkinson's disease, *Current Biology*, Vol. 15, No. 17, pp. 1572-1577, ISSN 0960-9822

Mitsumoto, A. et al. (2001). Oxidized forms of peroxiredoxins and DJ-1 on two-dimensional gels increased in response to sublethal levels of paraquat, *Free Radical Research*, Vol. 35, No. 3, pp. 301-310, ISSN 1071-5762

Natale, G. et al. (2010). MPTP-induced parkinsonism extends to a subclass of TH positive neurons in the gut, *Brain Research*, Vol. 1355, No. pp. 195-206, ISSN 1872-6240

Ng, C. H. et al. (2009). Parkin protects against LRRK2 G2019S mutant-induced dopaminergic neurodegeneration in Drosophila, *Journal of Neuroscience*, Vol. 29, No. 36, pp. 11257-11262, ISSN 1529-2401

Nicklas, W. J. et al. (1985). Inhibition of NADH-linked oxidation in brain mitochondria by 1-methyl-4-phenyl-pyridine, a metabolite of the neurotoxin, 1-methyl-4-phenyl-

1,2,5,6-tetrahydropyridine, *Life Sciences*, Vol. 36, No. 26, pp. 2503-2508, ISSN 0024-3205

O'Leary, K. T. et al. (2008). Paraquat exposure reduces nicotinic receptor-evoked dopamine release in monkey striatum, *Journal of Pharmacology and Experimental Therapeutics*, Vol. 327, No. 1, pp. 124-129, ISSN 1521-0103

Pals, P. et al. (2004). alpha-Synuclein promoter confers susceptibility to Parkinson's disease, *Annals of Neurology*, Vol. 56, No. 4, pp. 591-595, ISSN 0364-5134

Pankratz, N. et al. (2009). Genomewide association study for susceptibility genes contributing to familial Parkinson disease, *Hum Genet*, Vol. 124, No. 6, pp. 593-605, ISSN 1432-1203

Park, J. et al. (2005). Drosophila DJ-1 mutants show oxidative stress-sensitive locomotive dysfunction, *Gene*, Vol. 361, No. pp. 133-139, ISSN 0378-1119

Park, J. et al. (2006). Mitochondrial dysfunction in Drosophila PINK1 mutants is complemented by parkin, *Nature*, Vol. 441, No. 7097, pp. 1157-1161, ISSN 1476-4687

Perez, F. A. & Palmiter, R. D. (2005). Parkin-deficient mice are not a robust model of parkinsonism, *Proceedings of the National Academy of Sciences of the United States of America*, Vol. 102, No. 6, pp. 2174-2179, ISSN 0027-8424

Polymeropoulos, M. H. et al. (1997). Mutation in the alpha-synuclein gene identified in families with Parkinson's disease, *Science*, Vol. 276, No. 5321, pp. 2045-2047, ISSN 0036-8075

Przedborski, S. et al. (1995). Dose-dependent lesions of the dopaminergic nigrostriatal pathway induced by intrastriatal injection of 6-hydroxydopamine, *Neuroscience*, Vol. 67, No. 3, pp. 631-647, ISSN 0306-4522

Przedborski, S. et al. (2001). The parkinsonian toxin 1-methyl-4-phenyl-1,2,3,6-tetrahydropyridine (MPTP): a technical review of its utility and safety, *Journal of Neurochemistry*, Vol. 76, No. 5, pp. 1265-1274, ISSN 0022-3042

Przedborski, S. & Vila, M. (2003). The 1-methyl-4-phenyl-1,2,3,6-tetrahydropyridine mouse model: a tool to explore the pathogenesis of Parkinson's disease, *Annals of the New York Academy of Sciences*, Vol. 991, No. pp. 189-198, ISSN 0077-8923

Ramsay, R. R. & Singer, T. P. (1986). Energy-dependent uptake of N-methyl-4-phenylpyridinium, the neurotoxic metabolite of 1-methyl-4-phenyl-1,2,3,6-tetrahydropyridine, by mitochondria, *Journal of Biological Chemistry*, Vol. 261, No. 17, pp. 7585-7587, ISSN 0021-9258

Richfield, E. K. et al. (2002). Behavioral and neurochemical effects of wild-type and mutated human alpha-synuclein in transgenic mice, *Experimental Neurology*, Vol. 175, No. 1, pp. 35-48, ISSN 0014-4886

Rockenstein, E. et al. (2002). Differential neuropathological alterations in transgenic mice expressing alpha-synuclein from the platelet-derived growth factor and Thy-1 promoters, *Journal of Neuroscience Research*, Vol. 68, No. 5, pp. 568-578, ISSN 0360-4012

Ross, O. A. et al. (2006). Lrrk2 and Lewy body disease, *Annals of Neurology*, Vol. 59, No. 2, pp. 388-393, ISSN 0364-5134

Sacchetti, P. et al. (2001). Nurr1 enhances transcription of the human dopamine transporter gene through a novel mechanism, *Journal of Neurochemistry*, Vol. 76, No. 5, pp. 1565-1572, ISSN 0022-3042

Saha, S. et al. (2009). LRRK2 modulates vulnerability to mitochondrial dysfunction in Caenorhabditis elegans, *Journal of Neuroscience*, Vol. 29, No. 29, pp. 9210-9218, ISSN 1529-2401

Satake, W. et al. (2009). Genome-wide association study identifies common variants at four loci as genetic risk factors for Parkinson's disease, *Nat Genet*, Vol. 41, No. 12, pp. 1303-1307, ISSN 1546-1718

Saigoh, K. et al. (1999). Intragenic deletion in the gene encoding ubiquitin carboxy-terminal hydrolase in gad mice, *Nature Genetics*, Vol. 23, No. 1, pp. 47-51, ISSN 1061-4036

Sakaguchi-Nakashima, A. et al. (2007). LRK-1, a C. elegans PARK8-related kinase, regulates axonal-dendritic polarity of SV proteins, *Current Biology*, Vol. 17, No. 7, pp. 592-598, ISSN 0960-9822

Sang, T. K. et al. (2007). A Drosophila model of mutant human parkin-induced toxicity demonstrates selective loss of dopaminergic neurons and dependence on cellular dopamine, *Journal of Neuroscience*, Vol. 27, No. 5, pp. 981-992, ISSN 1529-2401

Sauer, H. & Oertel, W. H. (1994). Progressive degeneration of nigrostriatal dopamine neurons following intrastriatal terminal lesions with 6-hydroxydopamine: a combined retrograde tracing and immunocytochemical study in the rat, *Neuroscience*, Vol. 59, No. 2, pp. 401-415, ISSN 0306-4522

Schluter, O. M. et al. (2003). Role of alpha-synuclein in 1-methyl-4-phenyl-1,2,3,6-tetrahydropyridine-induced parkinsonism in mice, *Neuroscience*, Vol. 118, No. 4, pp. 985-1002, ISSN 0306-4522

Schmidt, N. & Ferger, B. (2001). Neurochemical findings in the MPTP model of Parkinson's disease, *Journal of Neural Transmission*, Vol. 108, No. 11, pp. 1263-1282, ISSN 0300-9564

Schober, A. (2004). Classic toxin-induced animal models of Parkinson's disease: 6-OHDA and MPTP, *Cell and Tissue Research*, Vol. 318, No. 1, pp. 215-224, ISSN 0302-766X

Setsuie, R. et al. (2007). Dopaminergic neuronal loss in transgenic mice expressing the Parkinson's disease-associated UCH-L1 I93M mutant, *Neurochemistry International*, Vol. 50, No. 1, pp. 119-129, ISSN 0197-0186

Sherer, T. B. et al. (2003). Subcutaneous rotenone exposure causes highly selective dopaminergic degeneration and alpha-synuclein aggregation, *Experimental Neurology*, Vol. 179, No. 1, pp. 9-16, ISSN 0014-4886

Shimizu, K. et al. (2003). Paraquat induces long-lasting dopamine overflow through the excitotoxic pathway in the striatum of freely moving rats, *Brain Research*, Vol. 976, No. 2, pp. 243-252, ISSN 0006-8993

Sidransky, E. et al. (2009). Multicenter analysis of glucocerebrosidase mutations in Parkinson's disease, *N Engl J Med*, Vol. 361, No. 17, pp. 1651-1661, ISSN 1533-4406

Silvestri, L. et al. (2005). Mitochondrial import and enzymatic activity of PINK1 mutants associated to recessive parkinsonism, *Human Molecular Genetics*, Vol. 14, No. 22, pp. 3477-3492, ISSN 0964-6906

Simon-Sanchez, J. et al. (2009). Genome-wide association study reveals genetic risk underlying Parkinson's disease, *Nat Genet*, Vol. 41, No. 12, pp. 1308-1312, ISSN 1546-1718

Singleton, A. B. (2005). Altered alpha-synuclein homeostasis causing Parkinson's disease: the potential roles of dardarin, *Trends in Neurosciences*, Vol. 28, No. 8, pp. 416-421, ISSN 0166-2236

Singleton, A. B. et al. (2003). alpha-Synuclein locus triplication causes Parkinson's disease, *Science*, Vol. 302, No. 5646, pp. 841, ISSN 1095-9203

Song, D. D. et al. (2004). Enhanced substantia nigra mitochondrial pathology in human alpha-synuclein transgenic mice after treatment with MPTP, *Experimental Neurology*, Vol. 186, No. 2, pp. 158-172, ISSN 0014-4886

Springer, W. et al. (2005). A Caenorhabditis elegans Parkin mutant with altered solubility couples alpha-synuclein aggregation to proteotoxic stress, *Human Molecular Genetics*, Vol. 14, No. 22, pp. 3407-3423, ISSN 0964-6906

Tanner, C. M. (2003). Is the cause of Parkinson's disease environmental or hereditary? Evidence from twin studies, *Advances in Neurology*, Vol. 91, No. pp. 133-142, ISSN 0091-3952

Taylor, K. S. et al. (2005). Screening for undiagnosed parkinsonism among older people in general practice, *Age and Ageing*, Vol. 34, No. 5, pp. 501-504, ISSN 0002-0729

Thiruchelvam, M. et al. (2000a). Potentiated and preferential effects of combined paraquat and maneb on nigrostriatal dopamine systems: environmental risk factors for Parkinson's disease?, *Brain Research*, Vol. 873, No. 2, pp. 225-234, ISSN 0006-8993

Thiruchelvam, M. et al. (2000b). The nigrostriatal dopaminergic system as a preferential target of repeated exposures to combined paraquat and maneb: implications for Parkinson's disease, *Journal of Neuroscience*, Vol. 20, No. 24, pp. 9207-9214, ISSN 1529-2401

Thiruchelvam, M. J. et al. (2004). Risk factors for dopaminergic neuron loss in human alpha-synuclein transgenic mice, *European Journal of Neuroscience*, Vol. 19, No. 4, pp. 845-854, ISSN 0953-816X

Ungerstedt, U. (1971). Postsynaptic supersensitivity after 6-hydroxy-dopamine induced degeneration of the nigro-striatal dopamine system, *Acta Physiologica Scandinavica. Supplementum*, Vol. 367, No. pp. 69-93, ISSN 0302-2994

Uversky, V. N. (2004). Neurotoxicant-induced animal models of Parkinson's disease: understanding the role of rotenone, maneb and paraquat in neurodegeneration, *Cell and Tissue Research*, Vol. 318, No. 1, pp. 225-241, ISSN 0302-766X

Velayati, A., Yu, W. H. & Sidransky, E. (2010). The role of glucocerebrosidase mutations in Parkinson disease and Lewy body disorders, *Curr Neurol Neurosci Rep*, Vol. 10, No. 3, pp. 190-198, ISSN, 1534-6293

Venderova, K. et al. (2009). Leucine-Rich Repeat Kinase 2 interacts with Parkin, DJ-1 and PINK-1 in a Drosophila melanogaster model of Parkinson's disease, *Human Molecular Genetics*, Vol. 18, No. 22, pp. 4390-4404, ISSN 1460-2083

Von Coelln, R. et al. (2004). Loss of locus coeruleus neurons and reduced startle in parkin null mice, *Proc Natl Acad Sci U S A*, Vol. 101, No. 29, pp. 10744-10749, ISSN 0027-8424

Wang, C. et al. (2007). Drosophila overexpressing parkin R275W mutant exhibits dopaminergic neuron degeneration and mitochondrial abnormalities, *Journal of Neuroscience*, Vol. 27, No. 32, pp. 8563-8570, ISSN 1529-2401

Wang, D. et al. (2008). Dispensable role of Drosophila ortholog of LRRK2 kinase activity in survival of dopaminergic neurons, *Mol Neurodegener*, Vol. 3, No. pp. 3, ISSN 1750-1326

Whitworth, A. J. et al. (2005). Increased glutathione S-transferase activity rescues dopaminergic neuron loss in a Drosophila model of Parkinson's disease, *Proceedings of the National Academy of Sciences of the United States of America*, Vol. 102, No. 22, pp. 8024-8029, ISSN 0027-8424

Whitworth, A. J. et al. (2008). Rhomboid-7 and HtrA2/Omi act in a common pathway with the Parkinson's disease factors Pink1 and Parkin, *Dis Model Mech*, Vol. 1, No. 2-3, pp. 168-174; discussion 173, ISSN 1754-8411

Winkler, S. et al. (2007). alpha-Synuclein and Parkinson disease susceptibility, *Neurology*, Vol. 69, No. 18, pp. 1745-1750, ISSN 1526-632X

Wong, K. et al. (2004). Neuropathology provides clues to the pathophysiology of Gaucher disease, *Mol Genet Metab*, Vol. 82, No. 3, pp. 192-207, ISSN 1096-7192

Wonnacott, S. et al. (2000). Presynaptic nicotinic receptors modulating dopamine release in the rat striatum, *European Journal of Pharmacology*, Vol. 393, No. 1-3, pp. 51-58, ISSN 0014-2999

Wu, D. C. et al. (2002). Blockade of microglial activation is neuroprotective in the 1-methyl-4-phenyl-1,2,3,6-tetrahydropyridine mouse model of Parkinson disease, *Journal of Neuroscience*, Vol. 22, No. 5, pp. 1763-1771, ISSN 1529-2401

Yang, W. & Sun, A. Y. (1998). Paraquat-induced free radical reaction in mouse brain microsomes, *Neurochemical Research*, Vol. 23, No. 1, pp. 47-53, ISSN 0364-3190

Yang, Y. et al. (2005). Inactivation of Drosophila DJ-1 leads to impairments of oxidative stress response and phosphatidylinositol 3-kinase/Akt signaling, *Proceedings of the National Academy of Sciences of the United States of America*, Vol. 102, No. 38, pp. 13670-13675, ISSN 0027-8424

Yasuda, T. et al. (2009). Effects of UCH-L1 on alpha-synuclein over-expression mouse model of Parkinson's disease, *Journal of Neurochemistry*, Vol. 108, No. 4, pp. 932-944, ISSN 1471-4159

Yokota, T. et al. (2003). Down regulation of DJ-1 enhances cell death by oxidative stress, ER stress, and proteasome inhibition, *Biochemical and Biophysical Research Communications*, Vol. 312, No. 4, pp. 1342-1348, ISSN 0006-291X

Yun, J. et al. (2008). Loss-of-function analysis suggests that Omi/HtrA2 is not an essential component of the PINK1/PARKIN pathway in vivo, *Journal of Neuroscience*, Vol. 28, No. 53, pp. 14500-14510, ISSN 1529-2401

Zetterstrom, R. H. et al. (1997). Dopamine neuron agenesis in Nurr1-deficient mice, *Science*, Vol. 276, No. 5310, pp. 248-250, ISSN 0036-8075

Zhang, J. et al. (2003). Manganese ethylene-bis-dithiocarbamate and selective dopaminergic neurodegeneration in rat: a link through mitochondrial dysfunction, *Journal of Neurochemistry*, Vol. 84, No. 2, pp. 336-346, ISSN 0022-3042

Zhang, L. et al. (2005). Mitochondrial localization of the Parkinson's disease related protein DJ-1: implications for pathogenesis, *Human Molecular Genetics*, Vol. 14, No. 14, pp. 2063-2073, ISSN 0964-6906

8

Comparison of Normal and Parkinsonian Microcircuit Dynamics in the Rodent Striatum

O. Jaidar, L. Carrillo-Reid and J. Bargas
División de Neurociencias, Instituto de Fisiología Celular,
Universidad Nacional Autónoma de México,
Mexico City,
México

1. Introduction

Experimentally, depriving the basal ganglia (BG) from their dopaminergic innervation, dramatically changes the behavior of all their circuits, neurons, and synapses in multiple ways. Dopamine afferents are received by all BG nuclei (Rommelfanger and Wichmann, 2010). In the absence of DA, BG generate enhanced pathological oscillatory patterns in the external segment of the striatum: globus pallidus (GPe), internal segment of the globus pallidus (GPi), subthalamic nucleus (STN) and substantia nigra pars reticulata (SNr) (Blandini et al., 2000). These pathological oscillatory patterns are expressed as increased cortical beta frequency coherence (Costa et al., 2006; Fuentes et al., 2009; Kozlov et al., 2009; Walters and Bergstrom, 2009) and are reflected as the inability to select, change or initiate motor actions (Magill et al., 2001; Ni et al., 2001; Wilson et al., 2006), as though all neurons were trapped in a massive oscillation that does not allow the selection of any circuit or action. Behaviorally, circuit disfunction is accompanied by bradykinesia, akinesia, tremor and muscular rigidity (Brown, 2007; Hammond et al., 2007; Galvan and Wichmann, 2008; Fuentes et al., 2009; Walters and Bergstrom, 2009; Zold et al., 2009).

One question is what are the manifestations of these changes at the level of the striatal microcircuitry (Alexander and Crutcher, 1990; Middleton and Strick, 2002), given that its neurons are the principal entrance to the BG (Alexander and Crutcher, 1990; Middleton and Strick, 2002), and DA is particularly concentrated in this nucleus (striatum); more than in any other BG nuclei (Bjorklund and Dunnett, 2007). To answer this question, here we show how the striatal microcircuit functions before and after DA depletion. The changes observed may be fundamental to understand BG activity during Parkinsonism.

2. Activity in the striatal microcircuit

The striatum integrates inputs from the cortex, the intralaminar thalamic nuclei, the dopaminergic afferents from the *substantia nigra pars compacta* (SNc) and other nuclei (Smith et al., 1994; Parr-Brownlie et al., 2009). The basic elements that configure the striatal microcircuit are the medium spiny projection neurons (MSNs) and its interneurons (Kreitzer, 2009). MSNs are the major cell population commonly being in a resting state with a polarized membrane potential (ca., -80 mV) and relatively low input resistance (ca., 100

MΩ in adult neurons) (Bargas et al., 1988; Reyes et al., 1998). Upon depolarization, these neurons fire tonically due to persistent voltage-activated K+-currents (Galarraga et al., 1989; Nisenbaum and Wilson, 1995; Bargas et al., 1999), with a long latency to first spike due inactivating K+-currents (Surmeier et al., 1988; Bargas et al., 1989), inward rectification (Galarraga et al., 1994; Nisenbaum and Wilson, 1995), and interspike intervals partially dependent on Ca²⁺-activated K+-currents (Pineda et al., 1992; Bargas et al., 1999), among other outward currents (Nisenbaum and Wilson, 1995; Shen et al., 2005).

MSNs can be classified as striatopallidal or indirect pathway neurons and striatonigral or direct pathway neurons, based on their axonal projections, receptors and peptide expression (Gerfen et al., 1990; Smith et al., 1998). Striatopallidal fibers target the GPe and striatonigral axons target the output nuclei of the BG: GPi and SNr. Interneurons are divided into genres with much intrinsic, still not-well studied variation: i) the parvalbumin-immunoreactive (PV+) or fast spiking interneurons (FS), ii) the somatostatin (SS), neuropeptide Y (NPY), tyrosine hydroxylase (TH), nitric oxide synthase (NOS)-immunoreactive populations of cells that fire with a low threshold calcium spike (LTS), iii) large cholinergic or tonic active neurons (TANs), and iv) calretinin-immunoreactive neurons (Wilson et al., 1990; Kawaguchi et al., 1995; Tepper et al., 2004; Kreitzer, 2009; Ibáñez-Sandoval et al., 2010; Tepper et al., 2010). A challenge is to find out how all these neurons process striatal inputs into coherent spatio-temporal patterned outputs: what is their role in microcircuitry processing. Thus, as a first approach we decided to observe what characteristics of the microcircuit activity are plainly evident in order to establish top-down hypothesis and experimental designs to understand the role of each neuron class during microcircuit activity (Carrillo-Reid et al., 2008).

MSNs seldom fire in physiological conditions (without a motor behavior) (Crutcher and DeLong, 1984; Kimura, 1992; Carrillo-Reid et al., 2008; Liang et al., 2008; Vautrelle, 2009; Jaidar et al., 2010), due to their intrinsic inward rectifying K+ currents and strong depolarization-activated K+-currents (see above and Bargas et al., 1989; Galarraga et al., 1994; Nisenbaum and Wilson, 1995; Bargas et al., 1999; Tepper et al., 2004). Since MSNs are majority, this characteristic makes the striatum to be classified as a quasi-"silent" nucleus; very different from the neurons of other BG nuclei which exhibit firing all the time (e.g., Nakanishi et al., 1987; Kita and Kitai, 1991; Ibáñez-Sandoval et al., 2007). Either activity from the cortex, thalamus, or addition of NMDA in vitro, activates the striatal microcircuits so that groups of MSNs begin to fire in a persistent or recurrent way (Vergara et al., 2003; Mahon et al., 2006; Vautrelle, 2009).

Firing in MSNs is characterized by prolonged membrane potential transitions from a hyperpolarized "down"-state to a depolarized "up"-state where bursts of action potentials are displayed (Wilson and Kawaguchi, 1996; Vergara et al., 2003; Vautrelle, 2009). In vitro, this firing pattern occurs without overt stimulation and is due to an acquired conditional bistability (Vergara et al., 2003; Carrillo-Reid et al., 2008). Because burst firing can also be recorded using calcium-imaging that allow the recording of dozens of cells simultaneously (Cossart et al., 2003), the use of this technique resulted useful to observe how burst firing can extend to neighboring neurons, and how this firing generates network dynamics, that is, to a cell assembly type of processing (Hebb, 1949).

3. The Cell Assembly hypothesis

Cell Assemblies (CAs) have been posited as the building blocks or structures capable to give support and store neuronal representations, or coding, of perceptual, cognitive, and motor processes (Grinvald et al., 2003; Harris, 2005). However, although Hebbian and non-Hebbian types of learning have been formalized and used in artificial neuronal networks under different paradigms (Bowles, 2006), the demonstration of the existence of these structures in living circuits has not been trivial and they are mostly assumed to exist using indirect evidence, such as the correlation of the firing generated by a single, or a small group of neurons, with field or multiunitary population recordings (e.g., Sakurai, 1996; Costa et al., 2006; Zold et al., 2009), or with population activity as revealed by voltage dyes (Grinvald et al., 2003; Grinvald, 2005). Numerous evidences of correlated firing in neurons, using these techniques, are available. However, an inconvenience for cell physiology is that these techniques do not achieve single cell resolution. That is, these techniques cannot identify the elements that participate in a given activity of the microcircuit. If they cannot be identified, a role for them cannot be found or assigned. On the other hand, speculations about how a circuit may function, based on cell-focused studies, are abundant and utterly speculative. Between these two extremes: system and cellular neurophysiology, respectively, there is very little work. To fill the gap we need to make a proper description of network dynamics at the cellular level while recording many cells simultaneous with single cell resolution. In the following section we will describe how this is achieved as well as some properties of the striatal microcircuit that reflect cell assembly organization and dynamics. At the same time, we will describe how these properties change in a Parkinsonian microcircuit.

4. Recurrent bursting

The first property is recurrent burst firing. Striatal neurons fire in bursts of action potentials riding on top of depolarizing plateau potentials called "up-states". This firing mode has been shown in vivo and in vitro (Wilson, 1993; Stern et al., 1997; Vergara et al., 2003). Plateau potentials underlying bursts of spikes can arise from intrinsic nonlinear properties leading to bistability (Hounsgaard and Kiehn, 1989; Hsiao et al., 1998; Kiehn, 2006), from temporal summation of excitatory and inhibitory synaptic events (Sanchez-Vives and McCormick, 2000; Yanagawa and Mogi, 2009), or both (Destexhe and Pare, 1999; Tal et al., 2008). It is possible that the same neurons can generate plateau potentials of different origin depending on network situation (Hounsgaard and Kiehn, 1989; Alaburda et al., 2005; Vautrelle, 2009).

Interestingly, recurrent bursts of action potentials on top of sustained depolarizations (up-states or plateau potentials) resemble a basic property of certain microcircuits called Central Pattern Generators (CPGs) (Grillner, 2006). The main difference between CAs and CPGs is that CPGs activity is thought to be "innate", whereas CAs are supposedly to be "acquired" through synaptic plasticity. CPGs can display their electrical behavior in the absence of afferent inputs, and in isolated tissue maintained vitro, as long as an "excitatory drive" turns them on. In the case of fictive locomotion and swimming, a physiological excitatory drive can be generated pharmacologically: by the addition of micromolar NMDA into the bath saline, a maneuver that induces conditional bistability, plateau potentials and recurrent regular bursting (Grillner et al., 1981; Guertin and Hounsgaard, 1998).

In the striatal microcircuit robust recurrent bursting is induced by the same pharmacological manipulation in vivo (Herrling et al., 1983) and in vitro (Vergara et al., 2003) obtaining an electrophysiological patterned output from spiny neurons; similar to that previously recorded in both CPGs or suspected CAs. Furthermore, unilateral NMDA administration induces contralateral turning behavior directly relating recurrent burst firing in medium spiny neurons with a rhythmic and regular motor behavior (Ossowska, 1995). Then, we can say that the striatal bursting activity under these conditions codes for movement (e.g., Hikosaka et al., 2006).

What happens when the DA is absent? A "logical" common mistake is to think that if a Parkinsonian patient or animal cannot generate movements then, the striatal microcircuit should even be more "silent" that in control conditions. However, it has been shown, *in vitro* and *in vivo*, exactly the opposite: after DA depletion the spontaneous firing and synaptic activity of striatal neurons becomes more active and noisy (Galarraga et al., 1987; Tang et al., 2001; Tseng et al., 2001; Liang et al., 2008). That is, a more robust neuronal activity and bursting can be recorded in the DA-depleted striatum.

5. Correlated firing

The next property observed during CAs physiological behavior, and which can be observed in the striatal microcircuit, is the synchronous or correlated firing of pools of neurons that here will be called "neuronal aggregates". Synchrony or correlated firing (coherence, phase locking) between these auto-associated clusters of neurons make up network states as described in many circuits (e.g., Petersen and Sakmann, 2000; Doupe et al., 2004; Carrillo-Reid et al., 2008; Li et al., 2010). In some cases, the time scale of synchronization is fast: that of synaptic and action potentials duration (Diesmann et al., 1999; Leger et al., 2005; Robbe et al., 2006). However, in most physiological conditions, a great variability in the responses of neurons at the action potential time scale is found (Calvin and Stevens, 1968; Shadlen and Newsome, 1994; Grinvald et al., 2003; Kostal et al., 2007). Thus, synchronicity in the action potential time scale is hard to record in most central nervous system circuits (Shadlen and Newsome, 1994; Arieli et al., 1996) and simulations of that activity change with minimal perturbations (Izhikevich and Edelman, 2008).

Notwithstanding, recurrent burst firing of individual neurons has been found to be synchronized and correlated among several members of a neuronal aggregate (Carrillo-Reid et al., 2008), and also in population recordings of network conditions in which a given neuron participates: its "preferred condition" (Grinvald et al., 2003). Moreover, up-states and bursting have been found to be a reflection of an attractor-like network dynamics (Cossart et al., 2003) capable to recruit connected neurons into a preferred aggregate. Connections, internal to the aggregate, can in part explain the maintenance of bursts shared by the elements of the group (Lambe and Aghajanian, 2007). That is, the up-state is a product or reflection of the correlated firing of a group of interconnected neurons.

In the striatum, correlated firing has been inferred by recording local field potentials correlated with neuronal firing (Murer et al., 2002; Berke et al., 2004; Costa et al., 2006; Mahon et al., 2006; Walters et al., 2007; Zold et al., 2009). Also, the use of calcium imaging techniques, which records bursting behavior of several cells simultaneously, reveals spontaneous peaks of burst synchronization and correlated firing after the application of NMDA (Carrillo-Reid et al., 2008) (See Figure). That is, recurrent bursting recorded in single neurons (Vergara et al., 2003) has been demonstrated to be shared by sets of neurons that spontaneously synchronize their bursts in a particular condition (Carrillo-Reid et al., 2008). During Parkinsonism caused by DA-depletion, the recording of pathological bursting activity exhibit an increase in the number of synchrony peaks (Jaidar et al., 2010). Synchronizing events emerge spontaneously and regularly during recordings. Up-states are the manifestation of a network phenomenon linking neurons that sometimes are located far

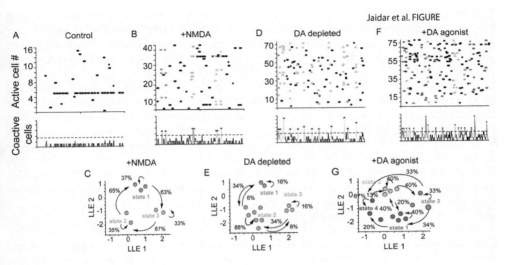

Fig. 1. Following the striatal microcircuit with calcium imaging.

A. Top: A raster plot showing the activity of a striatal slice in control conditions. It exhibits a few active neurons (y-axis = number of active neurons; files, x-axis = time = 3 min recording). No active neurons synchronized their bursting significantly with other neurons. Bottom: histogram representing activity displayed in the raster plot on top (sum of columns).

B. Top: After adding 8 µM NMDA to the bath saline more neurons become active (> 40). Colored dots shows peaks of significant spontaneous synchronization. Bottom: activity histogram shows the spontaneous peaks of synchronization (colored with asterisks) (P<0.05 dashed horizontal line).

C. Locally linear embedding (LLE) was used to reduce dimensions of the peaks of synchronization and to project the vectors in a two dimensional space. Column vectors representing similar neurons are represented by clusters of neighboring circles of the same color (network states). Note that neuronal aggregates follow a sequence when displaying their activity, that is, the microcircuit shows its dynamics as an activity cycle or phase sequence. This sequence of network states is robust and may repeat itself several times during about two hours of recording time (only one representative epoch = 3 min is shown).

D. Top: After dopamine depletion (DA-depletion) a striatal slice exhibits more active neurons than with NMDA (> 70). No NMDA is added to DA-depleted slices. That is, DA absence induces that more neurons in the microcircuit become active. Bottom: nevertheless, the same peak of synchrony repeats itself almost all the time during recording. That is, microcircuit dynamics is greatly lost. DA was lowered using the 6-OHDA model of Parkinsonism. The toxin was injected into the substantia nigra pars compacta and the experiments were done after observing turning behavior in lesioned animals.

E: LLE obtained from a DA-depleted slice shows that one network state becomes dominant impeding normal dynamics.

F: When a dopamine receptor agonist (1 µM SKF-81296) is administered in a slice with DA-depletion, diverse peaks of synchrony with high probability of occurrence return. However, the number of active neurons is still high.

G: LLE shows that microcircuit dynamics tends to be restored because the dominant network state is dissolved (see: Carrillo-Reid et al., 2008; Carrillo-Reid et al., 2009; Jaidar et al., 2010).

way from each other (Stern et al., 1997; Carrillo-Reid et al., 2008). Strikingly, in the striatal parkinsonian microcircuit all active neurons synchronize their bursts with one another (Jaidar et al., 2010). No matter what is the predominant component of an up-state: intrinsic, synaptic or both, the important feature is that up-states work as "windows" for synchronization and correlated activity (Yuste et al., 2005), while action potentials within the up-states need not be synchronized (Wickens and Wilson, 1998). A signature of a CAs is that its inputs do not determine all its outputs all the time, in a deterministic way. On the contrary, the spike trains are variable due to the simultaneous integration of inputs within internal circuitry states (Arieli et al., 1996; Grinvald et al., 2003; Harris, 2005).

As stated by the modified Hebbian learning theory, sets of neurons display synchronous or correlated firing because LTP has strengthened the connections among them: "neurons that fire together wire together", whereas LTD has weakened some synapses due to their uncorrelated firing leading to the separation of different neuronal aggregates. Thus, connections within a neuronal ensemble are non-random (Kozloski et al., 2001; Song et al., 2005; Planert et al., 2010). There are preferred pathways for the flow of activity (Markram et al., 1997; Ikegaya et al., 2004; Song et al., 2005) even if anatomically they seem intermingled (Grinvald et al., 2003; Harris, 2005; Song et al., 2005). In conclusion, recurrent bursting elicited in striatal neurons can be seen as the product of correlated firing among neurons belonging to groups or ensembles. The time window for synchronization is the up-state and the product of the ensemble is the same up-state shared by the neurons of the ensemble. Most probably, neurons sharing up-states do in fact maintain these plateau potentials along time due to their strong interconnections (Flores-Barrera et al., 2010).

6. Microcircuit dynamics as sequences of network states

In what follows, a peak of synchronized activity generated by the members of a neuron aggregate or cluster will be called a network state. Therefore, what is recorded using calcium imaging is sequences of network states. That is, different neuronal aggregates with correlated firing, alternate the activity among them following determined sequences (Figure). These sequences result in particular trajectories, sometimes following Hamiltonian or Eulerian rules (Carrillo-Reid et al., 2009). In the case of CPGs, it is clear that what flows through the circuit is the correlated activity of neuron pools that activate in a rhythmic, alternating and recurrent way, making up sequences of activity called "activity cycles" (Grillner, 2003). Activity cycles code for repetitive behaviors such as locomotion, deglutition, swimming, scratching and so on. Activity cycles can go on spontaneously even when the physiological stimulus is no longer active, such as in vitro "ficitive locomotion" (Guertin and Hounsgaard, 1998).

But recursive activity of this sort has also been postulated for CAs where they are called "phase sequences" by DO Hebb (1949), a term coined for chains of neuronal aggregates activated in sequence, each one displaying a network state (Harris, 2005).

In the striatum, the trajectories followed by active CAs may change as a result of the presence of particular modulatory neurotransmitters (Carrillo-Reid et al., 2008; Carrillo-Reid et al., 2009a). This quality allows the striatal circuit to generate diverse phase sequences that probably code for different behaviors while using the same neuronal aggregates.

Interestingly, in the absence of DA, phase sequences are lost. Almost all active neurons participate in the same, repetitive, network state, that apparently is not coding for a useful command or motor program (Jaidar et al., 2010). The normal dynamics of the microcircuit is gone (Figure). Addition of DA agonists under DA depleted states is capable to modify this state of affairs and partially restore a phase sequence (Jaidar et al., 2010).

To conclude, the striatal microcircuit generates phase sequences, activity trajectories, or cycles, that are lost during DA-depletion but that can be partially restored with DA receptor agonists. Because these methods allow the visualization of these phenomena with single cell resolution, they may be used to test anti-parkinsonian drugs and to search into the details of microcircuitry processing.

7. Final remarks

Over the last century two main visions of neuronal circuits have been generated from experimental data: First, the theory of Central Pattern Generators (CPGs) and, second, the theory of Hebbian Cell Assemblies. What we would like to stress here is that the time has come for a re-synthesis of both into a new microcircuit hypothesis, while new experimental evidence arrives. For instance, their requirements are very much the same. And since they were proposed somewhat independently, we have to conclude that biological evidence that put them forward is robust. Imaging technology used in conjunction with targeted recordings will allow the discerning of their operational rules in control and in pathological situations (Cossart et al., 2003; Grinvald et al., 2003; Carrillo-Reid et al., 2008 ; 2009a; Jaidar et al., 2010). It perhaps will be possible to record, compare and describe diverse pathological microcircuits. These microcircuits could then be challenged with therapeutic manipulations of potential value.

8. References

Alaburda A, Russo R, MacAulay N, Hounsgaard J (2005) Periodic high-conductance states in spinal neurons during scratch-like network activity in adult turtles. J Neurosci 25:6316-6321.

Alexander GE, Crutcher MD (1990) Functional architecture of basal ganglia circuits: neural substrates of parallel processing. Trends Neurosci 13:266-271.

Arieli A, Sterkin A, Grinvald A, Aertsen A (1996) Dynamics of ongoing activity: explanation of the large variability in evoked cortical responses. Science 273:1868-1871.

Bargas J, Galarraga E, Aceves J (1988) Electrotonic properties of neostriatal neurons are modulated by extracellular potassium. Exp Brain Res 72:390-398.

Bargas J, Galarraga E, Aceves J (1989) An early outward conductance modulates the firing latency and frequency of neostriatal neurons of the rat brain. Exp Brain Res 75:146-156.

Bargas J, Ayala CX, Vilchis C, Pineda JC, Galarraga E (1999) Ca^{2+}-activated outward currents in neostriatal neurons. Neurosci 88:479-488.

Berke JD, Okatan M, Skurski J, Eichenbaum HB (2004) Oscillatory entrainment of striatal neurons in freely moving rats. Neuron 43:883-896.

Bjorklund A, Dunnett SB (2007) Dopamine neuron systems in the brain: an update. Trends Neurosci 30:194-202.

Blandini F, Nappi G, Tassorelli C, Martignoni E (2000) Functional changes of the basal ganglia circuitry in Parkinson's disease. Prog Neurobiol 62:63-88.

Bowles R (2006) Investigating the Storage Capacity of a Network with Cell Assemblies. In. UK: Middlesex University.

Brown P (2007) Abnormal oscillatory synchronisation in the motor system leads to impaired movement. Curr Opin Neurobiol 17:656-664.

Calvin WH, Stevens CF (1968) Synaptic noise and other sources of randomness in motoneuron interspike intervals. J Neurophysiol 31:574-587.

Carrillo-Reid L, Tecuapetla F, Ibanez-Sandoval O, Hernandez-Cruz A, Galarraga E, Bargas J (2009) Activation of the cholinergic system endows compositional properties to striatal cell assemblies. J Neurophysiol 101:737-749.

Carrillo-Reid L, Tecuapetla F, Tapia D, Hernandez-Cruz A, Galarraga E, Drucker-Colin R, Bargas J (2008) Encoding network states by striatal cell assemblies. J Neurophysiol 99:1435-1450.

Cossart R, Aronov D, Yuste R (2003) Attractor dynamics of network UP states in the neocortex. Nature 423:283-288.

Costa RM, Lin SC, Sotnikova TD, Cyr M, Gainetdinov RR, Caron MG, Nicolelis MA (2006) Rapid alterations in corticostriatal ensemble coordination during acute dopamine-dependent motor dysfunction. Neuron 52:359-369.

Crutcher MD, DeLong MR (1984) Single cell studies of the primate putamen. II. Relations to direction of movement and pattern of muscular activity. Exp Brain Res 53:244-258.

Destexhe A, Pare D (1999) Impact of network activity on the integrative properties of neocortical pyramidal neurons in vivo. J Neurophysiol 81:1531-1547.

Diesmann M, Gewaltig MO, Aertsen A (1999) Stable propagation of synchronous spiking in cortical neural networks. Nature 402:529-533.

Doupe AJ, Solis MM, Kimpo R, Boettiger CA (2004) Cellular, circuit, and synaptic mechanisms in song learning. Ann N Y Acad Sci 1016:495-523.

Flores-Barrera E, Vizcarra-Chacon BJ, Tapia D, Bargas J, Galarraga E (2010) Different corticostriatal integration in spiny projection neurons from direct and indirect pathways. Front Syst Neurosci 4:15.

Fuentes R, Petersson P, Siesser WB, Caron MG, Nicolelis MA (2009) Spinal cord stimulation restores locomotion in animal models of Parkinson's disease. Science 323:1578-1582.

Galarraga E, Bargas J, Martinez-Fong D, Aceves J (1987) Spontaneous synaptic potentials in dopamine-denervated neostriatal neurons. Neurosci Lett 81:351-355.

Galarraga E, Bargas J, Sierra A, Aceves J (1989) The role of calcium in the repetitive firing of neostriatal neurons. Exp Brain Res 75:157-168.

Galarraga E, Pacheco-Cano MT, Flores-Hernández JV, Bargas J (1994) Subthreshold rectification in neostriatal spiny projection neurons. Exp Brain Res 100:239-249.

Galvan A, Wichmann T (2008) Pathophysiology of parkinsonism. Clin Neurophysiol 119:1459-1474.

Gerfen CR, Engber TM, Mahan LC, Susel Z, Chase TN, Monsma FJ, Jr., Sibley DR (1990) D1 and D2 dopamine receptor-regulated gene expression of striatonigral and striatopallidal neurons. Science 250:1429-1432.

Grillner S (2003) The motor infrastructure: from ion channels to neuronal networks. Nat Rev Neurosci 4:573-586.

Grillner S (2006) Biological pattern generation: the cellular and computational logic of networks in motion. Neuron 52:751-766.

Grillner S, McClellan A, Sigvardt K, Wallen P, Wilen M (1981) Activation of NMDA-receptors elicits "fictive locomotion" in lamprey spinal cord in vitro. Acta Physiol Scand 113:549-551.

Grinvald A (2005) Imaging input and output dynamics of neocortical networks in vivo: exciting times ahead. Proc Natl Acad Sci U S A 102:14125-14126.

Grinvald A, Arieli A, Tsodyks M, Kenet T (2003) Neuronal assemblies: single cortical neurons are obedient members of a huge orchestra. Biopolymers 68:422-436.

Guertin PA, Hounsgaard J (1998) NMDA-Induced intrinsic voltage oscillations depend on L-type calcium channels in spinal motoneurons of adult turtles. J Neurophysiol 80:3380-3382.

Hammond C, Bergman H, Brown P (2007) Pathological synchronization in Parkinson's disease: networks, models and treatments. Trends Neurosci 30:357-364.

Harris KD (2005) Neural signatures of cell assembly organization. Nature Rev Neurosci 6:399-407.

Hebb DO (1949) The organization of behavior. New York: Wiley.

Herrling PL, Morris R, Salt TE (1983) Effects of excitatory amino acids and their antagonists on membrane and action potentials of cat caudate neurones. J Physiol 339:207-222.

Hikosaka O, Nakamura K, Nakahara H (2006) Basal ganglia orient eyes to reward. J Neurophysiol 95:567-584.

Hounsgaard J, Kiehn O (1989) Serotonin-induced bistability of turtle motoneurones caused by a nifedipine-sensitive calcium plateau potential. J Physiol 414:265-282.

Hsiao CF, Del Negro CA, Trueblood PR, Chandler SH (1998) Ionic basis for serotonin-induced bistable membrane properties in guinea pig trigeminal motoneurons. J Neurophysiol 79:2847-2856.

Ibáñez-Sandoval O, Tecuapetla F, Unal B, Shah F, Koós T, Tepper JM (2010) Electrophysiological and morphological characteristics and synaptic connectivity of tyrosine hydroxylase-expressing neurons in adult mouse striatum. J Neurosci 30:6999-7016.

Ibáñez-Sandoval O, Carrillo-Reid L, Galarraga E, Tapia D, Mendoza E, Gomora JC, Aceves J, Bargas J (2007) Bursting in substantia nigra pars reticulata neurons in vitro: possible relevance for Parkinson disease. J Neurophysiol 98:2311-2323.

Ikegaya Y, Aaron G, Cossart R, Aronov D, Lampl I, Ferster D, Yuste R (2004) Synfire chains and cortical songs: temporal modules of cortical activity. Science 304:559-564.

Izhikevich EM, Edelman GM (2008) Large-scale model of mammalian thalamocortical systems. Proc Natl Acad Sci U S A 105:3593-3598.

Jaidar O, Carrillo-Reid L, Hernandez A, Drucker-Colin R, Bargas J, Hernandez-Cruz A (2010) Dynamics of the Parkinsonian striatal microcircuit: entrainment into a dominant network state. J Neurosci 30:11326-11336.

Kawaguchi Y, Wilson CJ, Augood SJ, Emson PC (1995) Striatal interneurones: chemical, physiological and morphological characterization. Trends Neurosci 18:527-535.

Kiehn O (2006) Locomotor circuits in the mammalian spinal cord. Annu Rev Neurosci 29:279-306.

Kimura M (1992) Behavioral modulation of sensory responses of primate putamen neurons. Brain Res 578:204-214.

Kita H, Kitai ST (1991) Intracellular study of rat globus pallidus neurons: membrane properties and responses to neostriatal, subthalamic and nigral stimulation. Brain Res 564:296-305.

Kostal L, Lansky P, Rospars JP (2007) Neuronal coding and spiking randomness. Eur J Neurosci 26:2693-2701.

Kozloski J, Hamzei-Sichani F, Yuste R (2001) Stereotyped position of local synaptic targets in neocortex. Science 293:868-872.

Kozlov A, Huss M, Lansner A, Kotaleski JH, Grillner S (2009) Simple cellular and network control principles govern complex patterns of motor behavior. Proc Natl Acad Sci U S A 106:20027-20032.

Kreitzer AC (2009) Physiology and pharmacology of striatal neurons. Annu Rev Neurosci 32:127-147.

Lambe EK, Aghajanian GK (2007) Prefrontal cortical network activity: Opposite effects of psychedelic hallucinogens and D1/D5 dopamine receptor activation. Neuroscience 145:900-910.

Leger JF, Stern EA, Aertsen A, Heck D (2005) Synaptic integration in rat frontal cortex shaped by network activity. J Neurophysiol 93:281-293.

Li X, Ouyang G, Usami A, Ikegaya Y, Sik A (2010) Scale-free topology of the CA3 hippocampal network: a novel method to analyze functional neuronal assemblies. Biophys J 98:1733-1741.

Liang L, DeLong MR, Papa SM (2008) Inversion of dopamine responses in striatal medium spiny neurons and involuntary movements. J Neurosci 28:7537-7547.

Magill PJ, Bolam JP, Bevan MD (2001) Dopamine regulates the impact of the cerebral cortex on the subthalamic nucleus-globus pallidus network. Neuroscience 106:313-330.

Mahon S, Vautrelle N, Pezard L, Slaght SJ, Deniau JM, Chouvet G, Charpier S (2006) Distinct patterns of striatal medium spiny neuron activity during the natural sleep-wake cycle. J Neurosci 26:12587-12595.

Markram H, Lubke J, Frotscher M, Roth A, Sakmann B (1997) Physiology and anatomy of synaptic connections between thick tufted pyramidal neurones in the developing rat neocortex. J Physiol 500 (Pt 2):409-440.

Middleton FA, Strick PL (2002) Basal-ganglia 'projections' to the prefrontal cortex of the primate. Cereb Cortex 12:926-935.

Murer MG, Tseng KY, Kasanetz F, Belluscio M, Riquelme LA (2002) Brain oscillations, medium spiny neurons, and dopamine. Cell Mol Neurobiol 22:611-632.

Nakanishi H, Kita H, Kitai ST (1987) Electrical membrane properties of rat subthalamic neurons in an in vitro slice preparation. Brain Res 437:35-44.

Ni ZG, Bouali-Benazzouz R, Gao DM, Benabid AL, Benazzouz A (2001) Time-course of changes in firing rates and firing patterns of subthalamic nucleus neuronal activity after 6-OHDA-induced dopamine depletion in rats. Brain Res 899:142-147.

Nisenbaum ES, Wilson CJ (1995) Potassium currents responsible for inward and outward rectification in rat neostriatal spiny projection neurons. J Neurosci 15:4449-4463.

Ossowska K (1995) Interaction between striatal excitatory amino acid and gamma-aminobutyric acid (GABA) receptors in the turning behaviour of rats. Neurosci Lett 202:57-60.

Parr-Brownlie LC, Poloskey SL, Bergstrom DA, Walters JR (2009) Parafascicular thalamic nucleus activity in a rat model of Parkinson's disease. Exp Neurol 217:269-281.

Petersen CC, Sakmann B (2000) The excitatory neuronal network of rat layer 4 barrel cortex. J Neurosci 20:7579-7586.

Pineda JC, Galarraga E, Bargas J, Cristancho JM, Aceves J (1992) Charybdotoxin and apamin sensitivity of the calcium-dependent repolarization and the afterhyperpolarization in neostriatal neurons. J Neurophysiol 68:287-294.

Planert H, Szydlowski SN, Hjorth JJ, Grillner S, Silberberg G (2010) Dynamics of synaptic transmission between fast-spiking interneurons and striatal projection neurons of the direct and indirect pathways. J Neurosci 30:3499-3507.

Reyes A, Galarraga E, Flores-Hernández J, Tapia D, Bargas J (1998) Passive properties of neostriatal neurons during potassium conductance blockade. Exp Brain Res 120:70-84.

Robbe D, Montgomery SM, Thome A, Rueda-Orozco PE, McNaughton BL, Buzsaki G (2006) Cannabinoids reveal importance of spike timing coordination in hippocampal function. Nat Neurosci 9:1526-1533.

Rommelfanger KS, Wichmann T (2010) Extrastriatal dopaminergic circuits of the basal ganglia. Front Neuroanat 4:139.

Sakurai Y (1996) Hippocampal and neocortical cell assemblies encode memory processes for different types of stimuli in the rat. J Neurosci 16:2809-2819.

Sanchez-Vives MV, McCormick DA (2000) Cellular and network mechanisms of rhythmic recurrent activity in neocortex. Nat Neurosci 3:1027-1034.

Shadlen MN, Newsome WT (1994) Noise, neural codes and cortical organization. Curr Opin Neurobiol 4:569-579.

Shen W, Hamilton SE, Nathanson NM, Surmeier DJ (2005) Cholinergic suppression of KCNQ channel currents enhances excitability of striatal medium spiny neurons. J Neurosci 25:7449-7458.

Smith Y, Bevan MD, Shink E, Bolam JP (1998) Microcircuitry of the direct and indirect pathways of the basal ganglia. Neuroscience 86:353-387.

Smith Y, Bennett BD, Bolam JP, Parent A, Sadikot AF (1994) Synaptic relationships between dopaminergic afferents and cortical or thalamic input in the sensorimotor territory of the striatum in monkey. J Comp Neurol 344:1-19.

Song S, Sjostrom PJ, Reigl M, Nelson S, Chklovskii DB (2005) Highly nonrandom features of synaptic connectivity in local cortical circuits. PLoS Biol 3:e68.

Stern EA, Kincaid AE, Wilson CJ (1997) Spontaneous subthreshold membrane potential fluctuations and action potential variability of rat corticostriatal and striatal neurons in vivo. J Neurophysiol 77:1697-1715.

Surmeier DJ, Bargas J, Kitai ST (1988) Voltage-clamp analysis of a transient potassium current in rat neostriatal neurons. Brain Res 473:187-192.

Tal Z, Chorev E, Yarom Y (2008) State-dependent modification of complex spike waveforms in the cerebellar cortex. Cerebellum 7:577-582.

Tang K, Low MJ, Grandy DK, Lovinger DM (2001) Dopamine-dependent synaptic plasticity in striatum during in vivo development. Proc Natl Acad Sci U S A 98:1255-1260.

Tepper JM, Koos T, Wilson CJ (2004) GABAergic microcircuits in the neostriatum. Trends Neurosci 27:662-669.

Tepper JM, Tecuapetla F, Koos T, Ibanez-Sandoval O (2010) Heterogeneity and diversity of striatal GABAergic interneurons. Front Neuroanat 4:150.

Tseng KY, Kasanetz F, Kargieman L, Riquelme LA, Murer MG (2001) Cortical slow oscillatory activity is reflected in the membrane potential and spike trains of striatal neurons in rats with chronic nigrostriatal lesions. J Neurosci 21:6430-6439.

Vautrelle N, Carrillo-Reid, L., Bargas, J. (2009) Diversity of up-state voltage transitions during different network states. In: Cortico-Subcortical Dynamics in Parkinson Disease (Tseng KY, ed), pp 73-85. New York: Humana/Springer.

Vergara R, Rick C, Hernandez-Lopez S, Laville JA, Guzman JN, Galarraga E, Surmeier DJ, Bargas J (2003) Spontaneous voltage oscillations in striatal projection neurons in a rat corticostriatal slice. J Physiol 553:169-182.

Walters JR, Bergstrom DA (2009) Basal ganglia network synchronization in animal models of Parkinson's disease. In: Cortico-Subcortical Dynamics in Parkinson Disease (Tseng KY, ed), pp 117-142. New York: Humana/Springer.

Walters JR, Hu D, Itoga CA, Parr-Brownlie LC, Bergstrom DA (2007) Phase relationships support a role for coordinated activity in the indirect pathway in organizing slow oscillations in basal ganglia output after loss of dopamine. Neuroscience 144:762-776.

Wickens JR, Wilson CJ (1998) Regulation of action-potential firing in spiny neurons of the rat neostriatum in vivo. J Neurophysiol 79:2358-2364.

Wilson CJ (1993) The generation of natural firing patterns in neostriatal neurons. Prog Brain Res 99:277-297.

Wilson CJ, Kawaguchi Y (1996) The origins of two-state spontaneous membrane potential fluctuations of neostriatal spiny neurons. J Neurosci 16:2397-2410.

Wilson CJ, Chang HT, Kitai ST (1990) Firing patterns and synaptic potentials of identified giant aspiny interneurons in the rat neostriatum. J Neurosci 10:508-519.

Wilson CL, Cash D, Galley K, Chapman H, Lacey MG, Stanford IM (2006) Subthalamic nucleus neurones in slices from 1-methyl-4-phenyl-1,2,3,6-tetrahydropyridine-lesioned mice show irregular, dopamine-reversible firing pattern changes, but without synchronous activity. Neuroscience 143:565-572.

Yanagawa T, Mogi K (2009) Analysis of ongoing dynamics in neural networks. Neurosci Res 64:177-184.

Yuste R, MacLean JN, Smith J, Lansner A (2005) The cortex as a central pattern generator. Nat Rev Neurosci 6:477-483.

Zold CL, Belluscio M, Kasanetz F, Pomata PE, Riquelme LA, Gonon F, Murer MG (2009) Converging into a unified model of Parkinson's disease pathophysiology. In: Cortico-Subcortical Dynamics in Parkinson Disease (Tseng KY, ed), pp 143-156. New York: Humana/Springer.

9

Neuroprotective Effects of Herbal Butanol Extracts from *Gynostemma pentaphyllum* on the Exposure to Chronic Stress in a 6-Hydroxydopamine-Lesioned Rat Model of Parkinson's Disease Treated with or Without L-DOPA

Myung Koo Lee[1] et al.[*]
[1]College of Pharmacy and Research Center for Bioresource and Health,
Chungbuk National University, Cheongju
Republic of Korea

1. Introduction

Parkinson's disease (PD), which is characterized by the degeneration of dopaminergic neurons in the substantia nigra pars compacta, is accompanied by symptoms of muscular rigidity, bradykinesia, rest tremor, and loss of postural balance (Fearnley & Lees, 1991). Mitochondrial dysfunction by reactive oxygen species (ROS)-induced oxidative stress has also been suggested to be important in the loss of dopaminergic neurons in PD (Ozawa et al., 1990). Therefore, the degeneration of the dopaminergic nigrostriatal tracts in PD results in a corresponding decrease in the levels of dopamine and its metabolites, including 3,4-dihydroxyphenylacetic acid (DOPAC), homovanillic acid (HVA), and norepinephrine (Hornykiewicz, 1982).

3,4-Dihydroxyphenylalanine (L-DOPA), the precursor of dopamine, is the most prescribed therapy for the symptomatic relief of PD (Neil & David, 2008; Marsden, 1994). However, chronic prolonged therapy for PD with L-DOPA results in a loss of drug efficacy and irreversible adverse effects, and subsequently leads to the development of motor complications, such as fluctuation and dyskinesia (Jankovic, 2005). L-DOPA and dopamine can accelerate the degenerative process in the residual cells in patients with PD and induce oxidative stress-induced neurotoxicity by generating ROS in primary dopaminergic neurons and dopaminergic cell lines (Cheng et al., 1996). ROS generation leads to neuronal damage and apoptotic or non-apoptotic cell death (Walkinshaw & Waters, 1995). Dopaminergic neurons are in a perpetual state of oxidative stress, and this imbalance may lead to reduced levels of endogenous antioxidants (Merad-Boudia, 1998). In addition, chronic treatment with L-DOPA

[*]Hyun Sook Choi[1], Chen Lei[1], Kwang Hoon Suh[1], Keon Sung Shin[1], Seung Hwan Kim[2],
Bang Yeon Hwang[1] and Chong Kil Lee[1]
[2]College of Physical Education, Kyunghee University, Youngin, Republic of Korea

leads to the production of a specific dopaminergic neurotoxin, 6-hydroxydopamine (6-OHDA), in the striatum of rodents (Borah & Mohanakumar, 2010). These results fuel the search for new agents for PD that are anti-oxidative substances or non-dopaminergic alternatives that can relieve the L-DOPA-induced cytotoxicity.

Various stressful stimuli can induce the production of many ROS and activate both the sympathetic nervous system and the hypothalamic-pituitary-adrenal-axis (Ganong, 2001), which increases the release of dopamine, norepinephrine, epinephrine, glucocorticoids, glutamate, and corticotropin releasing factor in the brain and peripheral circulation (Kandel et al., 2000). Chronic stress-induced adverse reactions are increased in neurodegenerative diseases, including anxiety disorders, depression, schizophrenia, stroke, Alzheimer's disease, and PD (Amanda et al., 2002). For example, the tremor in PD may be worsened by anxiety or anger (Schwab & Zieoer, 1965). In addition, a decrease in dopamine levels and an enhancement of dopamine turnover have been observed in 1-methyl-4-phenyl-1,2,3,6-tetrahydropyridine (MPTP)-treated mice after immersion immobilization stress, resulting in the mice being remarkably akinetic (Urakami et al., 1988). Repeated or relatively prolonged exposure to stress can also change central dopamine biosynthesis and extracellular dopamine levels in rat models (Ahmed et al., 1955), and changes in the cellular characteristics in the prefrontal cortex, such as dendritic atrophy and neuronal loss, have been found in response to stress (Rajkowska, 2000).

The stereotaxic injection of 6-OHDA into the substantia nigra, medial forebrain bundle, and striatum of the brain has been commonly used to produce experimental animal models of PD. These injections selectively injure dopaminergic neurons through the formation of various ROS (Perese et al., 1989). In addition, anti-oxidants, such as glutathione, catalase, and N-acetylcysteine, have been shown to be protective against 6-OHDA-induced cytotoxicity in PC12 and dopaminergic cells (Przedborski et al., 1995; Paxinos & Watson, 1986).

Gynostemma pentaphyllum (Cucurbitaceae; GP) is usually used as an herbal tea, and it is widely believed to result in various protective and functional improvements in diabetes, depression, anxiety, fatigue, hyperlipidemia, immunity, oxidative stress, and tumors (Razmovski-Naumovski et al., 2001). The major constituents of GP, which have been isolated, are a number of gypenoside derivatives (Razmovski-Naumovski et al., 2001). The gypenoside-rich fraction shows neuroprotective effects in the MPTP-induced mouse model of PD (Wang et al., 2010). The ethanol extract from GP has been found to have anti-stress and immunomodulatory functions in mice (Choi et al., 2008; Im et al., 2009). GP ethanol extract also exhibits protective effects against neurotoxicity by reducing tyrosine hydroxylase (TH) neuronal cell death and by normalizing dopamine levels in the 6-OHDA-lesioned rat model of PD (Choi et al., 2010). These results suggest that GP may function as a potential therapeutic and antioxidant in PD. The ethanol extract of GP was partitioned to obtain the butanol extract (GP-BX). GP-BX has been shown to have gypenoside-rich components, which were identified as gypenoside derivatives, and these include gynosaponin TN-1, gynosaponin TN-2, gypenoside XLV, and gypenoside LXXIV (Choi et al., 2010; Razmovski-Naumovski et al., 2005; Nagai et al., 1981; Takemoto et al., 1984; Yoshikawa et al., 1987).

The purpose of the present study was to investigate whether orally administered GP-BX obtained from the leaves of GP had protective effects against chronic stress in the 6-OHDA-lesioned rat model of PD with or without long-term L-DOPA treatment. Dopaminergic neuronal cell death induced by chronic stress in 6-OHDA-lesioned rats was blocked by the coadministration of GP-BX, and this was shown by histochemical (the number of surviving TH-immunopositive neuronal cells) and neurochemical (dopamine, DOPAC, HVA, and norepinephrine levels) techniques.

2. Experimental methods

2.1 Chemicals
L-DOPA, 6-OHDA, dopamine, norepinephrine, DOPAC, HVA, benserazide hydrochloride, apomorphine, and L-ascorbic acid were purchased from Sigma-Aldrich Co. (St. Louis, MO, USA). TH antibody was obtained from Millipore (Temecula, CA, USA). Anti-mouse IgG, Vectastain diaminobenzidine (DAB), and avidin/biotin complex (ABC) kits were purchased form Vector Laboratories, Inc. (Burlingame, CA, USA). All other chemicals were of analytical grade.

2.2 Preparation of GP-BX
GP was obtained from Geochang (Gyungnam, Korea), and a voucher specimen of the herbal leaves of GP was deposited at the herbarium of the College of Pharmacy, Chungbuk National University (Cheongju, Korea). The air-dried leaves of GP (10 kg) were extracted with ethanol (80%, v/v), and then the ethanol extracts were evaporated to dryness (GP ethanol extract, 1.05 kg; yield, 10.5%, w/w). The dry GP ethanol extracts (1 kg) were suspended in water and portioned subsequently with n-hexane, ethylacetate, and n-butanol. The final butanol extracts were evaporated to dryness under reduced pressure and temperature (GP-BX, 155 g; yield, 15.5%, w/w).

2.3 Animals
Rats (Sprague-Dawley, male, 200–250 g) were purchased from Samtako Co. (Animal Breeding Center, Osan, Korea). Animals were housed two per cage in a temperature-controlled environment with a 12-h light/dark cycle (lights on at 07:00) and with *ad libitum* access to standard rat food and water. All procedures were performed according to the guidelines of the Animal Ethics Committee of College of Pharmacy (Chungbuk National University).

2.4 Preparation of 6-OHDA-lesioned rats
The rats were anesthetized intraperitoneally with Zoletil 50 (100 mg/kg, Virbac, Carros, France) and placed in a stereotaxic stand (David Kopf Instruments, Tujunga, CA, USA). The coordinates for the striatum were measured accurately (antero-posterior, AP: -5.3 mm; lateral, ML: +1.9 mm; dorso-ventral, DV: -7.5 mm; relative to bregma). Next, 6-OHDA (8 µg/2 µL in saline solution containing 0.1% of L-ascorbic acid) was injected into the left substantia nigra pars compacta at 1 µL/min using a Hamilton syringe. After the injection, the needle was left in place for 5 min before being retracted in order to allow for complete diffusion of the medium. The rats were left until they had recovered from the anesthesia. Two weeks after the surgery, rats were challenged with apomorphine (0.5 mg/kg, s.c.), and the contralateral rotation was monitored. Rats showing fewer than 150 rotations per 30 min were excluded from further studies.

2.5 The exposure to chronic stress

Two weeks after the 6-OHDA lesions, the rats were placed individually in the electrified shock chamber for the exposure to chronic stress, and they received unavoidable electric footshock (EF) (intensity, 0.2 mA; duration, 10 s; interval, 10 min) at 14:00 every other day for 28 days using a shock generator (Seil Electric Co., Taejeon, Korea).

2.6 Drug treatment

Rats were divided into four groups with each group containing 7–10 rats. GP-BX (30 mg/kg), which was freshly prepared every day with water, was administered to 6-OHDA-lesioned rats orally (p.o.) once a day for 28 days. L-DOPA (10 mg/kg, i.p.) was treated with benserazide (15 mg/kg, i.p.) prepared in saline in order to prevent the peripheral decarboxylation of L-DOPA. The rats were sacrificed the day after the last exposure to stress and GP-BX administration. The experimental design was described as follows.

Experiment I:

Group I (normal rat groups): received 3 µL of saline containing 0.1% L-ascorbic acid by stereotaxic injection into the substantia nigra.
Group II (6-OHDA-lesioned rat groups): received 6-OHDA (8 µg/2 µL in saline solution containing 0.1% of L-ascorbic acid) by stereotaxic injection into the left substantia nigra.
Group III (6-OHDA-lesioned rat groups + chronic EF stress): exposed to EF stress for 28 days two weeks after receiving 6-OHDA (8 µg/2 µL).
Group IV (6-OHDA-lesioned rat groups + chronic EF stress + GP-BX): administered GP-BX (30 mg/kg) for 28 days to EF stress-exposed 6-OHDA-lesioned rat groups (Group III).

Experiment II:

Group I (L-DOPA-treated 6-OHDA-lesioned rat groups): treated with L-DOPA (10 mg/kg) for 28 days two weeks after receiving 6-OHDA (8 µg/2 µL).
Group II (L-DOPA-treated 6-OHDA-lesioned rat groups + chronic EF stress): exposed to EF stress for 28 days in L-DOPA (10 mg/kg)-treated 6-OHDA-lesioned rat groups (Group I).
Group III (L-DOPA-treated 6-OHDA-lesioned rat groups + GP-BX): administered GP-BX (30 mg/kg) for 28 days in L-DOPA-treated 6-OHDA-lesioned groups (Group I).
Group IV (L-DOPA-treated 6-OHDA-lesioned rat groups + chronic EF stress + GP-BX): administered GP-BX (30 mg/kg) for 28 days in L-DOPA-treated 6-OHDA-lesioned groups exposed to chronic EF stress (Group II).

2.7 TH-immunohistochemistry staining

For the immunohistochemical study, the rats were sacrificed 28 days after 6-OHDA lesioning and then perfused intracardially with saline, which was followed by 4% paraformaldehyde of the fixative solution. The brain was removed from the skull and placed in 30% sucrose solution. Sections of 35-µm thickness were cut with a Vibratome (Leica Microsystems GmbH, Wetzlar, Germany). The tissue sections were incubated with primary anti-TH antibody raised in rabbits and diluted in PBS containing 0.3% Triton X-100 (1:200, AB152, Millipore) overnight at 4°C. A 1:250 dilution of biotinylated anti-rabbit IgG was used as a secondary antibody, and the sections were then incubated with an ABC kit. TH immunoreactivity was visualized using a DAB kit (Vector Laboratories, Inc.). Photomicrographs of TH and digitized bright-field images were captured using a Zeiss Axiophot microscope (Carl Zeiss MicroImaging GmbH, Jena, Germany) (100X magnification). Cell counting was done using a computerized image analysis system (Axiovision software, Carl Zeiss MicroImaging GmbH). Analysis values obtained on the ipsilateral side (6-OHDA-lesioned side) were expressed as a percentage of those on the intact contralateral side (intact side).

2.8 Biochemical analysis

The brains were removed quickly, and the striatum was dissected in cold conditions. The samples were homogenized in 300 μL $HClO_4$. The homogenates were immediately centrifuged at 50,000 × g at 4°C for 20 min, and then, the supernatants were filtered using pore filters (0.45 μm). The levels of dopamine, DOPAC, HVA, and norepinephrine in the striatum were measured with a high-performance liquid chromatography (HPLC) system. The HPLC system consisted of a solvent delivery pump (Model 1525, Waters, Milford, MA, USA), an electrochemical detector (+0.85 V, Ag/AgCl reference electrode; Model 2465; Waters), and a Waters 120 ODS-BP column (5 μm, 50 × 4.6 mm). The mobile phase consisted of 10 mM citric acid, 0.13 mM Na_4EDTA, 0.58 mM SOS, and 10% methanol, and a flow rate of 1 mL/min. The results were expressed in terms of ng/g tissue.

2.9 Statistical analysis

All data were expressed as means ± S.E.M. Data were analyzed with an one-way analysis of variance (ANOVA) followed by a Tukey's test. P values <0.05 were considered statistically significant.

3. Results

3.1 TH-immunopositive neuronal cell survival in the substantia nigra of 6-OHDA-lesioned rats exposed to chronic EF stress and administered GP-BX

TH-immunopositive neuronal cell death by 6-OHDA lesions in the substantia nigra was ameliorated by the administration of GP-BX at 30 mg/kg (p.o.) for 28 days (Figure 1). TH-immunopositive neurons were observed consecutively in both the substantia nigra compacta and lateralis. TH-immunostained nerve fibers in the substantia nigra were tangled into a net, and the cells were either poly- or ovoid-shaped in the normal areas (Figure 1, A-I). The substantia nigra regions near the 6-OHDA-lesioned areas displayed drastic reductions in TH-immunopositive neuronal cells, and the staining intensity was decreased compared with the intact sides of the control rat groups (Figure 1, A-II). After exposure to chronic EF stress, TH-immunopositive neuronal cells were decreased in the substantia nigra of both the normal and the 6-OHDA-lesioned rats, even though the color was uneven, compared to the 6-OHDA-lesioned rat groups without chronic EF stress (Figure 1, A-II and III). However, the administration of GP-BX at 30 mg/kg (p.o.) for 28 days ameliorated the loss of TH-immunopositive neuronal cells induced by the exposure to chronic EF stress in both the intact and 6-OHDA-lesioned sides of 6-OHDA-lesioned rats (Figure 1, A-IV).

The number of TH-immunopositive neuronal cells on the ipsilateral sides (6-OHDA-lesioned sides) was analyzed as a percentage of those in the intact contralateral sides (intact sides) of 6-OHDA-lesioned rat groups. In the 6-OHDA-lesioned rat groups, 6-OHDA lesions caused a marked decrease in the number of TH-immunopositive neuronal cells in the intact and 6-OHDA-lesioned sides to 79.1% and 35.8%, respectively, compared to the normal rat groups (Figure 1, B-I and II). In addition, the exposure to chronic EF stress in the 6-OHDA-lesioned rat groups further decreased the number of TH-immunopositive neuronal cells in the intact and 6-OHDA-lesioned sides to 45.9% and 19.9%, respectively, compared to the 6-OHDA-lesioned rat groups (Figure, B-II and III). However, in the 6-OHDA-lesioned rat groups exposed to chronic EF stress, GP-BX administration (30 mg/kg) for 28 days showed a protective effect on the loss of the number of TH-immunopositive neuronal cells in the intact and 6-OHDA-lesioned sides to 63.0% and 38.1%, respectively (Figure 1, B-III and IV).

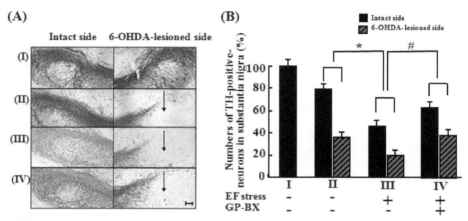

Fig. 1. Photomicrographs of tyrosine hydroxylase (TH) immunoreactivity on substantia nigra tissue sections from representative rats of each group (A), and the number of surviving TH-immunopositive neuronal cells in the ipsilateral substantia nigra [6-hydroxydopamine (6-OHDA)-lesioned side] was analyzed as a percentage of that in the intact contralateral side (intact side) (B). Normal rat groups (I), 6-OHDA-lesioned rat groups (II), 6-OHDA-lesioned rat groups + chronic electric foot (EF) stress (III), and 6-OHDA-lesioned rat groups + chronic EF stress + *Gynostemma pentaphyllum*-butanol extract (GP-BX) (IV). Rats were treated with GP-BX (30 mg/kg/day, p.o.) or vehicle (0.9% saline, p.o.) and then subjected to every-other-day sessions of EF stress (duration and interval of 10 s for 10 min, 2 mA). These data are representative of 7–10 animals per group, and the arrow indicates the 6-OHDA-lesioned side. TH-immunopositive neuronal cells were analyzed as a percentage of intact side. Scale bar is 100 μm. * $p < 0.05$ compared with 6-OHDA-lesioned rat groups; # $p < 0.05$ compared with 6-OHDA-lesioned rat groups + chronic EF stress (ANOVA followed by Tukey's test).

3.2 The levels of dopamine, DOPAC, HVA, and norepinephrine in the striatum of 6-OHDA-lesioned rats exposed to chronic EF-stress and administered GP-BX

The levels of dopamine, DOPAC, HVA, and norepinephrine in the striatum of GP-BX-administered normal rats (those without 6-OHDA lesions) were not altered compared to the GP-BX-untreated rat groups (data not shown). In addition, no differences were seen on the intact side of normal rats, 6-OHDA-lesioned rat groups, and 6-OHDA-lesioned rat groups administered GP-BX (30 mg/kg, 28 days).

A significant decrease in the levels of dopamine, DOPAC, HVA, and norepinephrine by 47.0%, 44.3%, 38.6%, and 40.5% in the 6-OHDA-lesioned sides of the 6-OHDA-lesioned rat groups, respectively, was observed (Figure 2, I and II). Chronic EF stress-exposed 6-OHDA-lesioned rat groups had a more marked decrease in the levels of dopamine, DOPAC, HVA, and norepinephrine to 71.7% and 28.2%, 66.9% and 28.3%, 61.0% and 25.3%, and 71.6% and

27.4%, respectively, in both the intact and 6-OHDA-lesioned sides, compared with 6-OHDA-lesioned rats without chronic EF stress (Figure 2, II and III). However, GP-BX administration (30 mg/kg) for 28 days resulted in an improvement in the reduced levels of dopamine, DOPAC, HVA, and norepinephrine by chronic EF stress to 84.6% and 47.8%, 79.7% and 47.9, 72.8% and 46.0%, and 88.6% and 46.8%, respectively, in the intact and 6-OHDA-lesioned sides of the 6-OHDA-lesioned rat groups (Figure 2, III and IV).

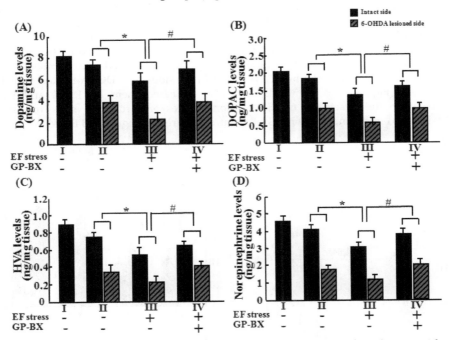

Fig. 2. Effects of GP-BX on the levels of dopamine (A), 3,4-dihydroxyphenylacetic acid (DOPAC; B), homovanillic acid (HVA; C), and norepinephrine (D) in the striatum of 6-OHDA-lesioned rats. Normal rat groups (I), 6-OHDA-lesioned rat groups (II), 6-OHDA-lesioned rat groups + chronic EF stress (III), and 6-OHDA-lesioned rat groups + chronic EF stress+ GP-BX (IV). Rats were treated with GP-BX (30 mg/kg/day, p.o.) or vehicle (0.9% saline, p.o.) and then subjected to every-other-day sessions of EF stress (duration and interval of 10 s for 10 min, 2 mA). After 4 weeks, the brains were removed, and the levels of dopamine, DOPAC, HVA, and norepinephrine were determined by a high-performance liquid chromatography (HPLC) method. Results represent means ± S.E.M. for 7–10 animals per group. * $p < 0.05$ compared with 6-OHDA-lesioned rat groups; # $p < 0.05$ compared with 6-OHDA-lesioned rat groups + chronic EF stress (ANOVA followed by Tukey's test).

3.3 TH-immunopositive neuronal cell survival in L-DOPA-treated 6-OHDA-lesioned rats exposed to chronic EF stress and administered GP-BX

Treatment with L-DOPA (10 mg/kg) for 28 days in 6-OHDA-lesioned rats slightly increased the number of TH-immunopositive neuronal cells in the 6-OHDA-lesioned sides compared to the L-DOPA-untreated 6-OHDA-lesioned rats (Figure 1-II and 3-I), indicating that a low dose of L-DOPA showed a protective and therapeutic activity. However, with exposure to chronic stress, the number of TH-immunopositive neuronal cells was significantly reduced in the substantia nigra in the L-DOPA-treated 6-OHDA-lesioned rat groups (Figure 3, A I and II). Furthermore, GP-BX administration (30 mg/kg) for 28 days protected against the loss of TH-immunopositive neuronal cells in L-DOPA-treated 6-OHDA-lesioned rat groups with or without chronic EF stress (Figure 3, A III and IV). Chronic EF stress induced the loss of a number of TH-immunopositive neuronal cells in both the intact and 6-OHDA-lesioned sides: the number of TH-immunopositive neuronal cells in the 6-OHDA-lesioned sides was decreased to 45.1% by the exposure to chronic EF stress in L-DOPA (10 mg/kg)-treated 6-OHDA-lesioned rat groups compared with those without chronic EF stress (Figure 3, A I and II). However, GP-BX administration (30 mg/kg) recovered the number of TH-immunopositive neuronal cells by 12.1% in the intact sides of L-DOPA-treated 6-OHDA-lesioned rats (Figure 3, B I and III) and also increased them by 18.6% and 36.7%, respectively, in the intact and 6-OHDA-lesioned sides of chronic EF stress-exposed 6-OHDA-lesioned rats compared with GP-BX-untreated groups (Figure 3, B II and IV).

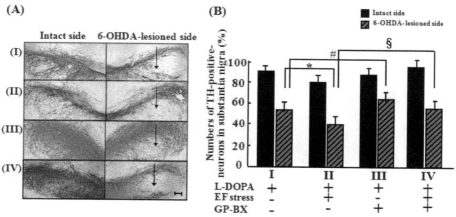

Fig. 3. Photomicrographs of TH immunoreactivity on substantia nigra tissue sections from representative rats of each group (A), and the number of surviving TH-immunopositive neuronal cells in the ipsilateral substantia nigra (6-OHDA-lesioned side) was analyzed as a percentage of that in the intact contralateral side (intact side) (B). L-DOPA-treated 6-OHDA-lesioned rat groups (I), L-DOPA-treated 6-OHDA-lesioned rat groups + chronic EF stress (II), L-DOPA-treated 6-OHDA-lesioned rat groups + GP-BX (III), and L-DOPA-treated 6-OHDA-lesioned rat groups + chronic EF stress + GP-BX (IV). Rats were treated with GP-BX (30 mg/kg/day, p.o.) or vehicle (0.9% saline, p.o.) and then subjected to every-other-day sessions of EF stress (duration and interval of 10 s for 10 min, 2 mA). L-DOPA (10 mg/kg/day, i.p.) was administered with benserazide (15 mg/kg/day, i.p.) prepared in saline. These data are representative of 7–10 animals per group, and the arrow indicates 6-OHDA-lesioned side. TH-immunopositive neuronal cells were analyzed as a percentage of intact side. Scale bar is 100 μm. * $p < 0.05$ compared with L-DOPA-treated 6-OHDA-lesioned rat groups; # $p < 0.05$ compared with L-DOPA-treated 6-OHDA-lesioned rat groups; § $p < 0.05$ compared with L-DOPA-treated 6-OHDA-lesioned rat groups + chronic EF stress (ANOVA followed by Tukey's test).

3.4 The levels of dopamine, DOPAC, HVA, and norepinephrine in the striatum of L-DOPA- treated 6-OHDA-lesioned rats exposed to chronic EF stress and administered GP-BX

The levels of dopamine, DOPAC, HVA, and norepinephrine were slightly increased in the striatal regions of the 6-OHDA-lesioned rat groups treated with L-DOPA (10 mg/kg), compared with those of the L-DOPA-untreated groups (Figures 2 and 4), but they were still decreased by 6-OHDA lesions (Figure 4, A-D I). The exposure to chronic EF stress in the L-

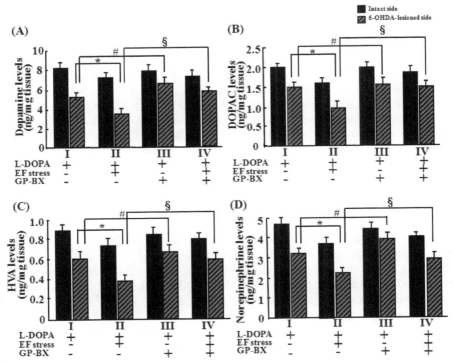

Fig. 4. Effects of GP-BX on the levels of dopamine (A), DOPAC (B), HVA (C), and norepinephrine (D) in the striatum of 6-OHDA-lesioned rats. L-DOPA-treated 6-OHDA-lesioned rat groups (I), L-DOPA-treated 6-OHDA-lesioned rat groups + chronic EF stress (II), L-DOPA-treated 6-OHDA-lesioned rat groups + GP-BX (III), and L-DOPA-treated 6-OHDA-lesioned rat groups + chronic EF stress + GP-BX (IV). Rats were treated with GP-BX (30 mg/kg/day, p.o.) or vehicle (0.9% saline, p.o.) and then subjected to every-other-day sessions of EF stress (duration and interval of 10 s for 10 min, 2 mA). L-DOPA (10 mg/kg/day, i.p.) was administered with benserazide (15 mg/kg/day, i.p.) prepared in saline. After 4 weeks, the brains were removed, and the levels of dopamine, DOPAC, HVA, and norepinephrine were determined by an HPLC method. Results represent means ± S.E.M. for 7-10 animals per group. * $p < 0.05$ compared with L-DOPA-treated 6-OHDA-lesioned rat groups; # $p < 0.05$ compared with L-DOPA-treated 6-OHDA-lesioned rat groups; § $p < 0.05$ compared with L-DOPA-treated 6-OHDA-lesioned rat groups + chronic EF stress. (ANOVA followed by Tukey's test).

DOPA (10 mg/kg)-treated 6-OHDA-lesioned rat groups showed a further significant decrease in the levels of dopamine, DOPAC, HVA, and norepinephrine in the 6-OHDA-lesioned sides of the striatal regions by 43.0%, 47.9%, 43.1%, and 47.4%, respectively, compared with those of the unstressed groups (Figure 4, A-D I and II). This was significantly recovered by 30 mg/kg GP-BX administration for 28 days (Figure 4, A-D I and III). In addition, 30 mg/kg GP-BX administration for 28 days resulted in an improvement in the levels of dopamine, DOPAC, HVA, and norepinephrine to 62.5%, 54.5%, 55.1%, and 31.7%, respectively, in the L-DOPA (10 mg/kg)-treated 6-OHDA-lesioned rat groups (Figure 4, A-D I and IV).

4. Discussion

The neurotoxin 6-OHDA is commonly used for animal models of PD, and it is believed to cause dopaminergic cell death with a unilateral destruction of the nigrostriatal system (Schober, 2004). Among the various bioactive functions of GP, it has been known to have anti-oxidant, anti-inflammatory, and immunostimulatory actions (Razmovski-Naumovski et al., 2005). In addition, GP ethanol extract has been found to have an anti-stress function against chronic EF stress in mice (Choi et al., 2008; Im et al., 2009). In this study, the neuroprotective functions of GP-BX on the exposure to chronic EF stress in the 6-OHDA-lesioned rat model of PD with or without long-term L-DOPA treatment were investigated by determining the quantities of TH-immunopositive neuronal cells surviving in the substantia nigra and the levels of dopamine, DOPAC, HVA, and norepinephrine in the striatum.

GP ethanol extracts at doses of 10–50 mg/kg/day for 28 days did not show toxic effects, such as weight loss or death in rats (Choi et al., 2008; Im et al., 2009), and the water extract (750 mg/kg) of GP also did not produce any significant toxic effects in rats during a 6-month period of treatment (Attawish et al., 2004). GP-BX (30 mg) was selected in this study, and its administration for 28 days did not exhibit adverse effects, such as weight loss, diarrhea, vomiting, or death.

The infusion of 6-OHDA into the CNS resulted in decreased rotational movements, including stereotypic behavior, by the change of monoamine contents (Deumens et al., 2002), which was recovered by GP-BX administration (data not shown). These findings suggest that GP-BX showed a preventive activity against 6-OHDA-lesioned rats.

The number of TH-immunopositive surviving cells showed a large decrease in the ventrolateral side of the substantia compacta (intact side), and their numbers were well maintained in the ventral tegmental area (VTA) of the ventral side (intact side). These findings were very similar to the pathological findings of PD. However, the number of TH-immunopositive neuronal cells in the VTA decreased slightly due to the passage of time with 6-OHDA (Figure 1, A I and II). The chronic exposure to EF stress every other day for 28 days enhanced the 6-OHDA-induced dopaminergic neuronal cell death in the 6-OHDA-lesioned rat groups used as a PD model system (Figures 1 and 2). The chronic EF stress also inhibited the therapeutic effects of L-DOPA (10 mg/kg) in the 6-OHDA-lesioned rats (Figures 3 and 4). However, GP-BX administration (30 mg/kg) for 28 days ameliorated the enhanced neurotoxic effects induced by the exposure to chronic EF stress in 6-OHDA-lesioned rats with or without L-DOPA: the number of surviving TH-immunopositive neuronal cells in the substantia nigra and the levels of dopamine, DOPAC, HVA, and norepinephrine in the striatum were recovered by GP-BX. In addition, GP-BX inhibited 6-OHDA-induced neurotoxicity in the brain regions of normal rats and 6-OHDA-lesioned rats (data not shown), which was similar to the findings with GP ethanol extract (Choi et al., 2010). These results indicate that oral administration of GP-BX exhibited a preventive and protective activity against the chronic EF stress- and/or 6-OHDA-induced dopaminergic neuronal cell death in rats.

Stressful stimuli induced the production of ROS and increased the release of catecholamines and glucocorticoids (Ganong, 2001; Kandel et al., 2000), which reduced the function of immune systems (Im et al., 2009). Immobilized stress inhibited the neuroprotective effects of free-running wheel exercise in a rat model of PD (Urakami et al,, 1988). The exposure to chronically repetitive stress also reduced dopamine levels in the rat brain, leading to decreased ambulatory activity (Ahmed et al., 1995; Rajkowska, 2000). ROS, which are generated by 6-OHDA by autoxidation, directly destroyed DNA, essential proteins, and cell lipid membranes to cause necrosis (Schober, 2004). In addition, 6-OHDA was detected in rat brain after L-DOPA treatment due to the high levels of dopamine and hydrogen peroxide (Maharaj et al., 2005), which induced dopaminergic neuronal cell death by inflammatory processes and oxidative apoptosis (Blum et al., 2004). L-DOPA treatment in MPTP-induced PD rodents increased the striatal 6-OHDA levels, which may be sensitized by monoamine oxidase inhibitor (Borah & Mohanakumar, 2010). Long-term treatment with L-DOPA caused disabling motor side effects in PD and alleviated oxidative stress-induced neurotoxicity by ROS formation against striatal dopaminergic neurons and PC12 cells (Basma et al., 1995; Walkinshaw & Waters, 1995; Migheli et al., 1999). Subchronic or chronic L-DOPA treatment resulted in increased levels of dopamine and hydroxyl-free radicals in the striatum (Pandey et al., 2009). L-DOPA also showed treatment dose-dependent dual functions, including protection and neurotoxicity, in the 6-OHDA-lesioned rat model of PD (Cenci, 2009). In addition, L-DOPA at low concentrations (3–10 µM) produced trophic or cell-protective effects on neuronal and differentiated PC12 cells (Mena et al., 1997). In this study, L-DOPA treatment of 10 mg/kg for 28 days showed a slightly protective effect by increasing TH-immunopositive surviving cells in 6-OHDA-lesioned rats. However, the TH-immunopositive surviving cells were decreased by chronic EF stress (Figures 1 and 3), suggesting that the function of L-DOPA in rat model of PD was aggravated by the exposure to chronic EF stress. Taken together, these results suggest that the formation of ROS by chronic stress can enhance dopaminergic neuronal cell death in 6-OHDA-lesioned rats with or without L-DOPA treatment. Therefore, it is proposed that antioxidants scavenging 6-OHDA- or L-DOPA-induced ROS are a key to the prevention and control of the symptoms of PD (Andrew et al., 1993).

Previously, we reported that GP ethanol extract had an anti-stress function by improving the loss of body weight and the reduction of grip strength in rodents, which was induced by chronic EF stress (Choi et al., 2008). The extract also showed an immunomodulatory activity by preventing dexamethasone-induced immunosuppression (Im et al., 2009). In addition, GP ethanol extract protected against 6-OHDA-induced neurotoxicity in 6-OHDA-lesioned rats (Choi et al., 2010). In this study, GP-BX exhibited a protective activity against chronic EF stress by reducing L-DOPA-induced neuronal cell death in 6-OHDA-lesioned rats treated with L-DOPA. These results suggest that the protective functions of GP-BX on chronic EF stress- and L-DOPA-induced neurotoxicity could be mediated by the modulation of the ROS formation and immune system in rodents.

The gypenoside-rich fraction, gypenosides, protected against oxidative neurotoxicity involving glutamate in primary cultures of rat cortical cells (Shang et al., 2006) and showed anti-inflammatory activity (Lin et al., 1993). Gypenosides also showed a protective effect on dopaminergic neuronal cell death in the MPTP-induced rat model of PD (Wang et al., 2010). It has been shown that GP-BX has several gypenoside derivatives, including gynosaponin TN-1, gynosaponin TN-2, gypenoside XLV, and gypenoside LXXIV (Choi et al., 2010; Razmovski-Naumovski et al., 2005; Nagai et al., 1981; Takemoto et al., 1984; Yoshikawa et al., 1987). These data further support that GP-BX can be applied for the prevention of the symptoms of PD by scavenging the formation of ROS.

Besides herbal GP, black tea extract exhibited neuroprotective and neurorescue effects against 6-OHDA-induced degeneration of the nigrostriatal dopaminergic system (Chaturvedi et al., 2004), and Yeoldahanso-tang, which is a Korean herbal formula containing 10 herbs, also protected against neurotoxicity in a MPTP-induced mice model of PD (Bae et al., 2011). Therefore, the comparative functions for PD among these herbal extracts, including drug interactions, adverse effects, and toxicity may need to be studied further.

5. Conclusion

GP-BX showed protective functions for dopaminergic neurons from chronic stress- and L-DOPA-induced neurotoxicity in 6-OHDA-lesioned rat model of PD. Considering our results, GP-BX may be helpful in preventing the L-DOPA-induced adverse or oxidative toxic effects for PD, especially with chronic stress, as well as slow down the progression of PD symptoms. Clinical trials for patients with PD using herbal GP extract and its bioactive components need to be studied further.

6. Acknowledgments

This work was supported by a grant of Research Center for Bioresource and Health, KIAT and MKE (2010).

7. References

Ahmed S.H.; Stinus, L., Moal, M.L. & Cador, M. (1995), Social deprivation enhances the vulnerability of male Wistar rats to stressor-and amphetamine-induced sensitization. *Psychopharmacology*, Vol.117, No.1, pp. 116-124, ISSN 0033-3158

Amanda D. S.; Sandra, L., Castro, Michael, J. & Zigmond. (2002). Stress-induced Parkinson's disease: a working hypothesis, *Physiology & Behavior*, Vol.77, No.4-5, pp. 527-531, ISSN 0031-9384

Andrew, R.; Watson, D.G., Best, S.A., Midgley, J.M, Wenlong, H. & Petty, R.K. (1993). The determination of hydroxydopamines and other trace amines in the urine of parkinsonian patients and normal controls. *Neurochemical Research,* Vol.18, No.11, pp. 1175–1177, ISSN 0364-3190

Attawish, A.; Chivapat, S., Phadungpat, S., Bansiddhi, J., Techadamrongsin, Y., Mitrijit, O., Chaorai, B. & Chavalittumrong, P. (2004). Chronic toxicity of Gynostemma pentaphyllum. *Fitoterapia,* Vol.75, No.6, pp. 539–551, ISSN 0367-326X

Bae, N.; Ahn, T., Chung, S., Oh, M.S., Ko, H., Oh, H., Park, G. & Yang, H.O. (2011). The neuroprotective effect of modified Yeoldahanso-tang via autophagy enhancement in models of Parkinson's disease. *Journal of Ethnopharmacology,* Vol.134, No.2, pp. 313–322, ISSN 0378-8741

Basma, A.N.; Morris, E.J., Nicklas, W.J. & Geller, H.M. (1995). L-DOPA cytotoxicity to PC12 cells in culture is via its autoxidation. *Journal of Neurochemistry,* Vol.64, No.2, pp. 825–832, ISSN 0022-3042

Blum, D.; Torch, S., Lambeng, N., Nissou, M., Benabid, A.L., Sadoul, R. & Verna, J.M. (2001). Molecular pathways involved in the neurotoxicity of 6-OHDA, dopamine and MPTP: contribution to the apoptotic theory in Parkinson's disease. *Progress in Neurobiology,* Vol.65, No.2, pp. 135–172, ISSN 0301-0082

Borah, A. & Mohanakumar, K.P. (2010). L-DOPA-induced 6-hydroxydopamine production in the striata of rodents is sensitive to the degree of denervation. *Neurochemistry International,* Vol.56, No.2, pp. 357-62, ISSN 0197-0186

Cenci, M.A. (2007). L-DOPA-induced dyskinesia: cellular mechanisms and approaches to treatment. *Parkinsonism & Related Disorders,* Vol.13, pp. S263–S267, ISSN 1353-8020

Cheng, N.; Maeda, T., Kume, T., Kaneko, S., Kochiyama, H., Akaike, A., Goshima, Y. & Misu. (1996). Differential neurotoxicity induced by L-DOPA and dopamine in cultured striatal neurons, *Brain Research,* Vol.16, No.743, pp. 278–283, ISSN 0006-8993

Chaturvedi RK.; Shukla, S., Seth, K., Chauhan, S., Sinha, C., Shukla, Y. & Agrawal, AK. (2006). Neuroprotective and neurorescue effect of black tea extract in 6-hydroxydopamine-lesioned rat model of Parkinson's disease. *Neurobiology of Disease,* Vol.22, No.2, pp. 421-34, ISSN 0969-9961

Choi, H.S.; Lim, S.A., Park, M.S., Hwang, B.Y., Lee, C.K., Kim, S.H., Lim, S.C. & Lee, M.K. (2008). Ameliorating effects of the ethanol extracts from Gynostemma pentaphyllum on electric footshock stress. *Korean Journal of Pharmacognosy,* Vol.39, No.4, pp. 341–346, ISSN 0253-3073

Choi H.S.; Park M.S., Kim S.H., Hwang B.Y., Lee C.K. & Lee M.K. (2010). Neuroprotective effects of herbal ethanol extracts from Gynostemma pentaphyllum in the 6-hydroxydopamine-lesioned rat model of Parkinson's disease. *Molecules,* Vol.15, No.4, pp. 2814-2824, ISSN 1420-3049

Deumens, R.; Blokland, A. & Prickaerts, J. (2002). Modeling Parkinson's disease in rats: an evaluation of 6-OHDA lesions of the nigrostriatal pathway. *Experimental Neurology,* Vol.175, No.2 pp. 303–317, ISSN 0014-4886

Fearnley, M. & Lees, A.J. (1991). Ageing and Parkinson's disease: substantia nigra regional selectivity. *Brain,* Vol.114, No.5, pp. 2283–2301, ISSN 0006-8950

Ganong, W. F. (2003). *Review of Medical Physiology*, 23th ed. pp. 359–384, McGraw-Hill, ISBN 0071287289, United States

Hornykiewicz, O. (1982). Imbalance of brain monoamines and clinical disorders. *Progress in Brain Research*, Vol.55, pp. 419–429, ISSN 0079-6123

Jankovic, J. (2005). Motor fluctuations and dyskinesias in Parkinson's disease: clinical manifestations. *Movement Disorders: Official journal of the Movement Disorder Society*, Vol.20, No.11, pp. S11–S16, ISSN 0885-3185

Im, S.A.; Choi, H.S., Hwang, B.Y., Lee, M.K. & Lee, C.K. (2009). Augmentation of immune responses by oral administration of Gynostemma pentaphyllum ethanol extract. *Korean Journal of Pharmacognosy*, Vol.40, No.1, pp. 35–40, ISSN 0253-3073

Kandel, E.R.; Schwartz, J. H. & Jessell, T.M. (2000) *Principles of Neural Science*, McGraw-Hill, ISBN 0071287289, United States

Lin, J.M.; Lin, C.C., Chiu, H.F., Yang, J.J. & Lee, S.G. (1993). Evaluation of the anti-inflammatory and liver-protective effects of Anoectochilus formosanus, Ganoderma lucidum and Gynostemma pentaphyllum in rats. *The American Journal of Chinese Medicine*, Vol.21, No.1 pp. 59–69. ISSN 0192-415X

Maharaj H.; Sukhdev Maharaj D., Scheepers M., Mokokong R. & Daya S. (2005). L-DOPA administration enhances 6-hydroxydopamine generation. *Brain Research*, Vol.1063, No.2, pp. 180-186, ISSN 0006-8993

Marsden, C.D. (1994). Parkinson's disease. *Journal of Neurology, Neurosurgery, and Psychiatry*, Vol.57, No.6, pp. 672–681, ISSN 0022-3050

Mena, M.A.; Davila, V., & Sulzer, D. (1997). Neurotrophic effects of L-DOPA in postnatal midbrain dopamine neuron/cortical historicity cocultures. *Journal of Neurochemistry*, Vol.69, pp. 1398-1408, ISSN 0022-3042

Merad-Boudia, M.; Nicole, A., Santiard-Baron, D., Saille, C. & Ceballos-Picot, I. (1998). Mitochondrial impairment as an early event in the process of apoptosis induced by glutathione depletion in neuronal cells: relevance to Parkinson's disease. *Biochemical Pharmacology*, Vol.56, No.5, pp. 645–655, ISSN 0006-2952

Migheli, R.; Godani, C., Sciola, L., Delogu, M.R., Serra, P.A., Zangani, D., De Natale, G., Miele, E. & Desole, M.S. (1999). Enhancing effect of manganese on L-DOPA-induced apoptosis in PC12 cells: role of oxidative stress. *Journal of Neurochemistry*, Vol.73, No. 3, pp. 1155-1163, ISSN 0022-3042

Nagai, M.; Izawa, K.; Nagumo, S.; Sakurai, N.; Inoue, T. (1981). Two glycosides of a novel dammarane alcohol from Gynostemma pentaphyllum. *Chemical & Pharmaceutical Bulletin*, Vol.29, pp. 779–783, ISSN 0009-2363

Neil, A. & David, B. (2008). Parkinson's disease, *Medicine*, Vol.36, No.12, pp. 630–635, ISSN 0025-7974

Ozawa, T.; Tanaka, M., Ikebe, S., Ohno, K., Kondo, T. & Mizuno, Y. (1990). Quantitative determination of deleted mitochondrial DNA relative to normal DNA in parkinsonian striatum by a kinetic PCR analysis. *Biochemical and Biophysical Research Communications*, Vol.172, No.2, pp. 483–489, ISSN 0006-291X

Paxinos, G. & Watson, C. (1986). *The Rat Brain in Stereotaxic Coordinates*, 2nd ed.; Academic
    Press, ISBN 0126930198, Australia

Pandey, A.; Borah, M., Varghese, P.K., Barman, K.P., Mohanakumar & R. Usha, R. (2009)
    Striatal dopamine level contributes to hydroxyl radical generation and subsequent
    neurodegeneration in the striatum in 3-nitropropionic acid-induced Huntington's
    disease in rats. *Neurochemistry International*, Vol.55, No.6, pp. 431–437, ISSN 0197-
    0186

Perese, D.A.; Ulman, J., Viola, J., Ewing, S.E. & Bankiewicz, K.S. (1989). A 6-
    hydroxydopamine-induced selective parkinsonian rat model. *Brain Research*,
    Vol.494, No.2, pp. 285–293, ISSN 0006-8993

Przedborski, S.; Levivier, M., Jiang, H., Ferreira, M., Jackson-Lewis, V., Donaldson, D. &
    Togasaki, D.M. (1995). Dose-dependent lesions of the dopaminergic nigrostriatal
    pathway induced by intrastriatal injection of 6-hydroxydopamine. *Neuroscience*,
    Vol.67, No.3, pp. 631–647, ISSN 0306-4522

Rajkowska G. (2000). Postmortem studies in mood disorders indicate altered numbers of
    neurons and glial cells. *Biological Psychiatry*, Vol.48, No.8, pp. 766-777, ISSN 0006-
    3223

Razmovski-Naumovski, V.; Huang, T.H-.W., Tran, V.H., Li, G.Q., Duke, C.C. & Roufogalis,
    B.D. (2005). Chemistry and pharmacology of Gynostemma pentaphyllum.
    Phytochemistry Review, Vol.4, pp. 197–219

Schober, A. (2004). Classic toxin-induced animal models of Parkinson's disease: 6-
    OHDA and MPTP. *Cell and Tissue Research*, Vol.318, No.1, pp. 215–224, ISSN
    0302-766X

Schwab, R.S. & Zieoer, I. (1965) Effect of mood, motivation, stress and alertness on the
    performance in Parkinson's disease. *Psychiatria et Neurologia*, Vol.150, No. 6, pp.
    345-357

Shang, L.; Liu, J., Zhu, Q., Zhao, L., Feng, Y., Wang, X., Cao, W. & Xin, H. (2006).
    Gypenosides protect primary cultures of rat cortical cells against oxidative
    neurotoxicity. *Brain Research*, Vol.1102, No.1, pp. 163–174, ISSN 0006-8993

Takemoto, T.; Arihara, S.; Yoshikawa, K.; Kawasaki, J.; Nakajima, T.; Okuhira, M. (1984).
    Studies on the constituents of Cucurbitaceae plants. XI. On the saponin constituents
    of Gynostemma pentaphyllum MAKINO. (7). *Yakugaku Zasshi*, Vol.104, pp. 1043–
    1049, ISSN 0031-6903

Urakami, K.; Masaki, N., Shimoda, K., Nishikawa, S. & Takahashi K. (1988). Increase of
    striatal dopamine turnover by stress in MPTP-treated mice. *Clinical
    Neuropharmacology*, Vol.11, No.4, pp. 360-368, ISSN 0362-5664

Walkinshaw, G. & Waters, C.M. (1995). Induction of apoptosis in catecholaminergic PC12
    cells by l-DOPA. Implications for the treatment of Parkinson's disease. *The Journal
    of Clinical Investigation*, Vol.95, No.6, pp. 2458–2464, ISSN 0021-9738

Wang, P.; Niu, L., Gao, L., Li, WX., Jia, D., Wang, XL. & Gao, G.D. (2010). Neuroprotective
    effect of gypenosides against oxidative injury in the substantia nigra of a mouse
    model of Parkinson's disease. *The Journal of International Medical Research*, Vol.38,
    No.3, pp. 1084-92.

Yoshikawa, K.; Arimitsu, M. Kuki, K. Takemoto, T.; Arihara, S. (1987). Studies on the constituents of Cucurbitaceae plants. XVIII. On the saponin constituents of Gynostemma pentaphyllum MAKINO. (13). *Yakugaku Zasshi*, Vol.107, pp. 361–366, ISSN 0031-6903